Praise for *Wild Remedies*

"I was intrigued and captivated from the very first paragraphs. Beautifully written, *Wild Remedies* abounds with plant lore, wisdom, and instruction. The authors have created a deeply thoughtful, insightful, and interactive book that enables readers to not only identify and forage wild foods but also to create a deepening relationship with nature and the world of plants."

— **Rosemary Gladstar,** herbalist

"*Wild Remedies* is a gorgeous book with tantalizing recipes for healthy foods and healing medicines. The authors go beyond mere consumption of herbs to nurture reciprocal relationships with plants and strengthen community connections. In effect, *Wild Remedies* is a prescription to heal people and planet together."

— **Thomas J. Elpel,** author of *Botany in a Day* and *Foraging the Mountain West*

"In *Wild Remedies*, **Emily Han** and **Rosalee de la Forêt** accomplish the most important thing a book exploring herbalism can do: framing it not as simply the *use* of herbs and supplements, but as a craft rooted in a direct relationship between people, plants, and the land they live upon. With this book in your hands, the plants at your feet will open into a whole new world."

— **jim mcdonald,** herbalist, www.herbcraft.org

"I've been studying wild edible and medicinal plants for decades, and I learned a lot reading this book. So if you want to use some of our best medicinal wild plants, this book is a great choice."

— **"Wildman" Steve Brill,** author of *Identifying and Harvesting Edible and Medicinal Plants in Wild (and Not So Wild) Places*

"**Rosalee de la Forêt** and **Emily Han**'s seasonal, carefully thought out, and practical approach to common backyard wild medicinals will inspire budding and established herbalists alike. It approaches backyard herbalism to a depth rarely covered in herbals. I can't wait to share this book with students as required reading in my herb courses."

— **Maria Noël Groves,** clinical herbalist at Wintergreen Botanicals and best-selling author of *Body into Balance and Grow Your Own Herbal Remedies*

"*Wild Remedies* reads like a joyous love poem to the earth and gives us the compass for a much-needed regenerative model of harvesting and working with medicinal plants."

— **Kami McBride,** author of *The Herbal Kitchen*

"*Wild Remedies* is a truly holistic and comprehensive map for the journey of nature connection, people connection, and ultimately ourselves."

— **Jon Young,** author, presenter, and founder of 8 Shields

"Rarely does a book take my breath away, but *Wild Remedies* had me in full swoon by the Table of Contents. With gorgeous illustrations, scintillating recipes, and detailed plant profiles, you'll be reaching for your harvesting basket with a newfound appreciation for the bounty and beauty of the green world. **Emily Han** and **Rosalee de la Forêt** have concocted an herbal tour de force, destined to deepen your connection to backyard plants."

— **Juliet Blankespoor,** director of the Chestnut School of Herbal Medicine

"*Wild Remedies* is an incredibly thoughtful, seasonally based forager's guide that empowers the reader to connect with plants and build a more reciprocal relationship with nature herself."

— **Susan Leopold,** executive director, United Plant Savers

"*Wild Remedies* couldn't come at a more important time, as humanity's connection to nature is essential not only for the health of the planet but also for ourselves. **Rosalee de la Forêt** and **Emily Han** have gone beyond simplistic laundry lists of what herbs are 'good for,' and instead paint a holistic picture for how the wholeness of the plant heals the whole person."

— **Sajah Popham,** author of *Evolutionary Herbalism*

"*Wild Remedies* is a wonderful book! Included are a host of activities to engage the reader in learning through a direct personal process. A focus on ethics and sustainability is woven throughout. The bulk of the text consists of in-depth treatments of mostly common plants set within a seasonal context and detailed with lovely illustrations while being paired with worldly delicious and inspiring recipes. Great addition to any library!"

— **Marc Williams,** executive director, Plants and Healers International

"*Wild Remedies* is a delightful blend of wildcrafting wisdom and social tutorial. In the pages of *Wild Remedies*, the authors show you how to start seeing and what to do once you recognize what you have seen. Nothing could be a greater gift."

— **Marie Viljoen,** author of *Forage, Harvest, Feast* and *66 Square Feet*

"**Rosalee de la Forêt** and **Emily Han** have taken the time, for each herb they introduce, to explore its connections to the surrounding ecology. In so doing, they've expanded our attention beyond the human sphere—what a gift! Mindful wildcrafting is a restorative practice in many ways: ecological, medical, spiritual, and deeply personal. *Wild Remedies* gently guides you through them all."

— **Guido Masé,** author of *The Wild Medicine Solution*

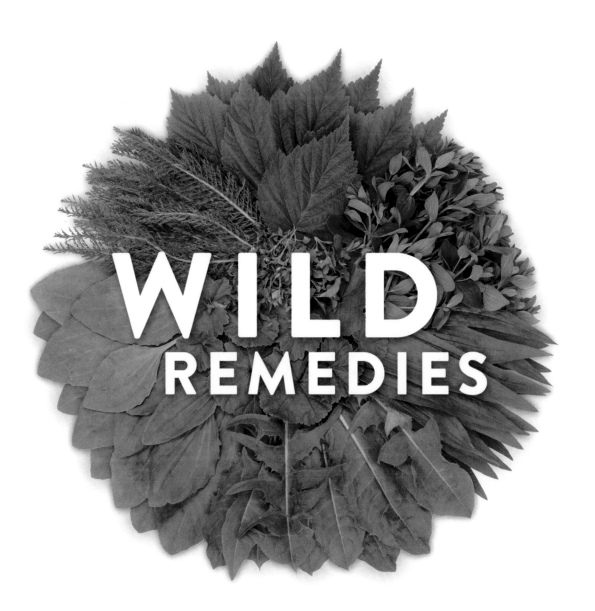

OTHER BOOKS BY THE AUTHORS

Rosalee de la Forêt

Alchemy of Herbs: Transform Everyday Ingredients into Foods and Remedies That Heal

Emily Han

*Wild Drinks and Cocktails: Handcrafted Squashes, Shrubs,
Switchels, Tonics, and Infusions to Mix at Home*

AVAILABLE THROUGH LEARNINGHERBS®

*Since 2005, LearningHerbs.com has empowered thousands of families to make simple, safe,
and reliable remedies using common herbs. Join the free online community on LearningHerbs.com
for recipes and trainings by Rosalee de la Forêt and Emily Han.*

Learning Experiences

Apothecary: The Alchemy of Herbs Video Companion: This beautiful video collection by
Rosalee de la Forêt takes you, step-by-step, through the creation of 15 core herbal remedies.
Transform your kitchen into a natural pharmacy.

HerbMentor®: The ultimate learning companion for anyone with a passion for healing herbs.
Courses, community, and curated resources, all trusted by the world's most reputable herbalists.

For Kids and Families

Wildcraft!® An Herbal Adventure Game: Cooperative board game exploring healing herbs, for ages 4+.

Herb Fairies®: This 13-book series and herbal learning system engages
kids through stories and offers exciting activities to encourage outdoor adventures.

Please visit:

LearningHerbs: www.LearningHerbs.com®
Rosalee's website: www.HerbsWithRosalee.com
Emily's website: www.EmilyHan.com
Hay House: www.HayHouse.com®

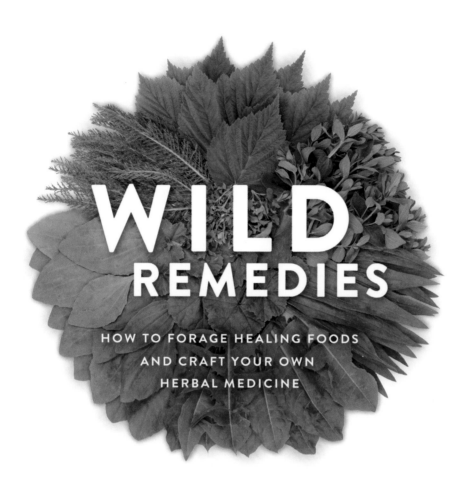

WILD
REMEDIES

HOW TO FORAGE HEALING FOODS
AND CRAFT YOUR OWN
HERBAL MEDICINE

ROSALEE DE LA FORÊT
AND EMILY HAN

HAY HOUSE, INC.

Carlsbad, California • New York City
London • Sydney • New Delhi

Published in the United States by: Hay House, Inc.: www.hayhouse.com® • *Published in Australia by:* Hay House Australia Pty. Ltd.: www.hayhouse.com.au • *Published in the United Kingdom by:* Hay House UK, Ltd.: www .hayhouse.co.uk • *Published in India by:* Hay House Publishers India: www.hayhouse.co.in

Cover design: Karla Baker • *Front-cover photo:* Emily Han • *Front-cover production:* Jan Bosman • *Interior design:* Julie Davison • *Indexer:* J S Editorial, LLC

All interior photos by Rosalee de la Forêt and Emily Han, except for the following:
Images used under license from Shutterstock.com: pages vii, 15, 23, 27, 36, 37, 40, 59, 69, 76–77, 128, 148–149, 175, 176, 180, 216–217, 230, 247, 248, 266, 269, 276–277, 280, 283, 284, 314, 317, 319, 322–323, 324, 329, 336, 344, 350, 351, 365, 366, 368
Ganna Tiulkina: pages viii–ix, xv, 49, 50, 51, 52, 83, 96, 107, 119, 133, 142, 154, 165, 174, 184, 200, 210, 222, 234, 246, 258, 270, 282, 296, 304, 316, 328, 338, 348, 364, 370–371, and chapter border illustrations
Ellen Hutchins, Fucus asparagoides (*now* Bonnemaisonia asparagoides), *1811, image courtesy of the Hutchins Family:* page x
Weymuller Photography: pages 5, 6, 11, 13, 21, 32, 48, 55, 56, 61, 401
Matt Burke: pages 88, 204, 205, 214, 262, 263
Tom Forker: page 315

Cataloging-in-Publication Data is on file with
the Library of Congress

Tradepaper ISBN: 978-1-4019-5688-2
E-book ISBN: 978-1-4019-5689-9
Audiobook ISBN: 978-1-4019-5867-1

10 9 8 7 6 5 4 3 2
1st edition, April 2020

Printed in the United States of America

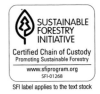

SUSTAINABLE FORESTRY INITIATIVE
Certified Chain of Custody
Promoting Sustainable Forestry
www.sfiprogram.org
SFI-01268
SFI label applies to the text stock

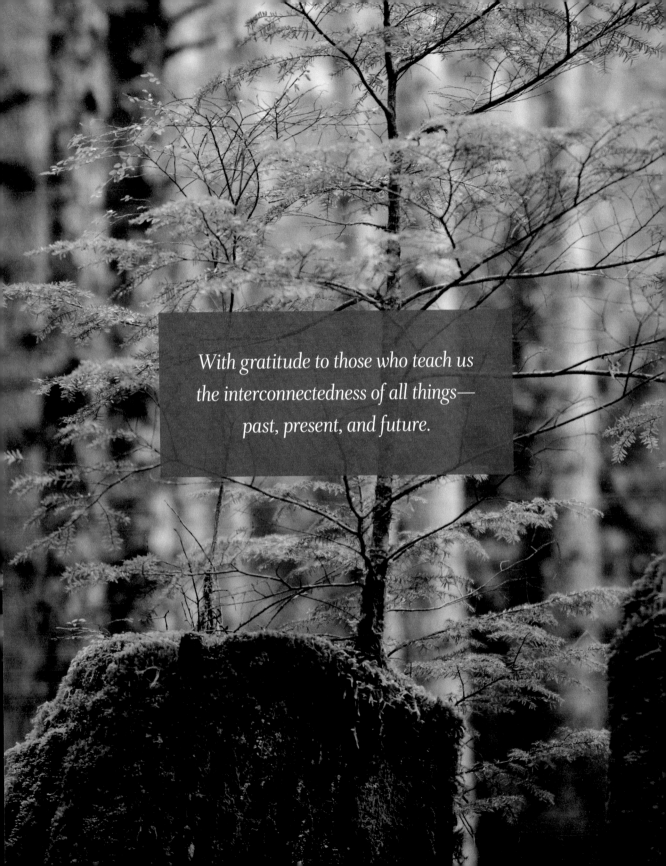

*With gratitude to those who teach us
the interconnectedness of all things—
past, present, and future.*

CONTENTS

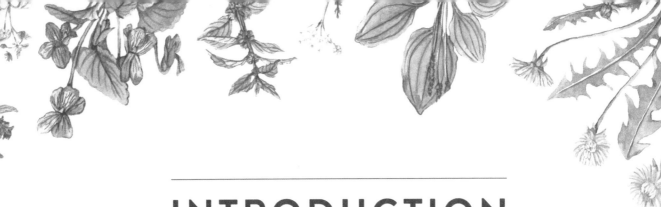

INTRODUCTION

Do you ever feel overwhelmed by the idea of healthy living?

Specialty drinks. Herbal powders. High-powered blenders. Superfruit smoothies. CrossFit. Earthing. Biohacking. Microdosing. Bulletproof Coffee. Spoonful of coconut oil . . . or was that apple cider vinegar? Green tea. Vegan diet. Paleo diet. Keto diet. Breatharianism?

These days it doesn't matter how many gadgets you've bought or how many handfuls of supplements you swallow; there's always a shiny new product on the horizon, promising to cure all your ills. Many of us live within a consumer culture that is trying to purchase its way to better health. Yet as the health industry grows, personal well-being isn't rising along with it. Statistics show that, as a society, we are as unhealthy as ever.

In a desperate race to have more energy, heal our digestive systems, and soothe our frazzled nerves, many of us have made an all too common error: we continue to chase the next big thing, the next great advance in wellness that should *finally* solve our issues. However, we can't solve our problems using the same tools that got us here in the first place. Instead we need to take a step back, and then perhaps 10 more. Or, more aptly, we need to start digging for the root cause. To peel back the layers until our fingernails are crusted with dirt, our faces glow with sunshine, and we emerge filled with wonder at the natural world that surrounds us.

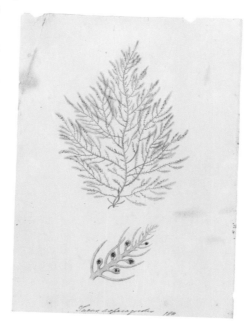

That's what Ellen did, and it forever transformed her life.

What Ellen loved most was feeling the ocean spray on her cheeks as she walked along the bay or the wind in her hair as she crested a peak to search for her favorite plants. But it wasn't always that way. As a child

Ellen was very sick. She was the youngest of six, raised by her mother after her father died when she was just two years old. By the time she was a teenager, her appetite was waning and her health quickly deteriorating. Finally a family friend and doctor took Ellen under his wing. He prescribed something that would dramatically change her life.

His prescription was not a fancy new drug. It wasn't even an herb. No, what he prescribed was far more radical: *botany*.

Ellen's doctor felt botanical studies would encourage her to spend time outdoors as she looked for plants, while also stimulating her mind indoors as she cataloged and drew the plants she found. Luckily this was the perfect prescription. As Ellen delved into the natural world around her, her appetite returned and her strength grew. Her newfound love of plants became her passion. Ellen realized she had a gift for finding plants in the wild and for growing her own garden. Her enthusiasm and joy for life were ignited as her relationship with nature grew.

If you think prescribing botany sounds a bit unconventional for a doctor, you're probably right. Ellen Hutchins was born in Ballylickey, Ireland, in 1785. Credited with being the first Irish female botanist, Ellen produced a body of work identifying and cataloging seaweeds and lichens that remains celebrated today. Museums around the world regularly display her beautiful plant pressings and watercolors, and many plants have been named after her.

The recognition that our good health and even our joy are intertwined with our connection to nature is as important today as it was in 1785. We could even argue that living in concrete jungles and spending our days working inside walls have made connecting with nature all the more urgent. Appreciating and participating in the natural world are often the key ingredients missing in the profit-driven natural health and wellness industry.

Author and journalist Richard Louv has written and lectured extensively on what he calls *nature-deficit disorder*, a term that describes "the psychological, physical and cognitive costs of human alienation from nature."[1] Louv is not alone in his theories; a growing body of research shows that a lack of nature connection may be causing many modern health problems, including anxiety, insomnia, and depression. In 2015 Stanford University researchers examined the brain activity of people who went on a local nature walk compared with those who walked on a high-traffic street. They concluded that walking in nature could lead to a lower risk for depression and other mental illnesses.[2] In another study, of nearly 1,000 residents of Sweden, researchers concluded that the more often people visit urban green spaces, the less often they will report stress-related illnesses such as burnout syndrome, insomnia and fatigue, depression, and feelings of panic.[3]

While these studies can offer objective evidence, the most powerful confirmation comes from going outside and spending time with nature, whether it's a park, garden, forest, or even the plants sprouting along a sidewalk. Having access to and regularly visiting a green space can fill you with joy and wonder. This offers a more profound experience than a superfood or specialized supplement ever could.

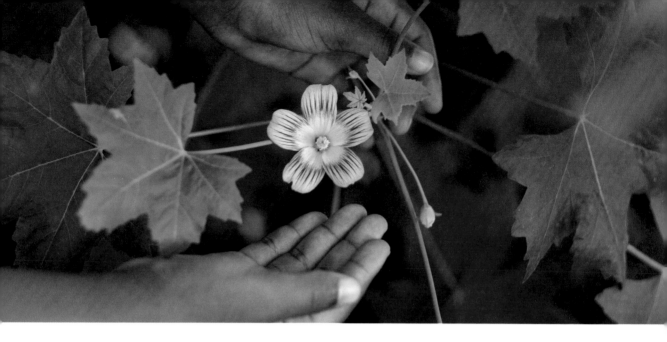

YOUR INVITATION

This book is your invitation to live a deeply joyful and powerfully connected life. A life that feels more vibrant, in which your senses are attuned to the rhythm of the seasons and you recognize the interdependence of all things. This is an opportunity to reclaim your life within nature, in which you play a positive role.

You will be empowered to make your own nourishing foods and plant medicines. Each day will offer new opportunities to meet the plants around you as you gain insights into their gifts. Your dinner table and herbal apothecary will form the basis for your health and well-being. This is your invitation to become a caretaker for this earth while cultivating community and sharing your love of the natural world with others.

We do not offer this invitation lightly. We live in troubled times. Turn on the news or scroll through your social media feeds, and you'll find out about everything from polluted oceans to corporate negligence to toxic spills to our own unprecedented levels of stress and chronic health challenges. Many of us don't need the news to tell us something is wrong. We notice it reflected in our personal health and the health of our wider community.

Witnessing the destruction and challenges we face is understandably overwhelming. It's common to feel helpless, wondering how we could possibly do anything to make a meaningful impact. It is hard to know how to get started. Many proposed solutions leave us feeling unsatisfied or even suspicious. We were once told that health would come in a pill, and experts offer contradictory advice that can spin us in circles and fill us with uncertainty.

We wrote this book as one small but powerful tool to use in responding to problems facing us today. While we acknowledge the troubled state of the world we live in, this invitation isn't about fear. Nor is it about suffering or taking anything away. Instead we invite you to add practices and tools to your life so you can live more deeply and richly. And by doing so, you will participate in a movement to transform our relationships with the earth and with each other.

What we propose takes time and energy, curiosity and commitment. We aren't offering a silver-bullet miracle cure or a feel-good tagline filled with false hopes. We aren't here to add to the dizzying confusion of short-term wellness fads. What we do offer is a transformational journey that strengthens your connections—and your health—by forming deep relationships to the plant world. We believe that a lack of connection to the natural world is what fuels the destruction around us. To reverse this path of destruction, we need to restore our relationship with the earth.

Like Ellen Hutchins, you will be going outside and getting to know the plants that grow around you. The title of this book, *Wild Remedies*, encompasses distinct yet interrelated dynamics. The first is the healing power of being in the wild, of spending time in nature. The second is the power of the remedies you can make by gathering and using local plants for food and medicine—a practice called wildcrafting or foraging. This is medicine that can promote healing ourselves, our families, and our planet.

Woven throughout this book are the ideals upon which *Wild Remedies* is based. As you move through the chapters, you will find information and exercises that bring these guiding principles to life.

WHO WE ARE

The ideals of *Wild Remedies* grew from our experiences with plant medicine and a desire to connect with nature more fully.

Rosalee became interested in natural health at a young age, but it wasn't until she attended an outdoor-living school that the ideas of holistic health and the natural world around her began to intertwine. During her apprenticeship Rosalee immersed herself in the plant world, learning everything from botany to foraging for wild foods to making tools like plant fiber cordage and baskets. However, shortly after beginning her studies, she suddenly came down with a strange illness that left her bedridden due to intense pain and fever. Doctors finally diagnosed a terminal autoimmune disease. Since Western science didn't have solutions for her, Rosalee turned to herbal medicine. Within six months of taking herbs and changing her diet, she was free from her debilitating symptoms.

This experience solidified Rosalee's desire to nurture her knowledge about medicinal plants as well as help others facing chronic illness. Rosalee went to herbal schools for many years, learning traditional ways alongside whole foods nutrition. She became a registered herbalist (RH) with the American Herbalists Guild (AHG) and a clinical herbalist. Always a teacher at heart, Rosalee also began sharing her herbal insights with others and eventually became the education director at LearningHerbs and author of *Alchemy of Herbs: Transform Everyday Ingredients into Foods and Remedies That Heal*.

Emily has always been interested in relationships between our food and drink and the world around us. When she was growing up, she loved running her fingers through the fragrant Vietnamese herbs in her family's garden and observing the caterpillars, snails, and other creatures there. With Zen teacher Thich Nhat Hanh, Emily practiced mindful eating and drinking, marveling at how a simple tangerine or cup of tea could contain an entire universe from sun and soil to bee and farmer. At the dinner table, she absorbed the concepts of food as medicine from her parents, practitioners of Traditional Chinese Medicine. And while marching with labor leader Cesar Chavez, she learned about the devastating effects of pesticides on farmworkers and the environment and the value of responsibility to one another.

Later, Emily became a writer, recipe developer, and educator focusing on nature, culture, and food. A passion for local ingredients merged with her love of being outdoors, sparking an interest in wild foods and drinks. Her search for models of ethical foraging eventually led her to wildcrafting herbalists and LearningHerbs, where she is now the communications director. Ever curious about plant–animal-microbial

relationships, Emily is an avid citizen scientist and Certified California Naturalist, and she weaves these perspectives into her work with herbs and food.

In writing *Wild Remedies*, we both wanted to share varying perspectives on wildcrafting since we live in such different cultures and bioregions—Rosalee in the rural Methow Valley in Washington State and Emily in the metropolis of Los Angeles. As we invite you on this journey, we acknowledge that we, too, are students! Nature is a perpetual teacher, and the ideals and practices in this book can grow and deepen over a lifetime.

journal:
YOUR FIRST STEPS

Throughout this book we will prompt you with journal exercises. These prompts, and ultimately the time you put into them, are the heart of *Wild Remedies*. As you will find, your own observations about the place where you live will be your best guide to foraging wild plants and connecting with nature.

You can use a blank journal to write down your reflections and answers. However, to make it easier, we've created a *Wild Remedies Journal* that you can download:

wildremediesbook.com/resources

REFLECT ON YOUR INTENTIONS: Begin your journal by reflecting on the following questions. Why are you here? Are you seeking to deepen your connections to the plants, animals, and world around you? Are you looking for answers to health challenges? Do you want to make delicious meals or herbal remedies? Write freely, recording anything and everything that comes to you.

CREATE YOUR AFFIRMATION: Based on your brainstorming, create an affirmation sentence or keywords for your intentions. Post it somewhere visible as a reminder that you are starting this journey. Here are some examples:

Curiosity & Resilience
Every day I am learning new ways to support my health.
I celebrate the earth's gifts and honor my connection to plants, animals, and people.

Wild Remedies Ideals

- **Awareness:** Form a deep connection to the natural world around you by practicing presence, wonder, and gratitude.

- **Interdependence:** Recognize interdependence among all beings.

- **Reciprocity:** Grow your reciprocal relationships with plants.

- **Caretaking:** Develop practices for self-care and care of the earth.

- **Seasonal Living:** Engage your senses and live in harmony with the seasons.

- **Empowerment:** Gain confidence to make your own nourishing foods and herbal remedies.

- **Community:** Cultivate community, listen to and learn from others, and work together to build a healthier world.

journal:
YOUR CHALLENGES

Sometimes when we start something new, we feel little doubts, worries, or even fear popping up. Where do you notice objections? Journal your reflections and look for ways to turn "I can't" into "How can I?"

WHAT TO EXPECT FROM THIS BOOK

Wild Remedies is an action guide to becoming deeply connected to the world around you. You will learn how to ethically gather local plants, whether you live in an urban, suburban, or rural environment. Even if you can't forage for wild plants where you live, we offer alternative ways to interact with and heal from nature.

At its core, this book will help reawaken your sense of wonder in the natural world and strengthen your reciprocal relationships within it. Throughout this book, we will give you the tools you need to get started. We also provide practical and inspiring ideas so you can share what you learn in these pages with your community.

We live in a world in which a zillion different things pull us in all directions. Immersing yourself in the natural rhythms of the earth is a powerful step. We also know that little by little is the most effective way to move forward. Going slowly allows you to more firmly and deeply introduce new traditions and habits into your life.

In Part I: Creating Your Foundation, we share the knowledge you will need to get started with gathering and making medicine from your local plants. We show you that it begins simply and easily—by getting to know where you live. You will find out how getting to know plants is a lot like getting to know people, and how ethical wildcrafting is strongly rooted not only in gathering but also in tending plants and their ecosystems. Throughout these chapters, you'll find community stories that highlight inspiring ways people are working with plant medicine. These stories also include tips for sharing your love of plants with your own community.

Parts II through VI feature chapters on two dozen plants. You'll learn about their medicinal gifts, how to identify and harvest them, and many simple recipes so you can bring these plants into your life. We chose these plants based on factors such as widespread availability and our own relationships with them. We have arranged them seasonally, following a general guideline for temperate regions. You may find that some of these plants don't live in your area or that our seasonal listings don't match up to yours. That's okay! An integral part of this book is tuning in to the natural rhythms where *you* live.

HOW TO GET THE MOST OUT OF THIS BOOK

We recommend reading all of Part I carefully, paying special attention to Chapter 2: Getting to Know Where You Live. You will find many powerful activities and observations throughout Part I, which will create your foundation for getting the most out of *Wild Remedies*. Once you're fully rooted in the principles of Part I, you can start with any of the seasons, depending on your current time of the year. Parts II through VI of *Wild Remedies* are divided into five seasons: spring, early summer, late summer, autumn, and winter. (While not often recognized in Western culture, late summer can be a notable time of year in the plant world.) Within each season are chapters devoted to particular plants. We recommend that you begin with the seasonal activities and exercises in Chapter 7 and then proceed with reading about the plants and recipes.

In traditional cultures, people have learned about plants in community while foraging and making food and medicine together. Right now it may feel like it's just you and this book. But community is an important part of the Wild Remedies Ideals, and throughout this book we'll show you ways to find and grow your own community of plant-minded friends.

Unlike wellness fads that come and go, your relationship with plants and nature will be everlasting, deepening with each new season, each new recipe, and each new breath. So let's get started!

journal:

YOUR COMMUNITY

Who in your community can support and assist your journey? These are people who can provide guidance, feedback, and encouragement—who will celebrate your successes and help you in times of difficulty. Brainstorm and research a list of the people and groups available to you. Here are some ideas to get you started:

- Family, friends, neighbors, elders
- Teachers and mentors
- Herbalists and plant medicine practitioners
- Gardeners
- Naturalists
- Meetup groups
- Mental health workers, counselors, coaches
- Religious and spiritual communities
- Online communities such as HerbMentor.com
- Nonhuman support such as a favorite tree or a spot by the river

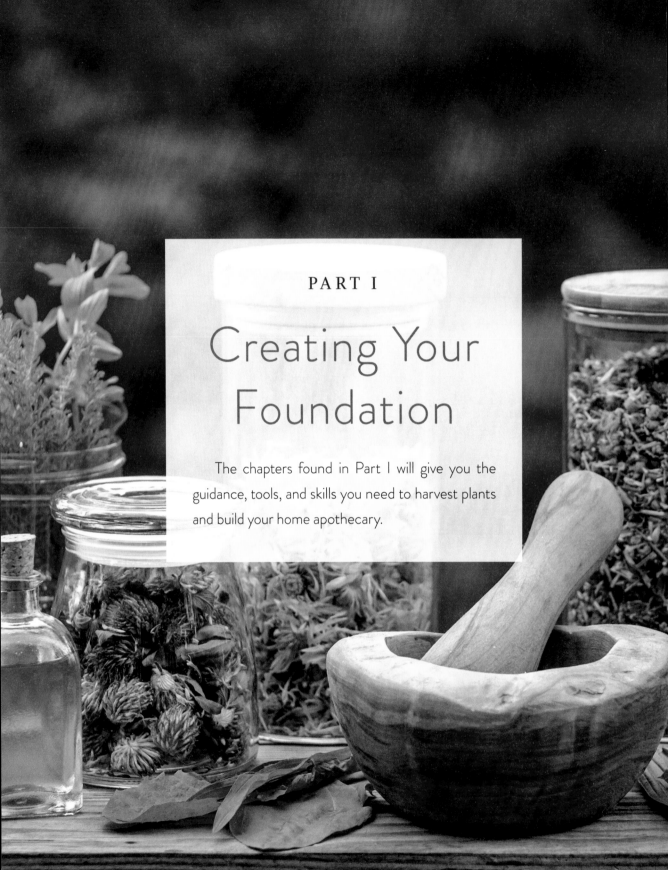

PART I

Creating Your Foundation

The chapters found in Part I will give you the guidance, tools, and skills you need to harvest plants and build your home apothecary.

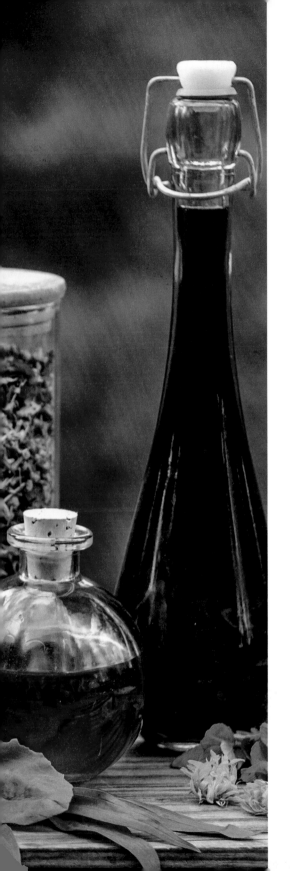

In Chapter 1 we begin to explore the power of plant medicine and many ways that plants can act as catalysts for your health. You'll see why phytonutrient deficiency is an increasing problem and how you can use herbal energetics to choose the best herbs for you.

While herbs from faraway places can be alluring, the most potent plants are often not far from your front door. In Chapter 2 you'll learn about your internal and external worlds and develop simple yet profound practices like your very own sit spot.

When done well, wildcrafting is an art, a skill, and a service. Chapters 3 and 4 illustrate wildcrafting principles and practice so you can learn how to ethically and safely forage for plants and tend their habitats.

We often hear beginning students share fears about harvesting the wrong plants. Chapter 5 shows you how easy it is to begin to recognize plant patterns. You can even start with the plants you find in the produce section of your grocery store.

Whether you love to spend hours in the kitchen or you have a more minimalist approach to cooking, *Wild Remedies* has many simple recipes to bring plants into your life. Chapter 6 outlines what you need to know to get your home apothecary started.

Using plants for food and medicine is a profound way to learn about the rhythms of the seasons, from the tender green leaves of spring and the bounty of summer berries to the deep roots of autumn and the precious gifts of trees in winter. In Chapter 7 you'll learn about living with the seasons and observing the natural rhythms where you live.

Throughout Part I, you'll find community stories that highlight ways to share your love of plants and give back to your community. For example, you'll see how folks have planted community herb gardens, taught children about plants, created free herbal clinics, and helped to reduce harmful chemicals in the environment. Our hope is that these stories spark something of your own design!

CHAPTER 1

THE POWER OF PLANT MEDICINE

If we can see our body as a wonder, we also have the opportunity to see the Earth as a wonder, and healing can begin for the body of the Earth. When we go home and take care of ourselves, we heal not only our own bodies and minds, but we help the Earth as well.

— Thich Nhat Hanh

For as long as we can imagine, plants have given us medicine. Archaeologists have revealed that *Homo erectus* ate medicinal plants at least as long as 800,000 years ago![1] Throughout history and up to the present, plant medicine has woven its way into oral traditions, including stories, songs, and ceremonies. In cultures that created written languages, often some of the first things recorded were how to use plants as medicine.

Contemporary Western herbalists trace their roots to an eclectic mixture of medicine from the Greeks, Persians, African diaspora, and First Peoples of the Americas. Herbalists may also weave in healing practices from Traditional Chinese Medicine, Ayurveda, and other traditions. There has been a long lineage of plant medicine, and it's not uncommon to see people today relying on herbs in the same ways that our ancestors did hundreds or even thousands of years ago.

Yet even with this rich heritage, many of us were born into a society that not only fears nature but believes we are separate from it. It is perhaps this one myth that is doing the most damage to our earth today. A culture of corporations repeatedly puts profits, self-interest, and convenience above all else. As a result, toxicants flow through our rivers, plastics choke the oceans, and single-use disposables clog up landfills. The earth's climate is changing so quickly and so dramatically that by 2030, the United Nations Intergovernmental Panel on Climate Change (IPCC) predicts, we will no longer be able to stop these cataclysmic changes. We're on track to see even more widespread natural disasters like drought, intense wildfires, species die-offs, famines, and on and on.

These changes affect all of us because we are all a part of this earth. Leaked radioactive material doesn't see boundary lines; it flows freely through our oceans and air. The poisons your neighbors spray on their dandelions seep into your water supply. Endocrine disruptors like parabens and phthalates created by the cosmetic and medical industries are found in breast milk all over the world. The truth is, we are deeply connected to this earth, and our personal health cannot be separated from the health of our planet. In order to heal the wound that is fueling environmental destruction, we must reintegrate ourselves into nature. We must rightfully see ourselves within this world and not separate from it.

Plants offer us a powerful way to restore this connection. Through interacting with plants, we can take practical steps that are healing while also being transformative and joyful. Connecting with plants and nature doesn't require us to travel to a far-off wilderness. In fact, the most powerful connections can happen simply and daily, through our food and medicine and by noticing the world around us. How we interact with these plants matters. If we approach plants with the perspective that this "free" food or medicine is ours for the taking, we will throw away much of their healing wisdom. If we harvest plants hastily, without awareness of how best to tend them, we will harm the plants, future harvests, even the greater ecosystem and ourselves.

The strongest relationships we form are based in reciprocity. We know that human relationships that are all-give or all-take are the most fragile. One of the most powerful ways to renew our connection to the earth is to practice both reciprocity and gratitude with beings beyond humans. Plants make it easy to instill this practice. We can easily feel gratitude for the beauty of a flower, the delicious food on our plate, and the healing we experience with herbal medicine. Out of this gratitude, a desire to reciprocate often blooms.

As we shift our awareness to see ourselves as *part* of nature, as we gratefully experience the bounty offered and recognize our important roles, we become empowered. We see that the health of this planet and future generations depends on our actions today. Imagine what this world would look like if we all stepped into our roles as caretakers of the earth, if we worked to strengthen our communities in solidarity with the soil, water, and all beings.

Throughout this book, you will learn ways to work with plants as food and medicine. By the time you finish, you will be able to rely on herbs to relieve many digestive complaints, address minor first-aid situations, soothe a variety of cold and flu symptoms, support natural detoxification, rejuvenate healthy skin, support oral health, relieve musculoskeletal pain, and more. You'll also see how simple it is to incorporate different plants as food and drink in your everyday life. When you have a hand in making your own medicine—from gathering to processing, infusing to straining—your sense of empowerment becomes an important part of the healing process, too.

WILDCRAFTING: A NEW FOCUS ON WILD AND LOCAL PLANTS

In our globalized society, it is easy to use plants from all over the world. In a single day, you might use hibiscus from Burkina Faso in your tea, cinnamon from Sri Lanka in your pastries, and lavender from France in your laundry detergent. Using a variety of herbs and spices to enliven your meals is a delightful experience and may provide an important conection to your ancestral roots. The most popular spices are often also renowned for their abilities to dramatically support your health. For instance, black pepper, turmeric, and ginger are well known for their anti-inflammatory properties.

While we are grateful for the gifts of these faraway plants, this book focuses primarily on common and easily identifiable plants that are safe to harvest. Many of the plants we chose are considered to be "weeds." We encourage you to learn which plants live and thrive near you so that you can directly participate in every aspect of your food and medicine. When you purchase plants from far-off places, you can't be certain of how they were grown and processed, nor can you develop a reciprocal relationship with them. Packaging and shipping plants around the world also requires the use of fossil fuels, contributing to climate change.

Tending, harvesting, and using local plants often provides the most meaningful gifts as well as the most vibrant food and medicine. In addition to cultivating plants in gardens, we can work with edible and medicinal plants that commonly grow in the wild—many of which are considered "weeds" by society at large. The practice of gathering and using wild plants is often called wildcrafting, or foraging. To practice ethical wildcrafting, we must be mindful of not just what we take but also how we approach the plant and the greater ecosystem. We will discuss Wildcrafting Principles in Chapter 3 and Wildcrafting Practice in Chapter 4.

Of course, we aren't expecting that everyone will wildcraft or forage all of their food or medicine. It begins with forming relationships with one or two plants. For some people, that may be enough. Others may not wildcraft at all. You can also get many herbs in this book from your garden, local farmers, apothecaries, and grocery stores. Whether or not you choose to wildcraft, this book will show you how to make foods and remedies, how to connect with joy and wonder to the world around you, and how to bring your senses alive and in tune with the natural rhythms of the seasons.

A LITTLE-KNOWN BENEFIT OF WILD PLANTS: PHYTONUTRIENTS

One reason for incorporating more plants, especially wild ones, into your food and medicine is for their abundant phytonutrients. While dietitians have long recognized the importance of macronutrients (carbohydrates, fats, proteins) and micronutrients (vitamins, minerals),

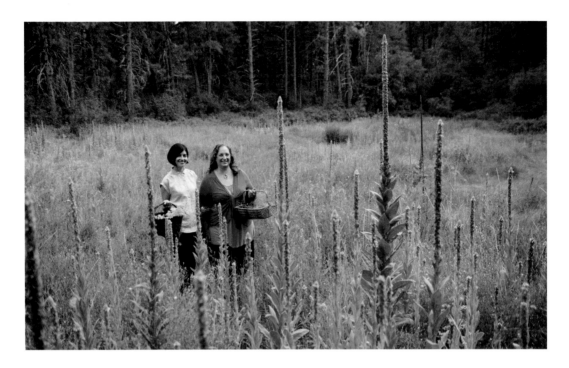

the importance of phytonutrients has caught on only recently. Phytonutrients are a variety of natural chemicals that plants have developed to deal with stressors such as sun exposure or being nibbled on by bugs. Because these compounds aren't directly involved with the normal growth of a plant, they are called secondary metabolites and include things like carotenoids, flavonoids, resveratrol, and phytoestrogens.

It's likely that throughout the year your ancestors ate hundreds of different plants that gave them a wide range of beneficial nutrients, the exact selection depending on where in the world they lived. Today modern humans who eat a standard American diet often consume no more than a couple dozen different plants, with most of their plant-based foods revolving around potatoes, tomatoes, corn, and lettuce. This monoculture diet has resulted in widespread phytonutrient deficiency. Many people are beginning to recognize that phytonutrient deficiency could be a contributing factor in chronic disease such as cancer and cardiovascular disease. Herbalist Kevin Spelman, Ph.D., reports that "your ancestors had 8 to 10 times—a conservative estimate; probably a more realistic estimate is maybe 100 times—more exposure to phytochemistry than we do today. And that [lack of phytochemical exposure] foments chronic disease."[2]

The more stress a plant experiences, the higher its phytonutrient content. This means that an apple growing on an old homestead, without receiving regular watering or fertilization, is often higher in nutrients than an apple grown with lots of coddling on a farm focused on high-yield produce. In other words, wild foods are often higher in nutrients than their

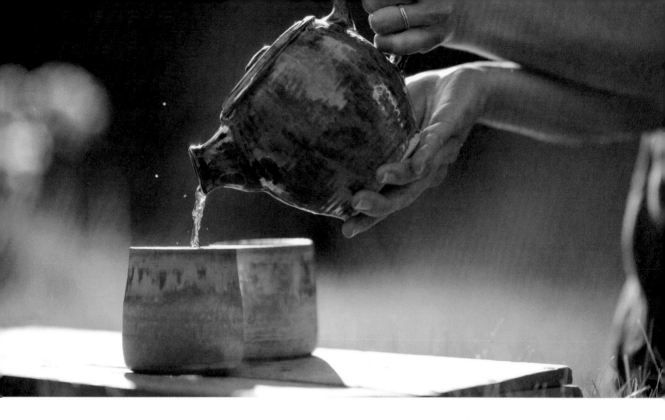

cultivated counterparts. By regularly eating, drinking, and making medicines with a variety of wild plants, you will add a wide range of phytochemicals to your diet.

GET TO KNOW PLANTS

With all that plants offer us as food, shelter, medicine, and more, it's surprising that many people today can identify only a handful of plants. Given that plants are beautiful and fascinating and offer many practical gifts, studying and interacting with them are wonderful ways to strengthen your relationship to the natural world. Plants grow everywhere—all you have to do is get to know them!

Getting to know plants is a lot like getting to know people. When we first meet a person, we often begin with a name. Just as people have lots of names—first names, second names, nicknames, etc.—so do plants. The more you get to know a person, the more names you may find, from Jennifer to Honeycakes to Mama to Mrs. Anderson. And the same goes for plants. Their names and nicknames include their formal genus and species names, which you will learn more about in Chapter 5: Botany Basics.

However, learning a person's name is only the very beginning of a relationship. The more we get to know people, the more we learn about their family, where they live, how they spend their time, what they like, what they don't like, and what their gifts and talents are. We may become aware of their prickly sides, their soft sides, their generous sides. The same is true for plants. With time, we learn where and how they like to grow, the common characteristics of their plant family, how they look and change through the seasons. As we become more acquainted, we also get to know their gifts. Do they provide food, medicine, and shelter to people and animals? Can their fibers be made into clothing or rope? Do their flowers bring us joy?

When you first meet someone, you don't typically ask, "What can you do for me?" within moments of meeting. Which is not to say that some people don't think this way! But we can often see right through people who are only out for themselves, and our first instinct can be to avoid them. Have you ever been in a one-sided relationship where you felt like you were constantly giving without getting anything in return (or vice versa)? These are often brittle relationships just waiting to snap.

When getting to know a plant, it can be easy for someone to think, "What is this plant good for? What can it give me?" But just as that is not a healthy way to approach human relationships, it's also a poor way to enter into a plant relationship. Instead, the most fulfilling and resilient relationships are built on trust and reciprocation. And as evidenced all over the globe, when we attempt to take and take and

take from the natural world without fully tending and reciprocating, we end up with a disaster, whether it be a clear-cut forest, an oil spill, or simply a pile of trash littering a green space.

We propose using your highest social skills when encountering plants. Avoid rushing into the relationship and instead get to know each plant over time. Be interested and curious about what these plants are. As your relationship deepens, constantly ask yourself, "How can I help this plant?" rather than simply jumping to ways the plant can serve you.

In your own life, you probably have close friends as well as acquaintances. Perhaps there are people you admire as well as people you aren't all that into even though you encounter them often. Sometimes closer relationships develop slowly over time. Sometimes it's love at first sight. The same goes for plants! You may find there are plants that you instantly are enamored with while others don't even catch your attention (yet!).

journal:

RECIPROCITY WITH PLANTS

Brainstorm the ways plants show up in your life. What gifts do they offer? For example, air to breathe, food, medicine, shelter, beauty, tools, etc.

Then, brainstorm the ways you are giving back to plants. What gifts do you offer? For example, gardening, picking up litter, helping to conserve habitat.

HOW TO CHOOSE PLANTS FOR YOU

All over the world, people approach using plants as medicine in many ways, and for thousands of years we have explored how to best choose a plant for a person or a condition. In other words, just as Western medicine has its own systems for diagnosing and prescribing, herbalists have their own unique ways of matching herbs to people.

One of these methods is using herbal energetics. Although the term *energetics* may sound esoteric, it's actually a very grounded way of experiencing herbs and one that you probably already observe every day. In a nutshell, herbal energetics is evaluating the qualities of hot, cold, moist, and dry in both plants and people. We then use opposing qualities to bring balance. For instance, if someone feels cold, we could use a warming plant to heat that person up.

community story:
HERB GARDENS IN THE CITY

For people who live in urban areas, finding access to plants can sometimes be difficult. In Boston, a grassroots group called Herbstalk came up with a solution. "We wanted to create ways that city folks could have more contact with healing plants in their daily lives," says Herbstalk founder Steph Zabel. Through its Community Gardens Project, the group places small container herb gardens in public and pedestrian spaces. Some of the plants they have grown are echinacea, marshmallow, and yarrow. Passersby can learn about traditional uses of the plants, and the gardens can also be used for teaching events and plant walks.

"Our purpose is to provide an interesting way for people to interact with plants, adding beauty, knowledge, and inspiration to their daily lives," says Steph. "In the long term, we aim to create a connected network of herbal gardens throughout the city of Boston and to facilitate an ongoing, interactive, educational display that will be a part of the urban landscape."

Would you like to start a similar project where you live? Steph recommends starting small and simple. To keep installation and maintenance manageable, focus on container gardens and herbs that are hardy and perennial (or that easily reseed themselves). Share the project with a group of like-minded and dedicated volunteers who can create each step together. And spread the word! Steph suggests inviting people to gather around the garden, to respectfully harvest herbs from it, and to create their own events and educational gatherings with the plants. "The more people who use and take an active interest in the garden, the more it—and the local community—will thrive," she says.

To learn more about Herbstalk's projects, visit herbstalk.org.

Here's an example. Think of a hot summer day. The heat is reflecting off every surface, and you can feel the heat building in you, too. Perhaps your face is flushed, your mouth is parched, and you feel a trickle of sweat down your back. You are starting to feel uncomfortably hot, and so you reach for a slice of watermelon. As you bite into that watermelon, does it seem hot or cold to you? Does it seem dry or moist? Judging that a watermelon is cooling and moistening is essentially herbal energetics as it relates to plants. Recognizing feelings of heat within yourself is one aspect of herbal energetics; using the cooling and moistening qualities of watermelon to relieve your sensations of heat and dryness is another. These are the basics of herbal medicine.

Whether we consciously recognize it or not, every day we experience qualities of hot, cold, moist, and dry in ourselves and in the foods and beverages we consume. These observations may shift dramatically from day to day, but they also shift more subtly with the changing of the seasons. Being aware of these qualities within yourself and in your food, drinks, and herbal remedies is a powerful way to be more present as well as to address your health needs.

Herbal energetics are woven throughout *Wild Remedies* as a way to encourage you to tap into a deeper sensory awareness. If you'd like to learn more about herbal energetics, see Rosalee's book *Alchemy of Herbs*.

journal:

ENGAGING YOUR SENSES

Here's a simple way to experience the qualities of hot, cold, moist, and dry. Take a bite or sip of a food or drink in each category, giving yourself some time to reflect after each one. What sensations do you notice in your mouth and body? How does your experience with each one compare with the others? We've provided some examples of common foods below, but feel free to try others, too.

- *Hot:* black pepper, ginger, thyme

- *Cold:* orange, cucumber, salad

- *Moist:* okra, watermelon, oatmeal

- *Dry:* cracker, coffee, black tea

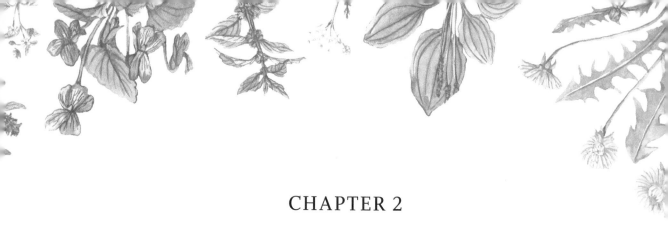

CHAPTER 2

GETTING TO KNOW WHERE YOU LIVE

Your wild paradise is not in some far-off land; it is in your own neighborhood. All you need is to discover it: see it, smell it, feel it, unveil its secrets, make it your own.

— Samuel Thayer

Where do you live?

This seemingly simple question crops up when we meet new acquaintances, fill out forms, and travel away from home. Yet one could answer in countless ways. The city of Los Angeles. Tongva land. The San Rafael Hills. Forty-six steps to the right of the elderberry tree. In the canyon where the towhee birds forage for insects in spring. Where the scent of orange blossoms permeates the nighttime air.

Some aspects of where we live remain fairly constant—the path of a local river or the geology underfoot, for instance. Others change with the seasons, such as the wildflowers or migratory birds that arrive annually, or a pattern of hot summers and cold winters. And some details shift day by day, like the sound of a squirrel scampering across the roof or the smell of soil after an unexpected rain.

If we rush through our days on autopilot, it can be easy to miss many of these things. Modern life can steer us into a rut of waking up, checking the notifications on our phones, commuting to work with headphones on, scrolling through lunch, and hurrying home to get in front of yet another screen. As a result, we might not know much about where we live beyond the names of our street and town. This lack of connection to the world around us—and our own bodies—can make us lonely (despite all those notifications!), sick, and unhappy.

However, if we slow down and engage our senses, the world opens up. We experience the richness of where we live and root ourselves in the here and now. We tune in to what we need to heal as individuals and what we can give back to others. This practice is essential if we want to forage plants for food and medicine. In order to know local plants, you need to know your local ecosystems, from the basics of your geography to the nuances of each season. Your first step as a wildcrafter is observation. From that observation, your ethics and practices will flow.

It is not difficult to rekindle your connection to the world around you. You are in fact already part of nature, and you have what you need. While getting to know where you live on a deeper level will take some research, much of your learning will arise from your own observations and your willingness to give it the attention it deserves.

GETTING TO KNOW YOURSELF

Before focusing on the outside world, however, take a moment to tune in to your internal world. Being able to listen to your body and recognize your own needs and patterns is an important part of living with the seasons and using plant medicine. By caring for yourself first, you can also be a much better caretaker for the plants, their ecosystems, and your family and community. Connecting with your unique self will help you understand how to truly care for your own well-being.

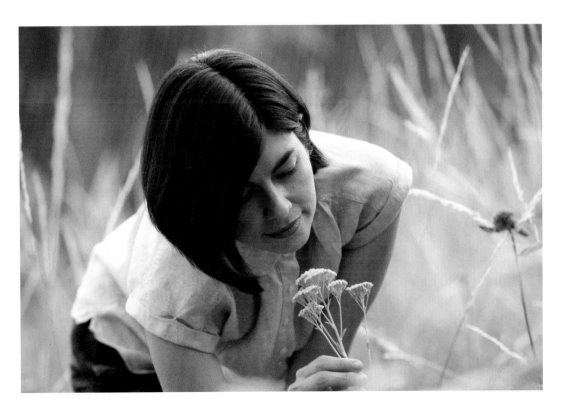

journal:
PRACTICING SELF-CARE IN TODAY'S HECTIC WORLD

Lexi Koch, an intuitive life coach, contributed this section of four practices to connect your needs, feelings, and inner voice. You can do this exercise as often as you wish. To deepen your practice, Lexi also offers a free audio meditation, a guided journey to connect with your inner voice at lexikoch.com/innervoice.

1. IDENTIFY YOUR NEEDS.

In modern life, we sit a lot and scroll a lot. We source answers from everywhere but within. Some of our most basic needs go unnoticed or ignored because we don't give ourselves permission to meet them. Simple needs get overlooked, like drinking water when we're parched or getting up to use the bathroom when we must. If we know our needs and believe they are worthy, a huge leap toward self-care begins.

See if you can notice your needs without downplaying or criticizing them. Five times throughout the day, write down your needs from the most simple to the most complex by writing, "Right now I need . . ."

2. ALLOW YOUR FEELINGS.

Have you ever taken the time to track your feelings through a day? Like waves, when you begin to watch, you see that each one passes, no matter how big or strong it is. When you name what you're feeling and honor that feeling, you show yourself greater respect and care.

Start to simply name and identify your feelings. Write down your feelings five times throughout the day: "Right now I am feeling [use one-word answers here]." See if you can also jot down how long it takes for the feeling to pass.

3. CONNECT WITH YOUR INTUITION.

Your intuition is the part of you that could not care less about "shoulds," cultural norms, or stories you inherited in childhood. Write down the question "What does self-care look like for *me*?" Listen for a quiet voice to whisper the answer to you. *Whatever* you hear, write that down. If you have a question about the answer, write it down and listen for your intuition to answer that as well. By listening to your inner guidance system, you find your individual voice as well as the unique way you need to care for yourself.

4. WATCH FOR SENSATIONS THAT ARE PLEASANT AND FEEL LIKE FLOW.

Flow happens when you are guided by the voice in your heart and not the critic in your mind. You feel in alignment with your whole being—body, mind, and soul—with no questioning and no doubting. Watching for flow moments will let you know a lot about what you love and what feels aligned for you. It also, conveniently, helps you to know what doesn't feel aligned and what doesn't feel like self-care.

Write about the last time you felt in flow, completely abandoned to the moment and at peace. What parts of that experience can you learn from and bring into your life today or tomorrow?

GAINING A SENSE OF PLACE

When we think of nature, we often imagine grand, wild places—dense rainforests, remote mountaintops, the locales highlighted in documentaries. But nature doesn't exist only in pristine reserves or faraway destinations. In fact, nature is everywhere, whether you live in the city, suburbs, or country. Where can you find nature where you live?

journal:
FINDING NATURE

Spend a day actively looking for nature in unexpected places. Highway medians, abandoned lots, bus stops, parking lots, and rooftops are just a few of the places you might find plant and animal life. At the end of the day, journal: What did this exercise teach you about the natural world? Did you learn anything about your own sense of observation?

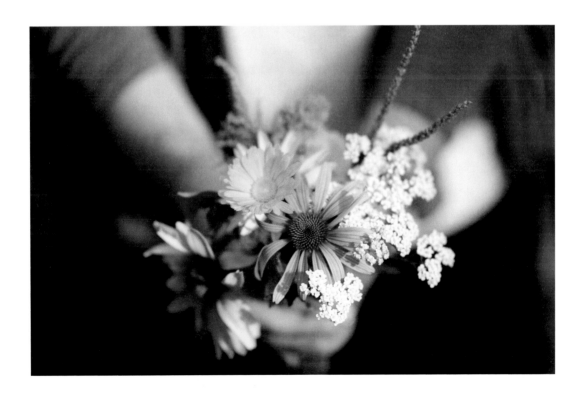

EXERCISE: SIT SPOT PRACTICE

One of the best ways to get in tune with your local habitat and seasonal rhythms is to have a safe spot outdoors where you can sit quietly, relax, and observe. This is often called a sit spot in naturalist teachings. Your sit spot can be in your yard, on a park bench, under a tree in a vacant lot, or in any other outdoor space. The more regularly you visit this place, the more powerful your observations will be. With that in mind, the easier your spot is to get to, the better.

There is no right or wrong way to use a sit spot, but the more you put into this exercise, the more you will get out of it. If you can spend only 5 minutes a week at your sit spot, then do it! If you are able to spend 20 minutes a day, awesome! The most important thing is consistency. It is far better to spend 5 minutes once a week than one hour once a season.

To find your sit spot, begin by making a list of potential locations. These may be very particular, such as a specific park bench, or they may be a general area, for example a botanical garden near your workplace. Some things to consider:

- Is the area safe?

- Is it easy for you to get to?

- Can you easily observe forms of nature, such as plants, animals, water, or the sky?

- Can you sit there comfortably, say on the ground, against a rock, or in a chair?

- Are you inspired to visit that spot regularly and consistently?

Once you have a prospective list of locations, visit them to narrow down your options. It's okay to have more than one sit spot. Maybe you'll visit one during the week and another on the weekend. Ideally you'll be able to visit your sit spot throughout the seasons, in all types of weather, and at varying times of day; however, if you move or travel frequently, then even that is not set in stone.

Starting any new practice can bring challenges. You can't erase those challenges, but you can make plans to overcome them. Brainstorm potential challenges and ways to get past them. For example, if time is a limiting factor, how can you choose a convenient sit spot that fits into your daily life? Perhaps there's a park where your children play, an area by your regular bus stop, or a spot you can get to on your lunch break.

UNDERSTANDING YOUR BIOREGION

Each of us lives in a bioregion—a unique geographic area that contains an ecosystem, a mosaic of natural features and communities of plants and animals (including people). As humans have moved around the world, they have transported plants and animals with them, both intentionally and accidentally. As a result, most bioregions have a mix of native, or original, plants and animals and nonnative species. Some introduced species may be considered invasive because they are able to spread easily without human help and disrupt existing ecosystems. The interplay of native and introduced plants can be nuanced; many so-called weeds, for instance, play a beneficial role in their environments.

An awareness of the natural features in your bioregion and their interconnected relationships will help you develop your Wildcrafting Principles (Chapter 3) and Wildcrafting Practice (Chapter 4). The questions in the journal prompt What's in Your Bioregion are designed to help you get to know your local area. It's okay if you don't know all the answers! You can jot down more information as your observations grow over time.

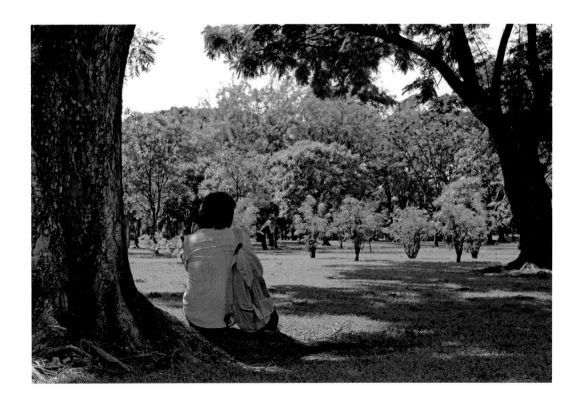

journal:
WHAT'S IN YOUR BIOREGION?

GEOGRAPHY

- From where you are, what direction is north, south, east, west?

- Where is the closest mountain range? Body of water?

- What geologic processes shaped the landscape?

- What type of soil is in your area?

- What watershed do you live in? Can you trace the path along which that water flows?

- What are the seasonal temperature and precipitation patterns in your region?

FLORA AND FAUNA

- What is your plant hardiness zone?

- What are the main plant communities or vegetation types where you live (for example, grassland, oak woodland, riparian)?

- Name some common trees or shrubs.

- Name some common annual plants.

- Name some common fungi or lichens.

- Name some common mammals.

- Name some common birds. Are they resident or migratory?

- Name some common reptiles, amphibians, or fish.

- Name some common insects or other invertebrates.

- Name some common pollinators. What plants do they pollinate?

- Are the plants and animals you listed native, introduced, invasive, endangered?

- Where in the food web does each of these species appear? Are they producers, consumers, scavengers, or decomposers?

HUMANS

- Who are the First Peoples in your area?

- What is the Indigenous name(s) for your area?

- What is your and your ancestors' relationship with this place?

- What is the history of land use and management in your area?

- What are some ways in which local people make a living in connection with nature (e.g., farming, fishing, logging)?

- Where does your drinking water come from? Where does your wastewater go?

- Who are your neighbors?

journal:
REFLECTION

It has been said that the more you know, the more you know you don't know! Likewise, becoming acquainted with where you live is an ever-evolving process. After participating in the exercises in this chapter, spend some time reflecting on your experience. Consider these questions:

- What do you already know about where you live?

- What don't you know about where you live?

- What examples of interdependent relationships have you noticed?

- No matter where you are in your journey, what are you excited to learn about next?

- How will you seek out information to learn more? Whom can you learn from?

SEARCHING FOR ANSWERS?

Many people, groups, and resources can help you learn about your bioregion and basic principles of ecology. Here are some you may want to check out:

- Local elders

- Indigenous educators

- Naturalists (many U.S. states have master naturalists)

- Farmers and gardeners (many U.S. states have master gardeners)

- Native plant nurseries and societies

- Field guides

- Local libraries

- Natural history museums

- Nature centers and interpretive centers

- Parks and preserves

- Environmental organizations (Audubon Society, Sierra Club, etc.)

- Citizen science websites and apps like iNaturalist

- Cooperative Extension Service offices and websites

- College and university science departments

- Massive Online Open Courses (Open University, edX, Coursera, etc.)

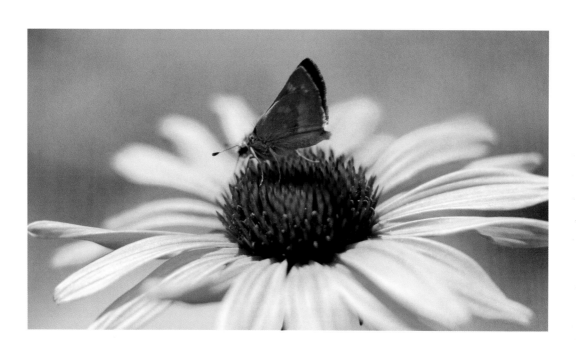

community story:
LAND AND LANGUAGE

Sandra Warriors Pistol Bullet spent the summer of 2018 interning at the Methow Valley Interpretive Center and at Methow Natives, a native plant nursery in Twisp, Washington. Her work involved learning about ecological restoration, including the transplanting and propagation of plants. She also began a language revitalization project to compile plant names in the Interior Salish language.

Sandra says, "I was inspired to do an interdisciplinary study that included both language work and the work being done toward restoration of land with indigenous plants because I believe they're interconnected. As someone from an Indigenous background, I believe there's a need to preserve culture and language and that this work has to center around healing the land and our relationship toward it."

Through Sandra's work, the Interior Salish language will continue to live on in the Methow Valley. There are plans to update plant signs in the Native Plant Garden to include Interior Salish. Sandra also worked with the local Methow Conservancy to create interpretive signs along a river valley hike.

Sandra's community projects honor the past as well as the present and future. "There are still Methow people who live in this valley and who have a connection toward the land and have their own way of life and their own language. The work being done has to not only tie in the past, but also tie in the present and look forward," she says. "I am hoping that the ecology restoration work with the indigenous plants helps those Indigenous [people] from Methow band connect with their ancestral territories through cultural practice and knowledge keeping, and that their narratives will be heard."

What ecological restoration projects are happening in your area? How can you learn about and support Indigenous cultures and languages where you live? How can you find out the names and stories of your local plants?

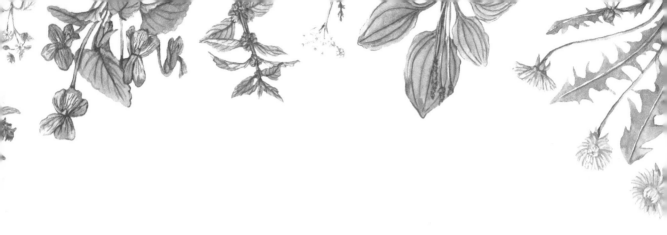

CHAPTER 3

WILDCRAFTING PRINCIPLES

*If we choose to use plants as our medicine, we then become
accountable for the wild gardens, their health, and their upkeep.
We begin a co-creative partnership with the plants, giving back what
we receive—health, nourishment, beauty, and protection.*

— ROSEMARY GLADSTAR

Gathering plants for food and medicine directly connects us to the earth and can be a powerful way to heal the detachment many of us feel in our modern lives. Sensing the sun on our faces as we pick tender leaves, smelling the damp soil while digging roots, listening to bees foraging alongside us—these experiences transform us from being a passive observer of nature into a participant.

So far, your *Wild Remedies* journey has included a deepened connection to your own body and the place where you live. Both of these are fundamental, but before we get to the practical how-tos of gathering plants, we need to root ourselves in the principles of ethical wildcrafting. As wildcrafters and foragers, our intention is to take care of the plants that take care of us and to gather them in a way that is not just sustainable but regenerative.

BE A CARETAKER

In the modern world, you'll find different perspectives on how humans should relate to their environment. Many people believe that the earth is ours to use without consideration for future generations. Others feel that the wilderness should remain "pure" and absolutely untouched by humans. Neither of these limited viewpoints reflects an inherent understanding of the natural world and our place within it.

Another perspective is recognizing both the ability and responsibility humans have to benefit their surroundings. In recent years scholars have challenged the idea that European settlers observed a pristine wilderness when landing in the New World. From the boreal forests down through the Amazon jungle, these lands were masterfully tended by Indigenous peoples. For example, as M. Kat Anderson writes of the California landscape in *Tending the Wild*, "Much of what we consider wilderness today was in fact shaped by Indian burning, harvesting, tilling, pruning, sowing, and tending." [1] This is not to say that we should all immediately start planting and pruning in wild spaces without first understanding the needs of an ecosystem. But we can work toward developing this awareness and learning from those who do know.

When you approach wildcrafting with a caretaking mentality, you can (and will) have a positive impact on your local ecosystem and your health. This is very different from setting out to harvest all the plants that you can. First and foremost, ethical wildcrafting goes beyond a "do no harm" approach. Instead, the intention is to create a more resilient ecosystem.

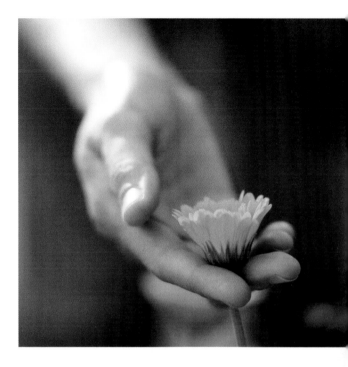

DEVELOP A RECIPROCAL RELATIONSHIP WITH THE LAND

Ethical wildcrafting begins with a mind-set of reciprocity and embodies the desire to give more than you take. This might mean spreading seeds when appropriate, pruning in a way that supports plant growth, or picking up litter. It can also mean being a voice in your area for a healthier and more resilient landscape, one that challenges practices like clear-cutting, dumping toxic waste, and spraying harmful pesticides and herbicides. If you rely on wild plants for food and medicine, know that they in turn rely on you to keep them from harm. Reciprocity also means that you show up regularly, and not just when you want something. This includes visiting areas in all seasons to observe the changes that natural cycles bring and to see how harvesting affects these areas.

As you form a relationship with your harvesting areas, carefully consider who you share them with. Wildcrafters are often secretive about their harvesting spaces. This isn't necessarily done out of a sense of ownership but rather comes from a commitment to the health of that place. Know that when you disclose your harvesting area—in person or on social media—those people may share it with others. If the area becomes overharvested, you cannot know whether the changes you witness are due to your own actions or those of others, making it difficult to adjust accordingly.

HARVEST WITH AWARENESS

Visiting your favorite wildcrafting spot can reveal a world of delight and intrigue. Did you notice that tiny mushroom growing out of the decaying tree? Is that a song from the first robin of the season? Notice how the air feels so fresh and crisp? So many joys await if you invest your full attention, from the moment you go out the door to the bottling of your herbal potion or the enjoyment of your foraged meal. This focus and awareness can be interrupted by the beep or buzz of digital devices. If it is possible for you, silence your phone when caretaking, wildcrafting, or processing plants.

Awareness also means avoiding falling into ruts or following oversimplified rules. Many foraging guides offer decrees about how many plants to take: "Pick 1 in every 10 plants" or "Harvest 30 percent of the total population." But these rules don't have a lot of value in a regenerative model. How much to harvest differs from plant to plant and changes from ecosystem to ecosystem, from season to season, and from year to year. Memorizing a set of numerical guidelines isn't helpful and can actually lead to overharvesting. Instead, practice awareness so you can ascertain what *is* and then adopt a harvesting strategy based on your actual situation.

journal:
YOUR LOCAL ENVIRONMENT

What are some current concerns in your area? For example:

- What kind of habitat loss (if any) is affecting your local ecosystems?

- Are rainfall (or snowpack) amounts lower than normal, normal, or higher than normal?

- Are invasive plants or animals taking a toll on native plants?

- Are there plants that are routinely overharvested?

Make a list of issues you are aware of. Contact people who may have a broader understanding of these topics (naturalists, herbalists, scientists, elders, etc.). Reflect on how your local issues affect the plant populations. What can you do to help?

emily's story:
CHANGING CLIMATE =
CHANGING FORAGING

For me, being a wildcrafter often means choosing *not* to harvest plants. From 2010 to 2017, a record 129 million trees died in California due to drought, bark beetle infestations, and rising temperatures. Countless other plants and animals suffered alongside them in the relentlessly dry, hot weather. As the drought persisted, I witnessed its devastation in places where I loved hiking and gathering plants. Foraging in these areas was no longer appropriate. Taking leaves, flowers, or berries from a drought-stressed plant wouldn't be respectful to that individual, the health of the plant stand, or the animals that depended on it for food. I would be taking more than I could give back.

As of this writing, the drought has ended, but its long-term effects, the acceleration of climate change, and habitat loss mean that my bioregion will continue to experience challenges. Rather than foraging in the wild, I focus on growing my own herbs, buying from local farmers, and planting native plants to support local wildlife. I still visit my former wildcrafting spots, and the plants continue to offer their gifts in different ways. Simply *being* with these plants can be profound medicine in itself.

How has climate change affected your bioregion and its plants and animals? What precautions might you need to take to support a resilient habitat?

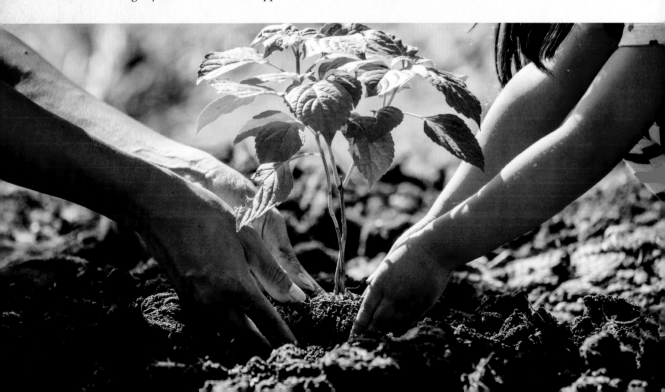

RECOGNIZE INTERDEPENDENCE

Harvesting plants is about forming relationships. At first glance it may seem that the relationship simply involves you and the plant, but we humans are just a small piece of the puzzle. A wider view reveals an intricate web of interdependence and reciprocity.

For instance, a wild rose bush doesn't live in isolation. Its ecosystem contains a multitude of elements all interacting with one another, from the sunlight and soil to the tallest trees and smallest microorganisms. It includes water that feeds roots and bees that pollinate blooms. Small mice that shelter in the brambles and birds that feast on the ripe hips, spreading the seeds to grow new roses.

Learning about these relationships enriches your experience of the world. It also helps you understand where and how plants grow and the potential effects of harvesting them. It's impossible to know all of this for every plant, but attention and curiosity ensure that you learn more each day.

ROOT YOURSELF IN SEASONAL CYCLES

Through refrigeration, fast global shipping, and indoor climate control, we can visit a grocery store and expect to find the same produce year-round, regardless of its growing season. This modern-day baseline of uniformity was created for comfort but also has

its downsides. Without the natural ups and downs of life, our experiences are dulled. Life is monotonous.

In contrast, living with the seasons enhances our lives. It's savoring the burst of flavor in each bite of freshly harvested fruit. It's embracing the weather. It's having experiences that make us feel more alive, from taking a sip of cool mint tea during summer to cuddling up with roasted-dandelion-root brew in the winter.

Seasonal living also means recognizing what is bountiful and what is not. Nothing is static within nature, and an abundant year of any plant is not a given. One year elderberries may droop heavily off their branches; another year conditions may change, creating meager clumps of dried-up fruits. Living seasonally means evolving your harvesting hopes and practices with the ebb and flow of the plants' offerings. These natural cycles teach us patience, resilience, and acceptance.

PRACTICE GRATITUDE, ALWAYS

Which do you think makes better food and medicine: mindfully walking through the park, taking time to connect with the world around you, carefully harvesting plants, and consciously choosing ways to support the health of the area? Or rushing to an area when you have 20 minutes on your lunch break, ripping up plants at will, stuffing them into your bag, and then hurrying back to work?

UNITED PLANT SAVERS
SPECIES AT-RISK LIST

United Plant Savers (unitedplantsavers.org) is an organization dedicated to promoting the preservation of North American native medicinal plants and their habitats. They publish lists of "At Risk" and "To Watch" plants to raise awareness of concerns regarding native plant populations. According to their work, these are the medicinal plants currently most sensitive to the impact of human activities:

- American ginseng (*Panax quinquefolius*)
- Bloodroot (*Sanguinaria canadensis*)
- Black cohosh (*Actaea racemosa* L.)
- Blue cohosh (*Caulophyllum thalictroides*)
- Echinacea (*Echinacea* spp.)
- Eyebright (*Euphrasia* spp.)
- False unicorn (*Chamaelirium luteum*)
- Goldenseal (*Hydrastis canadensis*)
- Lady's slipper orchid (*Cypripedium* spp.)
- Lomatium (*Lomatium dissectum*)
- Osha (*Ligusticum porteri, L.* spp.)
- Peyote (*Lophophora williamsii*)
- Sandalwood (*Santalum* spp., Hawaii only)
- Slippery elm (*Ulmus rubra*)
- Sundew (*Drosera* spp.)
- Trillium, beth root (*Trillium* spp.)
- True unicorn (*Aletris farinosa*)
- Venus flytrap (*Dionaea muscipula*)
- Virginia snakeroot (*Aristolochia serpentaria*)
- Wild yam (*Dioscorea villosa, D.* spp.)

Plants don't need to be on a designated list to be vulnerable, however. Be mindful of conditions in your local area and the plant's geographical range.

journal:
YOUR GRATITUDE PRACTICE

People all over the world have different ways of expressing their gratitude for the harvest. Some leave plant offerings, others leave a part of themselves like a lock of hair. Some sing, others pray, and still others silently offer their thanks. How will you express your gratitude to the plants? Journal ways that you will create a gratitude practice relevant to you. While it's natural to be influenced by others, strive to make this your own. This practice will undoubtedly shift with time and become more meaningful with repetition.

Your mind-set when gathering plants matters. The act of harvesting can be a continuous spiral of gratitude. There is gratitude for the plants themselves. There's consideration for all the people, pollinators, and seed spreaders who tended the plants before you and who will tend them after you. There's the appreciation of your own abilities to learn how to wildcraft, to show up with a full heart, to be present and physically able to harvest. And there is thankfulness for the many beings and influences that play roles in creating this earth, from the sun and the rain to the unseen microbes and fungi in the soils.

CULTIVATE COMMUNITY

Just as plants have interdependent relationships, humans too need community. Feeling connected not only strengthens your personal health but can also inspire you to work for the well-being of others. Throughout this book, you will read stories of how people have shared plant medicine with their communities. Consider ways you might contribute your unique interests and gifts. Perhaps you'll invite a stressed-out friend on a nature walk or host a brunch of seasonal foods. Maybe you'll volunteer at a school garden, donate herbal remedies to people in need, or work to increase equity in access to green spaces in your city. Remember, it's not all on your shoulders! Take the time to listen to and engage with others—there may be existing groups in your community that could use your help.

THE DOWNSIDES OF WILDCRAFTING

Wildcrafting can bring enormous gifts to you, your family, your community, and the areas you harvest. Unfortunately, when people approach harvesting with a human-centered mind-set, disaster often awaits. Plants like echinacea, goldenseal, and false unicorn have been all but lost in the wild. With wild plants trending, there are many examples of chefs, florists, and even herbalists who have ravaged ecosystems in their desire to harvest all that they find. This shortsighted approach destroys local areas, hurts individual plant populations, and cements the idea in people's minds that humans and the natural world shouldn't mix.

As ethical wildcrafters, we must take responsibility for how we portray wildcrafting to the wider world. When sharing activities and photos online, for example, consider whether you are glorifying the harvest of plants without discussing the principles and ethics involved.

While there are many examples of how humans have negatively impacted the plant world, the solution isn't a hands-off approach. If our interactions with plants are restricted to the produce section of the grocery store or highly manicured public spaces, our wild plants can easily be lost in an out-of-sight, out-of-mind situation. In addition, many plants have coevolved with human and nonhuman animals. Just as flowering plants rely on insects for pollination, root crops depend on diggers to aerate the soil and create spaces for seeds to fall into. Not fulfilling that responsibility to tend plants can lead to a decline in their populations. Deeper connections are formed with more intimate relationships. Harvesting plants and making them into healing foods and herbal remedies are among the most intimate interactions we can have with the plant world.

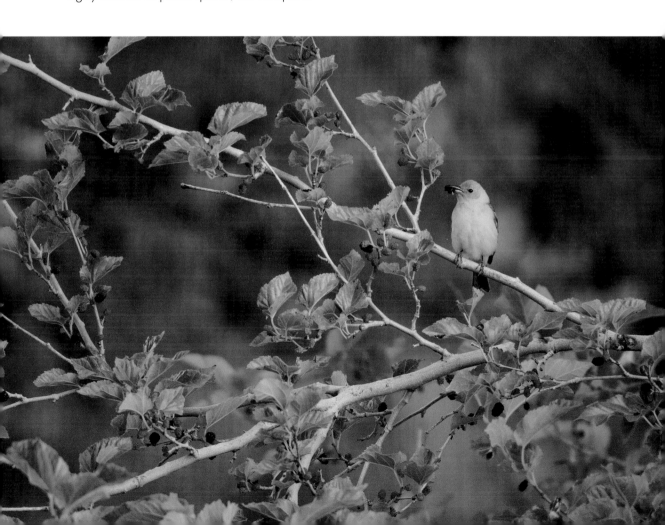

community story:
REDUCING ROADSIDE SPRAYING

Highways are prime areas for motivated local volunteers to make a difference. In many rural areas, roadsides are regularly sprayed with chemicals to stop the spread of "noxious" weeds. Volunteers can help prevent spraying by manually removing those plants and reestablishing a native plant ecosystem. This was the case with a small group of people from the Okanogan Chapter of the Washington Native Plant Society, who since 2008 have been transforming a stretch of busy highway. They meet in the spring and fall, rain or shine, to pull weeds and plant native seeds. Each year they sign a No-Spray Agreement with the Washington State Department of Transportation, which ensures their plot will remain herbicide-free.

More than a decade later, that stretch of the highway is a testament to a plant-loving community in action! Unlike other parts of the road regularly sprayed with herbicides, their area is filled with a colorful splash of native plants as a self-maintained ecosystem where little to no human intervention has been needed.

Are your local roads sprayed with herbicides? Would you like to start a similar undertaking? Joyce Bergen, the volunteer organizer of this project, has the following recommendations:

- Work with local native plant nurseries, which may be able to offer expertise as well as seed and plant donations.

- Look for local native plant experts to be advisers and oversee the process.

- Make sure you have a healthy number of volunteers before taking this on. Weeding a highway is hard work; it's not unusual to see some attrition in the number of workers. Consider whether you'll commit to a finite number of years or make it an ongoing project.

- If you live in the United States, you must interface with your regional department of transportation before beginning any work. If you wish to identify your site with a sign, the DOT can specify parameters for installing a sign that's legal and safe. It may also be able to lend you safety vests and warning signs to alert drivers to your presence.

- Start each work session with some sample weeds that are your target; not every volunteer will be familiar with every weed. A good mantra is: "If you're unsure, ask before you pull!" It's best to have a designated resource person to help volunteers with identification.

- For comparison, take photos of your site before you start and periodically thereafter.

- Each autumn, keep records of seeds and plants that are put in, so you can evaluate their success the following year.

journal:
REFLECTION

In this chapter, we have shared our wildcrafting ethics and principles. What are your own personal ethics and responsibilities in regard to wildcrafting? What concerns and fears do you have about it? How can you seek out existing communities that can advise you and support your inquiry into local sustainability issues? How can you share what you learn with others?

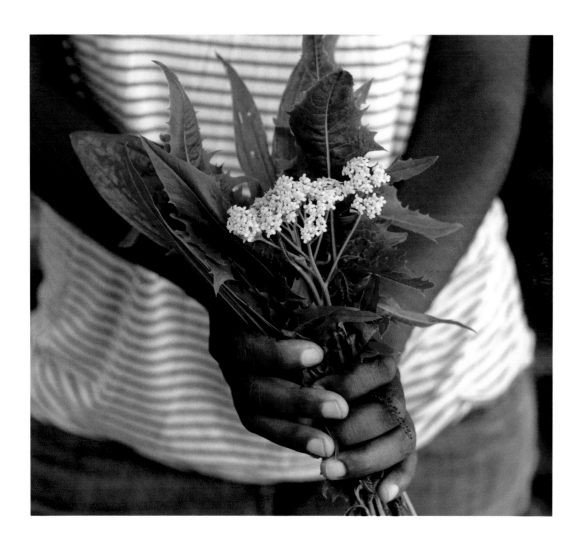

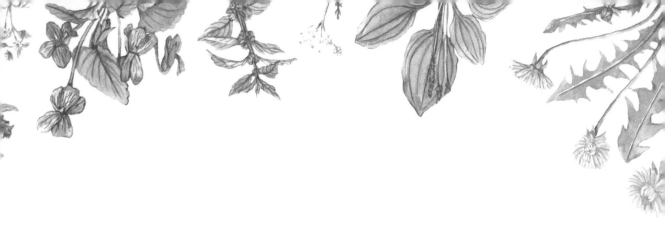

CHAPTER 4

WILDCRAFTING PRACTICE

You never take more than you can use to survive on Mother Earth. You always respect the plants, because without them, we wouldn't be here. And you always give back. So when we harvest these plants, we develop relationships with them.

— CRAIG TORRES

With our hearts full of caretaking intentions, we now set off to learn the practical skills of how to harvest plants. In Chapter 2, you took some steps to get to know your local environment. The next step is to focus on your specific harvesting areas.

CONSIDER THE WHOLE ECOSYSTEM

The more you know about an area's ecosystem, the more responsibly you can harvest within it. The questions and resources listed in Chapter 2: Getting to Know Where You Live are a good place to start. Although it's impossible to understand all the intricacies of an ecosystem, make an effort to observe, ask questions, and research the answers.

Is your harvesting area wild or cultivated? More precautions are needed when gathering plants from the wild rather than from a neighbor's garden, for example. Even places like vacant lots are part of an ecosystem. Before harvesting, look for the relationships in an area, including plants, animals, fungi, soil, and water. How sensitive are they to external forces, and how lightly do you need to tread? Examine the soil: Is there any erosion or compaction? Hillsides, stream banks, and other habitats can be vulnerable to erosion from human footsteps and plant harvesting.

Do at-risk plants grow in the area at any time of year? If so, how can you prevent having a negative impact on them? Unless you have received special training on regenerative methods for fragile habitats and at-risk plants, we recommend avoiding them. If you are interested in working with at-risk plants in wild lands, find experienced people who can mentor you closely. They can show you how to best approach a landscape and how to propagate plants successfully.

Even native plants that are not at risk should be approached with a caretaking attitude to ensure their stands remain healthy. Many of the plants in this book are so-called weeds, or invasive plants. These are ideal plants to begin harvesting, as they often have robust growing habits and may have negative impacts on native species and ecosystems. It is hard to adversely affect invasive plants, but it is not impossible. No matter what plant you harvest, keep in mind that even a weedy dandelion deserves as much respect as a loved native plant.

KNOW WHEN TO HARVEST

Herbalists traditionally harvest different plant parts at particular times of year. As a general guideline, harvest when the energy is in the part of the plant you'd like to use. For example, gather leaves while they are vibrant and fresh looking, before the plant flowers. Harvest flowers just before or shortly after they bloom.

Collect fruits when ripe, and seeds when ripe or dry. Dig roots when the energy of the plant has died back, between late summer and early spring. Harvest bark when the sap is running in late winter or spring and it is easy to separate from the inner woody layers.

Of course, exceptions can be made. For example, dandelion roots may be harvested in early spring, and the leaves attached to the roots may be a delicious addition to a spring salad. We have helped friends remove mullein plants from their gardens. The leaves were in prime condition but the roots, which also had to be pulled, worked well enough for medicine even though they were technically not in season. Sometimes we harvest plants out of necessity. If you cut yourself while hiking, an old, withered yarrow plant with green leaves is better than nothing!

NEVER HARVEST THE FIRST PLANT

The first individual plant you encounter is a sentinel. It is a clue to assess the area for that plant's abundance. You will find repeated across many cultures and ethical wildcrafting classes the precept to never harvest the first plant you find. There are many reasons for this, the first being respect. By not immediately grabbing that first plant from the earth, you can approach it with gratitude. If you find many plants grouped together, then greet the largest "grandparent" plant or another member of your choosing. Lay your appreciation at its feet and leave it to continue growing.

Not harvesting the first plant is also being a good caretaker. Some plants, like violet, may have both native and introduced species growing near you. A native plant may be part of an abundant stand, or it may be the only one for many miles. Never assume that finding one plant means you'll find many others nearby. Harvest begins only after a healthy plant population has been confirmed.

ASK PERMISSION

Wherever you gather, you need to have permission. Recognize and respect Indigenous tribal lands when looking for places to forage. Always ask before harvesting on private property. Don't be afraid to approach landowners—many people will welcome some extra weeding or tending. You can offer to prune old branches and clear debris while harvesting the elderberries from their backyard. If you want to harvest on public land, be aware of restrictions and necessary permits. Contact the appropriate local, state, or federal agency to find out how to proceed.

Many wildcrafters also ask the plant itself for permission. That may sound strange if you aren't accustomed to communicating with plants this way, but you may be surprised by what you find out! Some people receive an answer in words, images, or feelings. As plant ecologist Robin Wall Kimmerer describes it in *Braiding Sweetgrass*, "I must use both sides of my brain to listen to the answer. The analytic left reads the empirical signs to judge whether the population is large and healthy enough to sustain a harvest, whether it has enough to share. The intuitive right hemisphere is reading something else, a sense of generosity, an open-handed radiance that says take me, or sometimes a tight-lipped recalcitrance that makes me put my trowel away."[1]

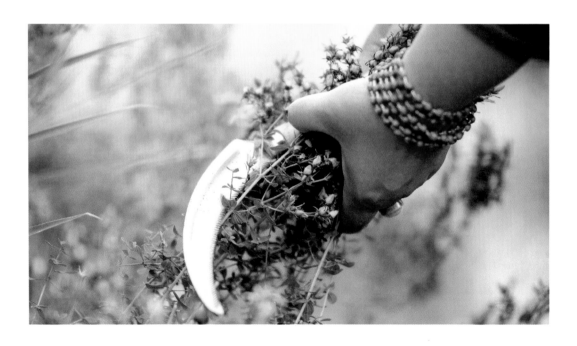

GIVE BEFORE TAKING

In Chapter 3 we explored the principles of caretaking and reciprocity with plants. Plan how you will put these into practice on the day of your harvest. This will look different for each person and the specific needs of that person's environment. For some it might be bringing an empty bag to pick up trash along the trail or a jug of water to feed drought-stressed plants. For others it might be arriving with a prayer or an offering. Having a ritual or practice helps to center you before you start picking and digging. And remember, these commitments go beyond the moment. In the long term, you might be planting seeds if appropriate, removing invasive plants to help native ones flourish, participating in environmental justice and protection efforts, and more.

HAVE A PLAN FOR YOUR HARVEST

Countless times we've seen beginners post photos of their harvest on social media and then ask for ideas about how to use it. "I harvested five pounds of yarrow—now what should I do with it?"

Don't let the excitement of the harvest preclude an actual plan! Harvesting first and figuring out your use afterward results in waste. Instead, make a list of the ways you want to use the plant, and determine how much you actually need for each purpose. Do you want to dry a pound for tea? Infuse some in oil or alcohol? Make dinner? Do you already have everything else you need, or do you have to buy vinegar first? Don't let your harvest rot because you were out of supplies.

Also consider how much you can realistically dry, process, and store. It can take a lot of time and energy to scrub roots, strip off seeds, or dehydrate leaves. When starting out you might have to guess on quantities, but over time you will get a better idea of the ratio of harvest to product. Keeping a record of your harvest helps you to track this.

Granted, having a plan isn't always possible. Maybe you head out to pick elderberries but instead find an abundant blackberry patch. However, you can still take a moment to realistically assess your needs and capabilities.

BE SAFE

For many people, interacting with nature brings up fear. If you have little or no experience with plants and the natural world, it's normal to be cautious. Safety begins with knowing your hazards. With knowledge, you can dispel fear of the unknown.

Most important is your personal safety. Whether you are in a city park or the wilderness, be aware of your surroundings at all times. It may be a good idea to tell someone where you are going and how long you expect to be there. Wear clothing and footwear suited for the weather and terrain. Depending on the trip, you may need to bring a small pack with water and a first-aid kit.

Know the potential dangers in your harvesting area, and show the appropriate caution. This may include things like incoming storms, slippery trails, poisonous plants, large predators, venomous snakes, or ticks. Also be aware of human-made factors such as the presence of hunters or illegal cannabis farms.

For some communities, being in wild areas can feel unwelcome or unsafe. Groups such as Diversify Outdoors, Outdoor Afro, Latino Outdoors, Native Womens Wilderness, and Pride Outside are some good resources for finding support and creating social change. TrailLink.com lists wheelchair-accessible trails in the United States; many cities and states also have lists.

Assess whether the area is safe to harvest from, especially in regard to the soil. Avoid areas regularly sprayed with pesticides or herbicides, areas that receive runoff or waste from agricultural or manufacturing operations, polluted waterways and floodplains, previously developed industrial land (brownfields), foundations of old buildings with lead-based paint, and locations with high animal traffic. Roadsides, railroad tracks, golf courses, and large-scale farms are all suspect. Learn to recognize the signs of recently sprayed chemicals on plants, such as oddly yellowed or deformed leaves and stems.

GET TO KNOW YOUR SOIL

It is common to view certain landscapes, particularly urban and industrialized ones, with suspicion. But Nance Klehm, an ecological systems designer and founder of Social Ecologies, advocates approaching your soil with curiosity and wonder instead. Among her many projects, she assists communities with soil assessment and bioremediation, "helping the soil help itself" using tools like plants, bacteria, and fungi to address contamination.

"There's a lot of fear and resistance around soil remediation, just like there's fear of foraging," Nance says. "But we *can* lean in and get curious about something that's ill and help heal it."

To learn about your soil, Nance suggests using your senses and asking questions. Below are Nance's suggestions to get you started.*

1. Conduct a thorough site assessment.

A site assessment is an on-site sensory process as well as a research-based process. Start by mapping and describing the structures and features of the site (trees, buildings, sources of water, etc.). Draw a wider arc encompassing adjacent properties, and note how they influence the site.

Refer to historical records and photos, if available; these can cast light on long-term dynamics at the site that might otherwise go unnoticed.

If you can, sit down with a longtime local resident or businessperson. Treating this person to a cup of tea or lunch and asking a few questions can reveal events or dynamics that would be impossible to know about otherwise. These "In Perts" (or local experts) can reveal clues as to the social and cultural use of the land and things that might have affected the land's integrity (demolition, reconstruction, car repair, vegetable gardening, etc.). Don't forget to ask them who else you should talk to!

*This section has been excerpted and adapted from Nance Klehm's "The Ground Rules Process" in *The Ground Rules: A Manual to Reconnect Soil and Soul*. We recommend going to http://socialecologies.net/tgrmanual and getting your own copy of this manual to learn more about site research, soil assessment, and remediation methods.

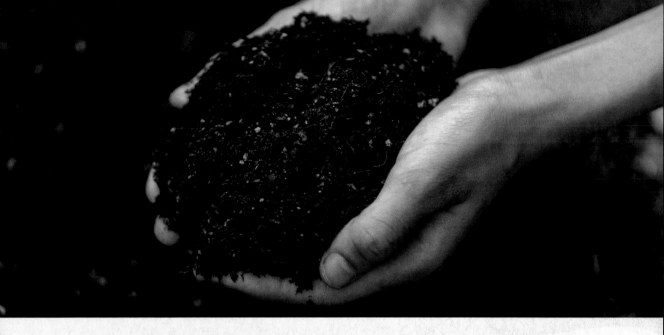

2. Explore the biology of the site.

Next, to understand the disturbances to and fertility of the land, try identifying the species and health of the site's cultivated and spontaneous vegetation. What species are there, and where? Which species or areas of the landscape seem healthy or struggling, and how?

Lift some soil up and smell it, look at its color and density, feel its texture between your fingers, and draw a ribbon. Do this in several different areas.

What traces of animals—wild or domestic—do you see?

How does water move through the site?

Are there obvious signs of pollution? How deep or widespread is it? What is the source? Is it current or historical, repeated or from a single event? Can you be specific in identifying the nature of contamination?

Using gloves, dig several test holes, each a foot deep, and look at the soil horizons. Conduct a shake test and percolation test to determine soil structure and composition. Collect enough soil to also conduct a chemical soil test at a local lab. (You can learn more about these soil tests in Nance Klehm's *The Ground Rules*.)

3. Develop a strategy for long-term neighborhood health.

Sit down with some key community people to discuss your findings, identify your goals, and develop a realistic and realizable strategy for proceeding with your soil remediation plan. In order to be successful, you need to work within your collective capacity!

4. Last but not least—get out and get digging!

caution:
COMMON POISONOUS PLANTS

Many plants are safe to handle and consume; some, however, can kill or at least cause a lot of discomfort. Except for the poisonous ones mentioned below, all the plants in this book have a long history of safe use. When identifying a new plant, you need to be 100 percent positive of your identification, so consult two or more local field guides in addition to this book. Know about any look-alikes that could be mistaken for the plant you seek. If in doubt, ask someone knowledgeable about local plants to verify what you've found. Native plant societies exist in many places and often have free meetings, outings, or online groups where you can ask for help. We also recommend taking classes with local herbalists, Indigenous educators, naturalists, and botanists.

In addition to the following common poisonous plants, familiarize yourself with any other toxic plants particular to your area. Field guides, foraging books, native plant societies, and Cooperative Extension Services can be good resources.

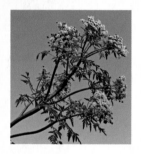

POISON HEMLOCK (*Conium maculatum*) is highly toxic; ingestion typically results in death, and some people get contact dermatitis from merely touching it. Growing along disturbed and riparian areas, this Apiaceae family plant has tall, hollow stems with purple spots; leaves that look like carrot greens; and umbrella-shaped clusters of tiny, five-petaled white flowers.

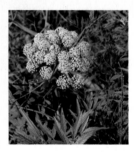

WATER HEMLOCK (*Cicuta* spp.) has been described as the most violently toxic plant in North America. Ingestion may cause vomiting, delirium, seizures, and death. Found in wet areas, this tall Apiaceae family plant has leaves and flowers similar to those of *Conium maculatum* and a bulbous, chambered root containing an oily yellow sap.

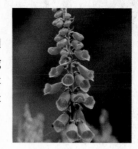

FOXGLOVE (*Digitalis purpurea*) can cause severe sickness and death when ingested. This common ornamental and wild-growing plant has a basal rosette of simple, coarse leaves and an upright stem with showy, bell-shaped flowers, usually purple or pink. It may be confused with plants like comfrey and mullein.

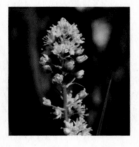

DEATH CAMAS (*Zigadenus* spp.) is a poisonous plant that can cause vomiting, convulsions, and death. Frequently mistaken for an onion plant, it grows from an onionlike bulb, is shaped like grass, and has small white flowers. It lives in habitats ranging from moist valleys to sandy plains.

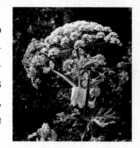

GIANT HOGWEED (*Heracleum mantegazzianum*) contains a sap that, on contact with skin, leads to a reaction called phytophotodermatitis, in which blisters and rashes occur when skin is exposed to sunlight. This towering (up to 15 feet tall) Apiaceae family plant grows in wet areas. It has white, umbrella-shaped flower clusters and thick, ridged stems with purple spots. Its relative cow parsnip (*Heracleum maximum*) can also cause skin irritation.

POISON IVY, POISON OAK, AND POISON SUMAC (*Toxicodendron radicans, T. diversilobum, T. vernix*) are Anacardiaceae family plants that contain a chemical called urushiol, which can cause rashes and blisters. Poison ivy and poison oak typically grow as bushes or vines in wooded areas and have clusters of three leaflets. Poison sumac is a large shrub or tree found in wet areas and has pinnate compound leaves on red stems.

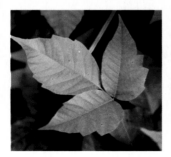
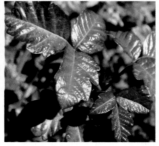
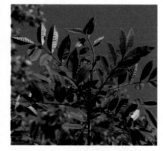

LOOK FOR THE WINDFALL

By following the cycles of nature, you can be the recipient of a windfall. Literally! High winds naturally prune trees. Go outside after a storm to find what can be gleaned. Cottonwood buds, willow branches, and evergreen needles are common examples of fallen bounty. Trees can fall by other means, too. One year Rosalee was walking along a river when she came across an area with heavy beaver activity. A huge cottonwood tree had recently been felled, and the branches were ripe with sticky cottonwood buds. That spring she harvested enough buds to make remedies for many years. When gathering windfall, do be mindful that fallen fruits and seeds can play an important ecological role for wildlife food and plant reproduction.

Sadly, human development can also provide abundant plant supplies. When a large tract of forest was set for development near Rosalee's mentor's house, the two of them visited the area regularly before it was bulldozed into flat land. They harvested many of the plants, and even moved some back to Rosalee's yard so they could continue living. Likewise, Emily spent months harvesting citrus and prickly pear from a lot that was scheduled for development into condos.

TOOLS OF THE TRADE

Below are some tools commonly used for wildcrafting. This is a thorough and extensive list and you may not need everything, at least not right away. Start simply and let your tool collection grow with time. Also consider borrowing from friends, family, or a tool-sharing program. (Look for "toolshares" and "timebanks" through social media, a simple online search, or by asking other folks in your area.)

Cutting, Clipping, and Digging

Your hands are among your best tools! Take care of them by wearing gloves when necessary. Simple kitchen scissors work well for harvesting herbaceous plants. Pruning shears are necessary for cutting woody stems and branches. For densely growing plants, a sickle comes in handy. Keep tools clean and sharp to prevent the spread of disease in plants. For root harvesting, a garden shovel or digging fork can help loosen the soil. In dry or rocky soil, a digging stick or *hori hori* (Japanese gardening knife) can be more convenient. Fruit pickers are useful for harvesting from tall trees.

Bringing Home the Harvest

For carrying your harvest, we recommend bags made of breathable materials such as mesh, paper, or cloth. (An old pillowcase works well.) Avoid plastic bags, which can trap heat and moisture, leading to wilting and spoilage. Baskets and harvesting aprons can keep your hands free for picking. For delicate flowers and berries, use sturdy containers to avoid crushing them. Whatever container you bring, bring extra! You never know what you'll find, and you don't want to have to store soil-encrusted roots with freshly picked berries.

Other Supplies

Other things you may want to pack in your foraging bag include water, a snack, first-aid kit, sun protection, insect repellent, and a device with GPS or a map and compass. Also consider bringing a field guide, hand lens or loupe for plant identification, camera/phone, and notebook.

HOW TO HARVEST

Each part of a plant requires a different harvesting method and has an optimal time to be harvested. Regenerative harvesting practices will give you the most potent plant medicines while ensuring healthy plant stands and future harvests. (You can learn more about plant parts in Chapter 5.)

Leaves

Leaves are usually gathered when young and fresh. Remember that plants have leaves to absorb sunlight and make food; without them, a plant can become stressed or even die. To minimize your impact, do not take many leaves from a single plant. When harvesting leaves (and buds) from trees, avoid taking them from the very end or terminal branch, unless you are pruning the entire branch. In some plants, such as nettle and mint, cutting can stimulate growth. These plants can be cut just above a leaf node, and they will grow back.

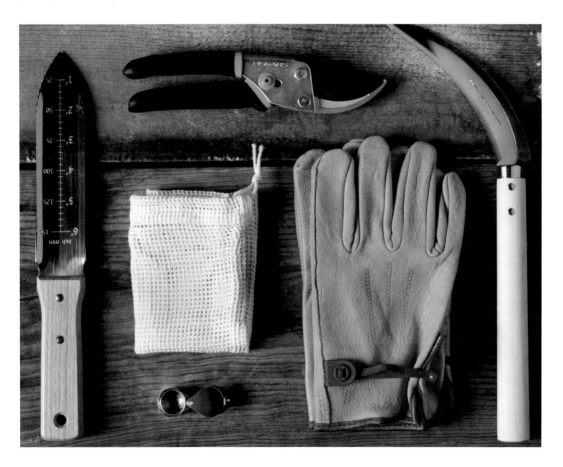

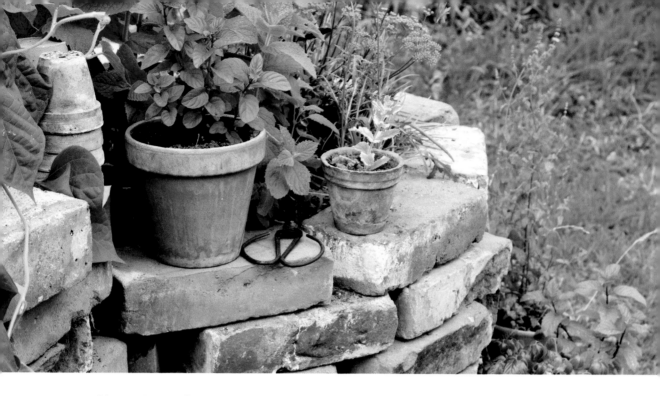

Harvest leaves after any dew or rainfall has evaporated. On hot days, pick leaves before they wilt. Using your fingers, scissors, or pruning shears, remove leaves and stems gently. Don't tug on the leaves, which can strip the stem or uproot the plant as you harvest. Gently shake the leaves to remove any bugs or dirt before placing them in your bag.

Flowers

Flowers are gathered as buds just before they bloom, or right after blooming. The plant you're harvesting and your desired use will dictate what is best. Note that many flowers from the Asteraceae family will turn into puff balls when dried; they are best harvested before fully flowering. Before harvesting, know the plant's life cycle and leave enough flowers so it can reproduce. Also consider whether insects or birds depend on nectar and pollen from the flowers.

For some plants, the more you pick their flowers, the more they will produce. However, a plant can eventually tire out, leading to poor fruits both that year and the next. One example of this is the elderberry; although harvesting its flowers stimulates the plant to produce more, if it is overly harvested, it won't flower or fruit as strongly the following year.

Gather flowers after any dew or rainfall has evaporated and before they wilt in the heat of the afternoon. Individual flowers or petals may be plucked at the base, or flowering stems may be clipped using your fingers, scissors, or pruning shears. Gently shake off any bugs or dirt.

Fruits and Seeds

Fruits and their seeds may be used in food and medicine and, when appropriate, to propagate a plant in the wild or in your garden. When harvesting, keep in mind that that fruits protect seeds, and seeds are necessary for the plant to reproduce. Animals may also depend on these for food.

Fruits can usually be gathered by hand or by using pruning shears or fruit pickers when they are ripe. Depending on the plant and your use, you might collect immature seeds or dried seeds. Dried seeds can be gathered by shaking them into a bag, or seed heads can be cut and dried at home.

Roots and Rhizomes

Harvesting roots and rhizomes can lead to the death of that particular plant and a decline in the plant population. First, ask yourself whether you really need the roots. Many plants have the same medicinal properties in their aerial portions. For other plants, aerial portions can be combined with roots to make whole plant medicine, using less root material.

Herbalists often dig roots in autumn or early spring. This is generally a good time for dividing and transplanting roots as well. Harvesting roots after a plant has gone to seed and died back for the year is the best time for root medicine, and it gives animals a chance to eat the seeds and the plant a chance to reproduce.

It's important to know the plant's needs so that you can harvest it appropriately. Some roots, such as echinacea, can be divided so the plant continues living. The crowns of some plants, like dandelion, can be replanted after the roots have been removed. Other hardy roots can continue to grow if some of the root is left in the ground (again, dandelion). Plants with rhizomes can be followed horizontally through the ground and the ends can be harvested, leaving the rest of the plant to continue growing. With plants that have deep, woody taproots as well as more succulent side roots, the side roots can be harvested, leaving the main plant deeply rooted in the earth.

Be aware that when you dig, you disturb not only the soil but nearby plants' roots, insects, and microorganisms as well. Yet by loosening the soil, you also help oxygenate it and create spaces for seeds to fall into. Dig patiently, and refill the hole before leaving.

Bark

Bark is best harvested in late winter or spring, when sap is flowing through the tree. This makes the outer bark easy to separate from the woody core (xylem). Generally the inner bark (phloem and cambium) is used for medicine. If harvesting young branches or twigs, then the thin outer bark may be used in addition to the inner bark.

Bark not only protects a tree from water loss and predators but also helps transport the sugars created in the leaves to the other parts of the plant. Improperly harvesting bark can damage or kill a tree. Avoid cutting bark from the trunk of a living tree, which is never necessary for medicine making.

The best way to harvest bark is either by gathering from a recently felled tree or by pruning branches. When pruning, use the correct size shears so that you can make a clean cut. Using shears that are too small or too dull can leave a rough and frayed cut that opens the plant to infections. When deciding which branches to prune, look for ways to help the overall growth of the tree or shrub. Branches that grow downward or that rub together are easy choices for pruning. You can also prune dead branches from the tree to help keep it strong and healthy.

GROWING AND BUYING PLANTS

Wildcrafting is not always possible or appropriate. For example, someone's physical limitations may render wild harvesting difficult. Local conditions ranging from habitat loss to lack of access to safe gathering areas may inhibit harvesting. However, even if you don't wildcraft, you can still work with plants for food and medicine. In many circumstances, growing your own plants or buying plants from others can be a better choice. (For a list of reputable companies to source your seeds, plants, and more, see the Recommended Resources on page 377.)

Growing Plants

Having a garden where you can dig your fingers into the soil, watch seeds sprout, and then harvest through the seasons enriches your relationship with plants. Even if you don't have a large space in which to grow all your own herbs, a small plot, a few containers on your balcony, or a community garden space can give you the opportunity to spend time with plants and learn more about them. Gardening can also benefit local wildlife.

To help you get started with gardening, we've included gardening tips in each plant chapter. You'll also want to find out what hardiness zone you live in. Then you can select the plants that best fit your climate. For U.S. residents, we recommend consulting with your state's Cooperative Extension Service to help choose regionally adapted varieties. Look for local sources of seeds at nurseries, seed growers, or community seed swaps. If local sources aren't an option, you can order medicinal herb seeds and starts from specialty companies.

If growing your own garden isn't for you, look for gardens or farms in your area that offer opportunities for harvesting. Many of the best herbs are disdainfully called "weeds" and are intentionally pulled from gardens. Ask friends, neighbors, or local farms if they would like some help "weeding."

Buying Plants

Several of the plants in this book are sold at grocery stores, health food stores, and farmers markets. For example, mint, apples, and citrus are widely available, and some markets carry cultivated dandelion and mustard greens. Prickly pear pads and fruits can often be found at Latin markets, and burdock roots at East Asian markets.

Local herbalists and herb farmers may offer plants that were grown or wildcrafted near you. Start a conversation to learn more about their approach to growing and harvesting plants, using Chapter 3: Wildcrafting Principles as a guide for your questions. For example, how do they consider their role as caretakers? Do they assess their impact on the areas they farm or harvest? Are they aware of local climate issues and ecological interdependence? Be critical of people selling large amounts of endangered plants.

You can also buy dried herbs from larger apothecaries and companies. Research these well to make sure the herbs they sell were harvested and processed ethically. Ecology-conscious companies should have that information prominently displayed or at least readily available upon inquiry.

Swapping Plants

Herb swaps, food swaps, and crop swaps can be great places to trade plants you've grown or wild harvested. Depending on the particular swap group, you may be able to exchange fresh and dried plants as well as seeds, foods, and remedies. These are also wonderful events for meeting like-minded people and sharing knowledge in your community. (You might find swaps in your area through online searches, social media, or asking local plant lovers.)

Visiting with Plants

Whether or not you choose to harvest your own plants, you can still visit them! You can learn a lot from plants simply by sitting with and observing them. Smell them, nibble them if appropriate, notice changes in their aromatics and taste depending on season or location. Watch how other beings interact with each plant. Above all, be a steward for plants while also basking in their wonder.

IT BEGINS WITH SMALL STEPS

With practice, many of the skills presented in this chapter will become second nature. You'll quickly be able to identify your favorite plants. Your senses will be attuned to assessing a local ecosystem, and you'll know how to best caretake and wildcraft to ensure future harvests. If you feel overwhelmed, take this as a signal to slow down. Savor the process. Remember that it all begins with visiting plants and practicing awareness.

There is admittedly a lot of work involved in wildcrafting. It's often touted as "free," but the reality is that it takes a lot of energy and time. And that is how it should be! The greatest rewards come from effort and bring a deep sense of joy and empowerment.

journal:
REFLECTION

Wildcrafting doesn't have to involve heading out into the far-off wilderness. Some of the best foraging is found close to home. Brainstorm in your journal:

- What areas could you consider for future harvesting?

- Do you have friends or family with yards full of edible and medicinal plants?

- Are there farmers nearby whom you could approach about helping with "weeding"?

- Do you have a garden, or are you interested in starting one?

- Are there community gardens in your area?

community story:
GROW A ROW

With the goal of providing accessible, "by the people, for the people" health care, Lorna Mauney-Brodek started the Herbalista Free Clinic in Atlanta in 2013. Operating from a camper van nicknamed the Herb Bus, the Herbalista crew offers free clinical care, a spot of tea, and herbal education. Today the Herbalista Health Network has evolved to include an Herb Bike, Self-Care Herb Stations, and other programming.

As part of its community-building mission, the Herbalista Health Network has also established a Grow a Row program. Through Grow a Row, Herbalista encourages people to cultivate sustainable, local medicinal plants in the Atlanta area. Working with farmers, schools, and individuals, the organization provides seeds, plants, and guidance in the craft of medicinal herb growing. In turn, growers donate a portion of their harvest to the free clinic. Locals have a list of 33 different herbs they can choose from; the most popular ones to grow are yarrow, milky oats, calendula, tulsi, and turmeric.

"We think the best remedy for the modern condition is to simply get involved!" Lorna says. "Build resiliency by building skill sets and then sharing them with others." To learn more about Herbalista and get resources for starting your own community herbalism project, visit herbalista.org.

Are you interested in "growing a row"? Are any local herb organizations looking for donations? How can you share your herbal bounty with others?

WILDCRAFTING CHECKLIST

❑ How are you harvesting with attention and gratitude?

❑ What practices do you have to ensure that you are giving back more than you are taking?

❑ Can you correctly identify the plant? Are you 100 percent sure?

❑ Do you know the best time of year to harvest? The best time of day?

❑ Are you dressed appropriately for the weather and conditions? Do you need to bring water? A first-aid kit?

❑ Do you have the proper tools?

❑ Do you have permission to gather?

❑ Is the area free from contamination?

❑ Are you in a fragile habitat? Are there rare or sensitive plants growing there at any time of the year? Will your actions cause soil erosion?

❑ Have you surveyed other areas to ensure this is an ideal location?

❑ How abundant or rare is the plant you want to harvest? Is it endangered, native, invasive?

❑ Is the plant population healthy in your region and in that particular stand?

❑ Do animals, birds, and insects depend on this plant for food or shelter?

❑ Will your actions kill a plant, prevent it from reproducing, or leave it vulnerable to disease? How can you mitigate this?

❑ What is your plan for how you will use the plants you harvest?

❑ Are you harvesting only what you need?

❑ Are you harvesting what you can realistically dry, process, and store?

❑ Are you prepared to keep records to track your harvest and asses your impact?

❑ After harvesting, how will you tend to any holes or other clean-up activities?

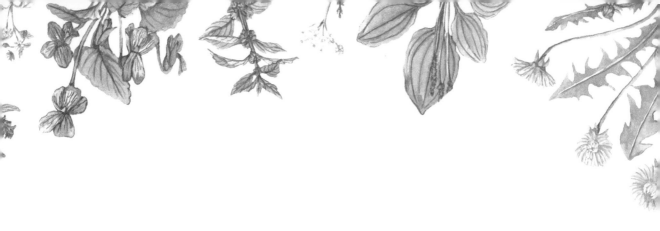

CHAPTER 5

BOTANY BASICS

Names are the way we humans build relationship,
not only with each other but with the living world.

— ROBIN WALL KIMMERER

When you encounter a plant, what comes to mind? Do you think of its common name, such as dandelion, or a Latin name, like *Taraxacum officinale*? Or perhaps you know it as "yellow flower" or "weed" or "bitter herb." As long as humans have had language, we have developed ways of naming and categorizing plants. This has helped us build relationships with plants, to differentiate among them, and to communicate information—including what's edible, medicinal, and poisonous—with others in our community. In today's Western science–based culture, plants are given Latin names and classified according to a system invented by Swedish botanist Carl Linnaeus in 1735.

It's important to note that there are many approaches to identifying plants. A person can learn to work with a plant without ever knowing its Latin name or what a "pinnately compound leaf" is. Your botanical knowledge may come from observation, experience, or traditional teachings, all of which have merit. That said, many works on plant identification and medicine incorporate Western science conventions. Familiarizing yourself with these concepts can help you get more out of this book and to forage safely. Using this shared language, you'll also be able to communicate with many other foragers, herbalists, gardeners, and plant people across the world.

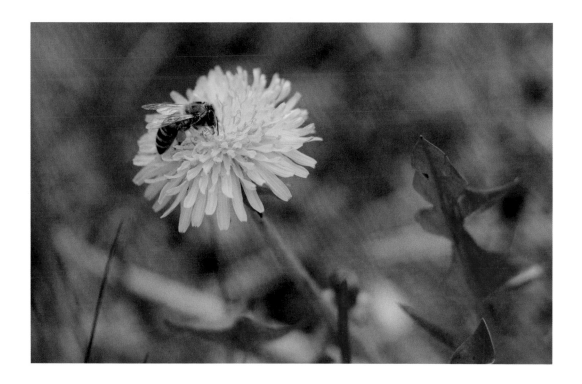

PLANT NAMES

In everyday life, people usually call plants by common names such as dandelion, bitterwort, or clockflower. Some plants have dozens of common names or share common names with other, completely different plants. Latin botanical names can help people avoid confusion. In Linnaeus's naming system, every plant has a unique two-part name, or binomial. (Additions to the binomial may include subspecies, varieties, cultivars, and hybrids.)

Plant names go from the general to the specific. Let's take a look at dandelion. Its botanical name is *Taraxacum officinale. Taraxacum* is the genus and *officinale* is the species. Whether you're communicating in English or Spanish or any other language, you can use the name *Taraxacum officinale* and a botanist will know exactly which plant you are referring to. In writing, once a genus name has been used in a paragraph, it may be abbreviated; thus, in subsequent references, it may be written as *T. officinale.*

In herbalism, sometimes a number of species within the same genus are used similarly. Rather than list a hundred species of rose, an herbalist might refer to them as *Rosa* spp., meaning several species in the genus *Rosa*. In other cases, like St. John's wort, medicinal use is very specific, so the entire botanical name is used: *Hypericum perforatum.*

How can you remember all these botanical names? We've found that writing them down on remedy labels and in field journals is a great way to commit them to memory.

PLANT IDENTIFICATION

Of course, knowing the name of a plant gets you only so far. You also need to be able to identify it. When foraging, this can be a matter of life and death, as plants occasionally have toxic look-alikes. The ability to identify plants can also help you learn new things about your ecosystem and the other beings that call it home. You can start to identify plants by learning some basics of plant biology.

Most plants have six parts, each of which plays a different role:

Roots anchor a plant to the ground and absorb water and nutrients from the soil. Some plants have a primary taproot (like a carrot). Others have a fibrous root system made of up many thin roots.

Stems or trunks support the plant above the ground, carry water and nutrients from the roots to the leaves, and transport food from the leaves to the rest of the plant. Some stems are herbaceous and bendable, while others are woody and hard. Some are round in cross-section, while others are square.

Leaves capture energy from the sun and convert water and carbon dioxide into food for the plant and oxygen. Leaves come in many shapes, sizes, and arrangements (see page 49).

Flowers are the reproductive parts of most plants, and they produce seeds. They are often brightly colored and fragranced to attract animals to help with pollination. Pollination occurs when insects, birds, bats, or even the wind carry pollen from one flower to another. Some flowers, like dandelions, can also self-pollinate.

Fruits protect developing seeds and may have a fleshy exterior, like an apple, or a hard exterior, like a walnut. Fruits like apples and rose

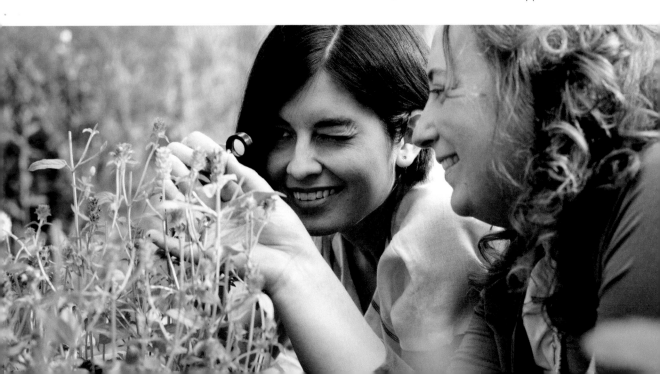

hips can entice animals to eat them and deposit the seeds elsewhere.

Seeds contain the material for new plants. They consist of an embryo and stored food covered with a protective coat. Seeds may be dispersed by gravity, wind, water, or animals, including people.

In addition to seeds, some flowering plants can reproduce asexually, producing genetic clones of the parent. Some common methods include bulbs (such as onions), rhizomes (such as ginger), stolons or runners (such as violets),

tubers (such as potatoes), and suckers or root sprouts (such as roses). Humans have also learned to propagate plants through methods like cutting, grafting, and layering.

In most cases, plants can be identified on the basis of their leaves and flowers. Sometimes descriptions of other parts (like seeds), growth habit, or habitat can also aid identification. You might not be able to identify a plant at all times of year; instead, you'll need to visit it through the seasons to examine its changing leaves and flowers. Here are some basic leaf and flower descriptors:

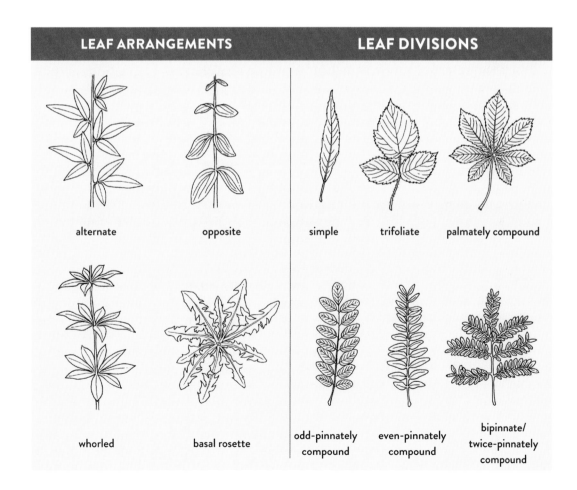

LEAF ARRANGEMENTS

alternate

opposite

whorled

basal rosette

LEAF DIVISIONS

simple

trifoliate

palmately compound

odd-pinnately compound

even-pinnately compound

bipinnate/ twice-pinnately compound

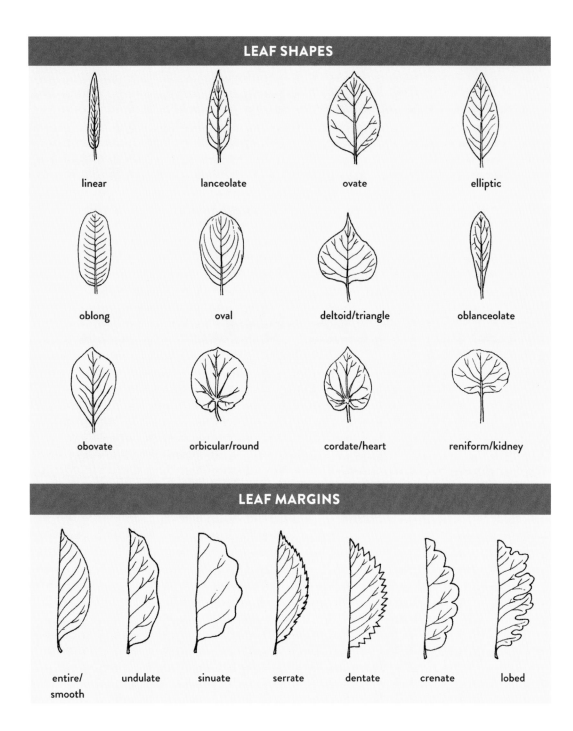

PARTS OF A LEAF

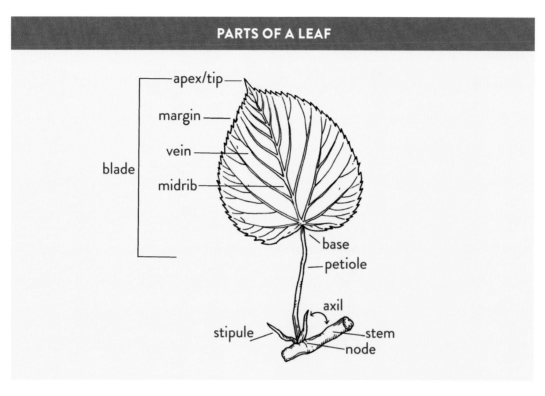

apex/tip

margin

vein

midrib

blade

base

petiole

axil

stipule

stem

node

PARTS OF A FLOWER

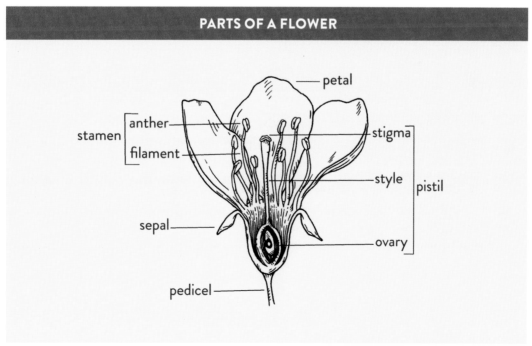

petal

stamen

anther

filament

stigma

style

pistil

sepal

ovary

pedicel

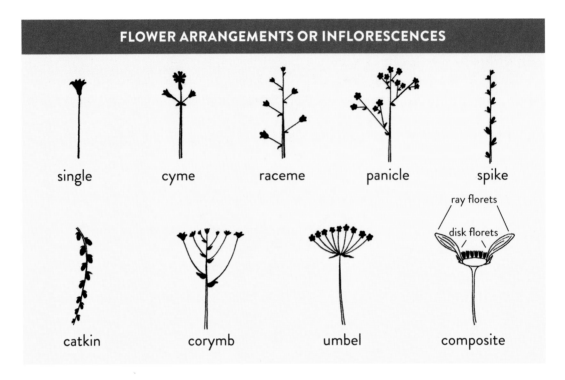

FLOWER ARRANGEMENTS OR INFLORESCENCES

single

cyme

raceme

panicle

spike

catkin

corymb

umbel

ray florets

disk florets

composite

PLANT FAMILIES

A plant's genus and species are actually just the last two groupings in Linnaeus's hierarchical classification system. Above the genus level is the family. Learning plant families is one of the best ways to observe patterns, which is what plant identification is really all about. Plants in the same family may have similar leaf, flower, fruit, or seed structures, so once you know the characteristics of a family, it can help you narrow down your search to identify a new plant. Members of a plant family may also share chemical constituents and medicinal properties.

Of the hundreds of plant families, these are some major ones we suggest learning. These families encompass many edible and medicinal plants as well as poisonous plants that require caution.

Apiaceae or Umbelliferae (parsley): Plants in this family are high in volatile oils, frequently cultivated for food, and often used to support digestion and treat fevers. However, this family also includes many toxic plants. Botanical characteristics include compound umbels and flowers with five sepals, five petals, and five stamens. Some species within this family are best identified by their seeds. Members include carrot, parsley, and poison hemlock.

Anacardiaceae (cashew or sumac): Many plants in this family contain resins and a chemical called urushiol, which can cause dermatitis. Botanical characteristics include alternate leaves and trifoliate or pinnate leaves, and flowers with five or three sepals united at the base. Flowers may have five, three, or zero petals and five or ten stamens. Members include cashew, mango, and poison ivy.

Asteraceae (aster): This is the largest family of flowering plants. They often have inulin-rich roots and are considered alteratives. Botanical characteristics include composite flower heads usually made up of smaller disk florets and ray florets. Members include dandelion, echinacea, and yarrow.

Rosaceae (rose): Medicinally, plants in this family are often astringent. Botanical characteristics include flowers with five petals and five sepals, many stamens, and ovate serrated leaves. Members include apple, blackberry, and rose.

Lamiaceae (mint): Plants in this family are frequently high in volatile oils, diaphoretic, emmenagogic, and carminative. Botanical characteristics include square stems, opposite leaves, and aromatic leaves. Members include mint, sage, and basil.

Fabaceae (pea): This family includes edible as well as toxic plants, and plants that can fix nitrogen in the soil. Botanical characteristics include irregular flowers, pealike pods, and pinnately compound leaves. Members include beans, clover, and vetch.

Brassicaceae (mustard): These plants tend to be spicy and acrid. Botanical characteristics include four petals and four sepals, six stamens (four tall and two short), and seed pods that grow in a radial pattern. Members include black mustard, broccoli, and cabbage.

To learn more about plant families, pick up the excellent guide *Botany in a Day* by Thomas J. Elpel.

journal:
GROCERY STORE BOTANY

Opportunities to learn about botany exist all over, not just in the wild. Try this exercise the next time you visit your local grocery store, farmers market, or anywhere fresh produce is sold. Journal about your observations.

- Find a vegetable that has leaves. How would you describe the leaf shape? Are the margins smooth or toothed? What pattern are the veins in? What do you notice about the color and texture?

- Find another vegetable with leaves. In what ways are these leaves similar to or different from the first?

- How many other leaf shapes can you find?

- What were you surprised to learn during this exercise?

On future trips to the store, you can repeat this exercise, looking for roots, fruits, and even flowers and seeds and comparing their appearances.

journal:
LOOKING AT A FLOWER

For this exercise, you will pay close attention to a flower. This can be any flower, from a dandelion growing through a sidewalk to a flower at the nursery. You don't even need to know its name—all you need is curiosity. (However, you do want to avoid touching poisonous plants; see Common Poisonous Plants on pages 36 to 37.) Journal about your observations.

- In what month is this flower blooming?
- What color(s) is it?
- Is there a single flower on the stem, or several? If more than one, how are they arranged (for example, in a cluster, spike, or umbrella shape)?
- How wide is the flower?
- What shape is the flower? What shape are its petals?
- How many petals are there? (Or are there too many to count?)
- What does the flower smell like?
- Are there any creatures on it?
- What details will you remember most?

PLANT LIFE CYCLES

Besides aiding identification, understanding a plant's life cycle can help you appreciate the rhythms of the seasons, time your harvests, and tend plants better. For instance, if you know that picking a flower will prevent a plant from reproducing, you can be mindful of where and how you harvest (and perhaps plant extra seeds). Through observation, you might learn how other creatures are intertwined with the life of the plant. Or perhaps you'll be able to recognize when a plant is not dead but merely dormant for the winter, and you can return to marvel at its new leaves unfurling in the spring.

Some plants live for a few months, while others live for years. Plant life cycles may be organized into broad categories:

Annuals complete their life cycle in one growing season. They germinate from seed; develop flowers, seeds, and fruits; and then die. Annuals include purslane and wild mustard.

Biennials complete their life cycle in two growing seasons. In the first year, they grow leaves, often in the form of a low-growing

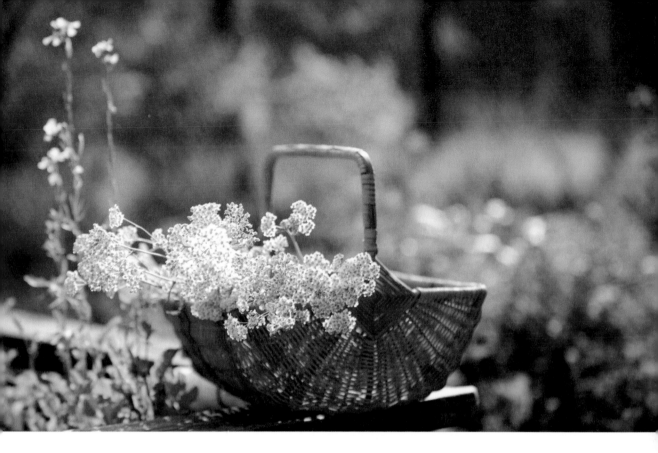

rosette. They may go dormant in autumn or winter. In the second year, they flower, seed, fruit, and die. Biennials include burdock and mullein.

Perennials live for more than two growing seasons. Herbaceous perennials have stems that typically die back to the rootstock in autumn or winter and then regrow the following spring. Examples include dandelion and nettle. Woody perennials have persistent stems or trunks. They may be deciduous, losing their leaves for part of the year, or evergreen, keeping their leaves for more than one growing season. Examples include mint and pine.

Ephemerals germinate when conditions are favorable, such as after a rain in the desert or a disturbance like the plowing of a field. They quickly complete their life cycles, producing many seeds. Ephemerals like chickweed may have several generations in one year.

PLANT COMMUNITIES

Plants rarely live alone. Whether in a field or forest or along the side of the road, they coexist with other plants (not to mention microorganisms, fungi, and animals). When you're learning to identify a plant, you may be concentrating on its individual features like leaf arrangement and flower shape. But don't overlook the world around the plant. Take note of other plants growing nearby, as well as the natural resources (water, sunlight, etc.) available to them. This information can help you learn about the ecosystem and locate and identify these plants in the future.

journal:
REFLECTION

At this point, you might feel like there's lots of new information swirling around in your head. Keep in mind that getting to know plants is an intimate process. And intimacy takes time! Practice observing plants little by little in your everyday life. Maybe you'll want to focus on just one plant, getting to know its leaves and flowers in minute detail. Or perhaps you'll enjoy looking at a wide variety of plants and comparing patterns. As you spend more time with plants, you will find the approach that works best for you. Write about the following in your journal:

- What excites you about learning how to identify plants?

- What do you find challenging about plant identification?

- How will you address your challenges? For example, will you give it time, practice more, find a mentor?

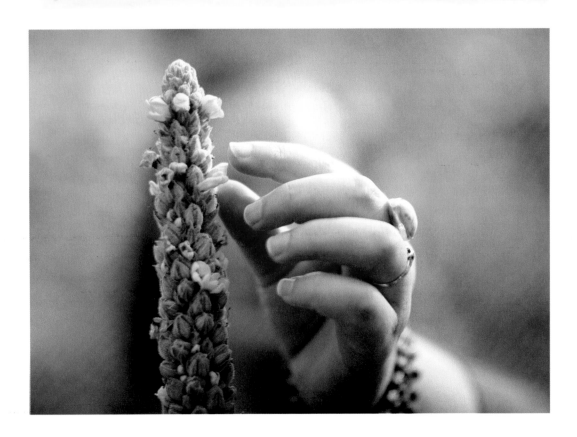

community story:
EARTHSEED DETROIT

What happens when herbalism, environmental activism, and food justice combine? Meet Earthseed Detroit (earthseeddetroit.com), a Michigan-based community outreach program founded by Lottie Spady in 2009. Earthseed Detroit is an umbrella service that hosts classes and projects geared toward sustainable living and community medicine-making. Lottie works closely with urban farms and community gardens to establish native Michigan medicinal gardens to use as outdoor classrooms and for community foraging.

"Today, many children growing up in an urban environment do not have any type of relationship with the earth," Lottie says. "Their time outside is very limited, and just the sight of a bumblebee is enough to send them running away shrieking. Some young people can't spend a lot of time outside due to environmental factors such as air quality, and others just don't find it appealing."

Here are some activities Lottie suggests for increasing community access to healthy and native medicinal herbs:

- Herbal education for youth and families: After-school, alternative-school, and home-school programs may be more receptive to herbal education. Children and their parents can participate in hands-on experiences that demystify how to make plant-based wellness supports for the family.

- Farm/garden/community partnerships: Create farm and community partnerships whereby an organically principled urban farm or garden that has been soil tested agrees to allocate some naturalized areas to go unmowed and untilled. These make the perfect outdoor classrooms for plant identification, foraging, seed saving, and medicine making.

- Seed saving and swapping: Consider creating a seed save-and-swap event where community members can share, trade, or receive donated seed and seedlings.

- Container gardening: Encourage folks to try growing a medicinal herb garden in containers. A whole garden can flourish in a few five-gallon buckets from the hardware store filled with clean soil and compost.

- Raised bed gardening: Create a barrier between potentially contaminated soil and clean soil with a raised bed. Place landscape fabric or newspaper on the bottom of the bed area and fill with at least 12 inches of clean soil and compost for growing.

How can you help increase community access to plant medicine? In what ways can you collaborate with existing programming in your community? Are there youth programs looking for volunteers or instructors?

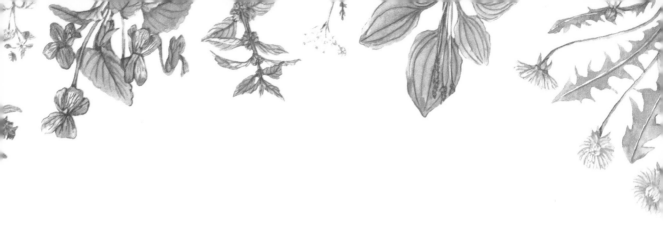

CHAPTER 6

PLANTS IN THE KITCHEN

*Using medicines collected and created by your own hands is an
experience entirely unlike using store-bought medicines, and
I am convinced the result is a much more potent remedy because
of the personal relationship that is developed while making it.*

— JIM MCDONALD

Once you've filled your basket with plants, it's time to bring them into your kitchen so you can make health-giving foods and remedies. Ideally, you want to process plants as soon as possible after harvesting them. You can eat fresh plants, dry them, freeze them, or make a variety of herbal remedies.

INSPECTING PLANTS

After harvesting, inspect the plants and remove any wilted or damaged parts. Do your best to shake off insects at your gathering spot, but don't be surprised if some remain, especially on flower heads. Give plants another shake before bringing them indoors. If there are numerous insects, spread the plants on a light-colored towel and wait for the critters to disperse. Take this opportunity to learn about the other creatures that are in relationship with this plant, and see if you can identify them.

TO WASH OR NOT TO WASH?

Washing plants can rinse away their aromatic components, so we typically wash them only if they are very dusty or dirty.

Flowers: Avoid washing flowers as they are delicate and can easily lose their aroma. Gently remove any dirt with a smooth cloth or small brush.

Fruits and berries: If necessary, rinse with cool water. Fragile berries, such as raspberries, can be gently swished in a bowl of water just before eating them.

Leaves: If necessary, rinse with cool water and dry with a clean towel or salad spinner.

Roots: Dislodge dirt by agitating roots in several changes of clean water. Gently scrub with a vegetable brush, leaving as much of the root sheath on as possible.

STORING FRESH PLANTS

Here is some guidance for short-term storage before eating or making remedies with plants:

Flowers: Store flower heads in a sealed container in the refrigerator for no more than a few days.

Fruits and berries: Most fruits can be stored in the crisper drawer of the refrigerator. Keep

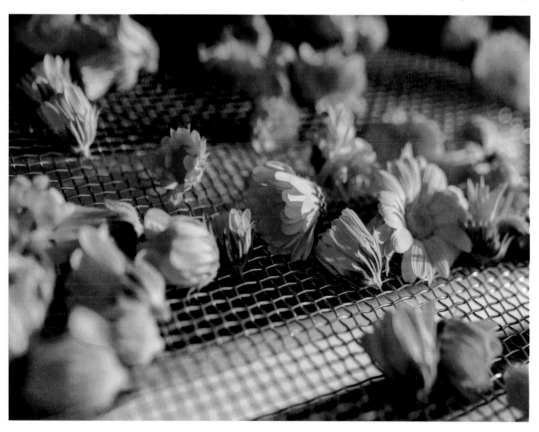

berries in the fridge in a shallow, towel-lined container with the lid slightly ajar.

Leaves: Treat tender herbs like a bouquet: place the stems in a glass of water, cover with a plastic bag (optional, but this can extend fresh-ness), and store in the refrigerator for no more than a few days. Leafy greens as well as woody herbs will keep for about a week when loosely wrapped in a damp towel and placed in a sealed container in the refrigerator.

Roots: Wrap roots in a dry towel and place in a sealed container in the refrigerator for no more than a week. Long, slender roots can also be wrapped in plastic or beeswax-coated food wrap.

DRYING PLANTS

Drying plants can extend the harvest and preserve them for future use. To maintain qual-ity, dry them as soon as possible after gathering. Pick leaves, flowers, and seeds after morning dew has evaporated and before the full heat of the sun arrives. Except for roots, do not wash plants unless absolutely necessary, as this will make it more difficult to dry them thoroughly. Roots and large fruits should be chopped or sliced before drying.

The ideal drying spot is a warm place out of direct sunlight, with low humidity and good air circulation. Drying time may take an hour, a few days, or up to a month depending on the method, the plant's moisture content, and cli-mate. (If you live in a humid climate, the use of a dehydrator or oven may be necessary.) Use your fingers to test for dryness: leaves and flowers should crumble and stems should snap easily. Roots and fruits must be completely dry in the center.

Here are four drying methods to consider:

Hanging: Tie herbs in small bundles and hang them upside down in a well-ventilated, shaded room. To protect bundles from dust, cover them with paper bags with holes punched in the sides for ventilation. This method also works well for seed heads, as the dried seeds can drop or be shaken into the bag.

Drying Rack: To make a drying rack, stretch wire mesh, nylon netting, muslin, or cheese-cloth over a wooden picture frame and staple it in place. Or purchase multi-tiered herb dry-ing racks or shallow baskets with good airflow. Spread herbs in a single layer, turning them as needed for even drying.

Dehydrator: A food dehydrator allows you to control temperature and air circulation, which can be especially useful in humid loca-tions. Spread herbs in a single layer and dehy-drate them at 95°F to 115 °F, checking regularly.

Oven: Use this method only if the oven can be set very low, about 100°F, or if you have a pilot light. Line a baking sheet with parchment paper and spread the herbs in a single layer. Place in the oven with the door ajar, checking regularly and turning the herbs as needed for even drying.

GARBLING PLANT PARTS

Garbling is the process of separating the part of the plant you want from the part you will discard. You can do this before or after plants have been dried. To garble dried leafy

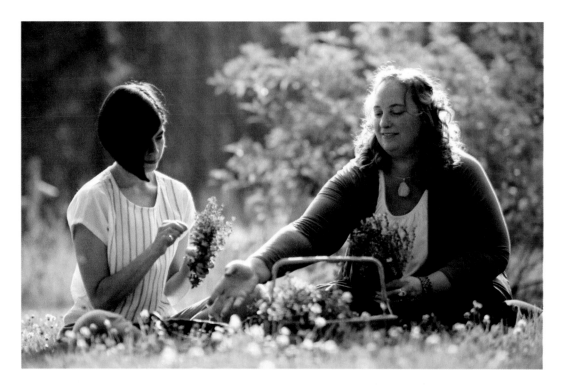

plants, place them in a large bowl or another container and use clean, dry hands to gently rub the leaves or flowers off the stems. A wire mesh can be used to garble and sift the herbs into finer pieces.

STORING DRIED PLANTS

Keep herbs and spices potent and flavorful by protecting them from moisture, light, heat, and air. Store dried plants in airtight containers such as glass jars or stainless steel tins in a cool, dry place. A cabinet, drawer, or shelf out of direct sunlight can work well; avoid locations like over the stove or dishwasher. Label containers with the name of the plant and other useful information like the date and place of harvest or purchase.

Example label:

> *Dandelion root*
> (*Taraxacum officinale*)
> Family: Asteraceae (aster)
> Harvest location: Mom's backyard
> Harvest date: 2/7/20

Most dried plants will keep for a year or two, with whole herbs lasting longer than those that are crushed or ground. To determine freshness, use your senses: do the herbs look vibrant, smell fragrant, and taste flavorful? If not, toss them in the compost or, if appropriate, use them in the bath or in a soup stock.

SUBSTITUTING DRIED AND FRESH PLANTS

Drying plants can concentrate their flavors. In general, if a recipe calls for fresh plants, you can substitute half the amount of dried plants. Conversely, if a recipe calls for dried, you may be able to substitute twice as much fresh. Keep in mind that in culinary recipes, making substitutions can affect the intended texture or consistency. Also be aware that moisture in fresh herbs may increase the likelihood of fermentation or spoilage in preparations like infused oil, honey, or low-percentage alcohol.

FREEZING PLANTS

Freezing is another way to preserve plants. Although their appearance and texture can change, they will retain flavor and will often be fine for juices, teas, syrups, or cooked dishes. Leafy greens can be blanched (briefly plunged into boiling water, then immersed in ice water) and frozen. Smaller quantities of herbs can be finely chopped, packed into an ice cube tray, and topped off with a little water or oil before freezing. Berries can be frozen on trays and then transferred to bags or containers. Remember to label and date frozen plants, which should keep for about a year.

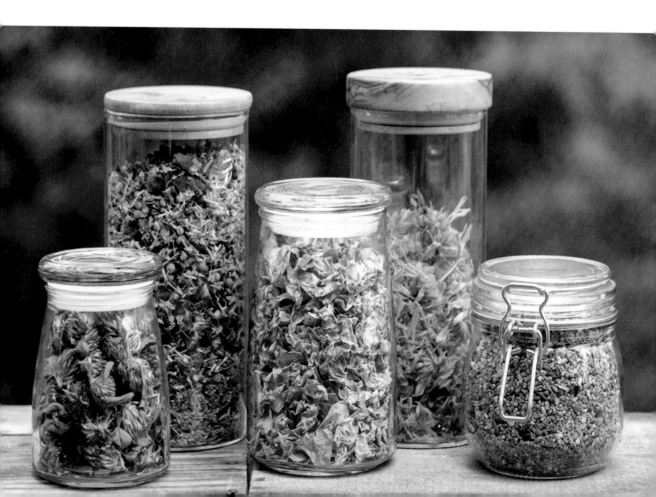

MEASURING

The recipes in this book use a mix of standard U.S. volume measurements and weight measurements. The latter are most accurate for herbs and spices that do not have a uniform size or shape. For example, a dried burdock root may be cut into large slices or finely minced. Stuffing those oddly shaped pieces into a measuring spoon or cup can yield very different results. When a recipe calls for weight measurements, we recommend using a digital scale that measures grams, kilograms, ounces, and pounds. For small amounts of herbs, we typically measure in grams, as that is easier to calculate than fractions of an ounce.

HERBAL PREPARATIONS

Throughout this book are many kinds of recipes for foods, drinks, and herbal remedies. Below are some of the types of preparations you will encounter, starting from simple water-based extracts to other solvents. By working through the recipes, you will gain experience with these solvents, or menstruums, each of which has different properties and uses. Besides extracting plant constituents, some of these solvents are natural preservatives. Thus you can extend the life of your seasonal harvest and create remedies that last for months or even years.

Water extracts: Water can extract most plant constituents except for resins. Leaves and other delicate plant parts are typically prepared as infusions, made by pouring boiling water over fresh or dried plant material. In some cases, cold water is used to extract a substance called mucilage from plants like mallow. Roots and other tough plant parts are typically prepared as decoctions, made by simmering the plant material in a pot of water. These various extractions may be consumed as teas, poured into herbal baths and steams, and used topically as washes. They should be used promptly, within a day or two.

Syrups: Syrups are made by combining an infusion or decoction with a sweetener such as honey or sugar. This can have medicinal benefits (think cough syrup) or be simply enjoyed in a glass of sparkling water or on pancakes. Store syrups in clean, airtight containers in the refrigerator. Syrups made with equal volumes of liquid and honey may last for up to a year, while those made with less honey or sugar may last only a week or two. Discard if you see any signs of mold or fermentation such as bubbling, cloudiness, or sliminess. For longer-term storage, syrups may be frozen.

Vinegars: Vinegar can extract minerals, trace elements, and alkaloids. It is also used for digestion and the respiratory system. You can mix herb-infused vinegars with honey to make oxymels, or include fruit in the blend to make shrubs. Store infused vinegars in a cool, dark place such as a cupboard or the refrigerator and use within a year for best flavor. Discard if you see any signs of mold or fermentation such as bubbling, cloudiness, or sliminess. Note that vinegar can corrode metal; if your jar has a metal lid, place a piece of parchment paper between the lid and the jar.

Alcohol extracts: Alcohol can extract most plant constituents except for minerals and trace elements. The percentage of alcohol used depends on personal preference, the plant material, and the constituents you wish to extract. For example, many dried leaves can be extracted in 40 percent alcohol, while resins, such as cottonwood buds, should be extracted in 95 percent alcohol. Alcohol-based plant extracts are commonly called tinctures. Other alcohol extractions include bitters, made with bitter-tasting herbs; liqueurs, which are sweetened; and elixirs, which are typically made with brandy and honey. Store all of these in a cool, dark place. Tinctures can last four to six years, while bitters, liqueurs, and elixirs may lose flavor after a year or two.

Glycerin extracts: Glycerin can extract tannins as well as some minerals and trace elements, alkaloids, acids, and mucilage. Glycerin extracts, called glycerites, are often used by those who want to avoid alcohol in tinctures. However, glycerites have a shorter shelf life, about one to two years. Glycerin can also be added to alcohol extracts to stabilize tannins from plant barks such as willow.

Oils: Oil can extract a plant's oils and resins. Herb-infused oils can be used as is or to make body care products like salves, lip balms, creams, and serums. If you will be ingesting the oil, be sure to infuse it with dried herbs; oils infused with fresh herbs have the potential for botulism. Oils and oil-based products have variable shelf lives; discard if they smell rancid.

KEEPING GOOD RECORDS

As the months pass and shelves fill up with remedies, it's easy to forget what some of the jars contain. Save yourself from guessing games and label everything! Labels can be fancy custom designs from your home printer or a simple roll of painter's tape and a permanent marker. Include details like the name of the plant, preparation strength, and when it was made or when you should strain.

Example labels:

> *St. John's wort* (Hypericum perforatum)
> Fresh herb in olive oil
> Made on: 6/21/19
> Strain on: 7/21/19

> *Dandelion root* (Taraxacum officinale)
> 1:5 tincture in 50% grain alcohol
> Made on: 4/7/20

In addition to labels, we like to keep a journal to record information such as dates, ingredient sources, alterations made to existing recipes, and tasting notes. Calendar apps or paper planners can also be used to set reminders for when to strain or check on remedies in progress.

COMPOSTING LEFTOVERS

Making herbal remedies like teas and tinctures often involves straining out used plant material, or marc. Keep these remnants out of landfills and in the natural cycle by composting, which returns nutrients to the soil and supports beneficial microorganisms. Even if you don't have a garden, you might still be able to compost. For many years Emily and her neighbors maintained a compost bin on a small patch of ground outside their apartment building. They used the compost for potted plants and gave it to gardener friends. Community gardens, schools, and local governments may also have composting programs.

PANTRY INGREDIENTS

We believe it's important to know where our food and medicine come from and to consider how an ingredient affects the well-being of other people, animals, plants, soils, and waterways. Whenever possible, we like to support our local economies and people who produce food organically and regeneratively. That said, access to ingredients varies, so use what is available to you. You can also find mail-order sources in the Recommended Resources on page 377.

Alcohol: We generally recommend using a midrange-quality alcohol; there's no need to splurge, but you do want it to be palatable. We prefer alcohol in glass bottles as opposed to plastic due to the possibility of flavors or chemicals leaching from the plastic into the remedy. The strength of a spirit is described as a proof or percentage. The percentage is half the proof. For example, a 100-proof spirit is 50 percent alcohol by volume (ABV). Most vodkas and brandies are 80 proof or 40 percent ABV. Some recipes call for a higher-proof spirit, such as Everclear or

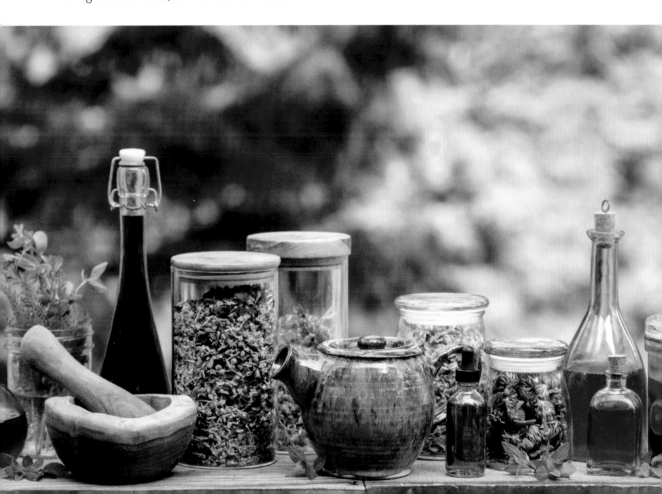

another brand of grain alcohol, which can range from 151 to 190 proof. High-proof alcohol can also be diluted with distilled water to the desired percentage.

Beeswax: Look for beeswax pastilles, or grate larger blocks of beeswax on a cheese grater (we have one dedicated to this purpose, as it can be difficult to clean). The smaller the pieces of beeswax, the more quickly they will melt for making salves and creams. Plant-based alternatives to beeswax include candelilla wax and carnuba wax, but these have different properties, so if using you may need to adjust quantities and techniques.

Carrier oils: These oils are used in body care recipes. We typically use olive oil, which is readily available and high in antioxidants; apricot kernel oil, which absorbs well and has a mild aroma; and jojoba oil, which mimics the skin's sebum and has a long shelf life. Feel free to experiment with the many other oils available.

Cooking oils: Look for expeller-pressed or cold-pressed oils, which have been physically extracted without the use of solvents like petroleum-derived hexane. We most often use delicious and heart-healthy olive oil. Be aware that many mass-market olive oils have been adulterated with lower-quality oils; purchasing from a reputable company or directly from an olive farm is often preferable.

Fruits and vegetables: Recently harvested, in-season fruits and vegetables are often more flavorful and nutritious than those shipped from far away. If possible, seek out produce from local gardens and farms. To save money at farmers markets, look for bruised or imperfect produce (called "seconds") sold at a discount.

Glycerin: Also spelled glycerine, this clear liquid can often be found at apothecaries, health food stores, and online. Be sure to use vegetable- or soy-based glycerin, not animal.

Herbs and spices: Bottled grocery store spices are often stale. Try to buy from places with high turnover, or look for opportunities to buy spices in bulk at grocery stores and spice shops. Also look for fair-trade herbs and spices that have been organically grown or sustainably wild harvested.

Honey: Mass-market honey is often adulterated or produced in unsustainable ways. When possible, look for locally produced, treatment-free honey (and beeswax) in order to support local beekeepers and bees. (Note that honey should not be given to children under one year old.) Plant-based alternatives to honey include brown rice syrup, maple syrup, and agave nectar, although these do not share the same medicinal or preservative properties and you may need to adjust quantities.

Lavender (Lavandula angustifolia) *essential oil:* This can often be purchased at health food stores and apothecaries. Although lavender is not an endangered plant, some plants used in essential oils are, so we prefer to buy all essential oils from ethical producers. If you don't have or don't like lavender essential oil, it can be omitted from most recipes.

Rosemary antioxidant: Sometimes called rosemary antioxidant CO_2 extract, this can often be purchased from apothecaries and suppliers of essential oils and body care ingredients.

Vinegar: Herbalists typically use raw, unfiltered apple cider vinegar or wine vinegar. For safe preservation, use vinegar with at least 5 percent acidity (this information should be on the label). Distilled white vinegar can be used but tends to have a very harsh taste.

Water: Teas and other preparations are best made with good-quality water such as filtered tap water or well water (or bottled water if necessary for safety). Some fermentation recipes call for water that is free of chlorine, which can destroy desirable yeast and bacteria. In those cases, use filtered or spring water, or leave a pitcher of chlorinated tap water on the counter for 24 hours to let the chlorine evaporate.

Witch hazel distillate: Also called distilled witch hazel extract, this can often be found at pharmacies, health food stores, and apothecaries. Avoid using an alcohol extract (tincture) of witch hazel.

USEFUL KITCHEN TOOLS AND SUPPLIES

Most herbal recipes can be made with simple kitchen tools. Below are some basic supplies that we recommend having on hand. Look for them in kitchen stores, hardware stores, thrift shops, and online.

Funnels: These are invaluable for filling bottles mess-free. We have several sizes, including a small funnel for filling dropper bottles, a funnel for larger bottles, and a wide-mouth funnel for jars.

Glass jars with tight-fitting lids: Jars are essential for storing dried herbs, making herbal remedies and recipes, and storing finished concoctions. Canning jars are especially durable, and

it's good to have an assortment of half-pint, pint, quart, and half-gallon sizes. Old food jars can be reused if they don't have any lingering odors (see Cleaning and Sterilizing on page 68). Note that vinegar can corrode metal; for vinegar infusions, swing-top jars with glass lids are handy.

Glass bottles: Small dropper bottles are great for storing and dispensing tinctures, bitters, and infused oils. A variety of bottles with tight-fitting caps or corks can be used to store syrups, liqueurs, vinegars, and more.

Kitchen appliances: Several recipes call for a food processor or blender. In some cases you can improvise with a mortar and pestle, kitchen

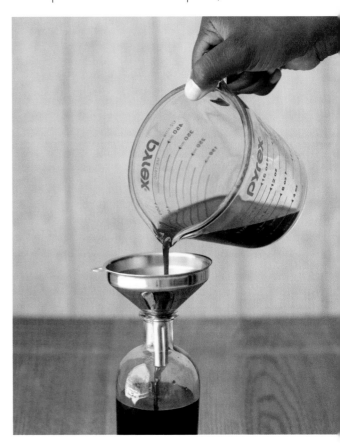

knife, or whisk, but a food processor or blender will make things much easier.

Measuring tools: A digital kitchen scale helps to accurately measure herbs and spices that do not have a uniform shape. Look for a scale that measures grams, kilograms, ounces, and pounds. You'll also want a set of measuring spoons and liquid and dry measuring cups.

Pots and pans: A small saucepan, medium saucepan, and larger pot will get you through most recipes. Use stainless steel, enamel, or glass pans, and avoid aluminum or other reactive metals. Some recipes call for a double boiler; we like the universal double boiler inserts that can fit over any pan and have a pouring spout. A metal mixing bowl placed over a saucepan of simmering water also works well.

Spice grinding tools: An inexpensive coffee grinder works well for grinding whole spices (keep it dedicated to herbs and spices so they don't flavor your coffee, and vice versa). A mortar and pestle or *suribachi* (Japanese grinding bowl) can be used to grind small amounts of herbs or spices.

Straining tools: For straining herbs from liquids, fine-mesh strainers are indispensable. Look for stainless steel strainers with a very fine mesh. We have multiple strainers, including a small one for teas and a larger one that can fit over a bowl. Cheesecloth, nut milk bags, or jelly bags are useful for straining and squeezing liquid out of plant material. A sprouting jar lid is also handy for straining liquids from mason jars.

CLEANING AND STERILIZING

When making herbal remedies and recipes, it's important to start with clean hands, tools, and containers. Jars and bottles should be thoroughly washed with hot, soapy water and rinsed well.

If desired, you can sterilize containers to prevent unwanted microorganisms and remove odors from previous contents. To sterilize a glass jar or bottle, place it in a deep pot and cover it with water. Bring the water to a full, rolling boil. Continue to boil for 15 minutes, then turn off the heat. Remove the container using tongs or a canning jar lifter, and shake out any excess water before filling it.

journal:
REFLECTION

What recipes and plant medicines are you excited to make? Dinners? Tinctures? Body care potions?

What tools or supplies do you already have? Do you need anything else to get started?

What challenges do you anticipate in regard to processing or preparing plants? What can you do to solve them?

WHAT'S YOUR COMMUNITY STORY?

Gathering with friends and family in your herbal kitchen is a great way to share your love of plants and continue learning with others. This could be anything you want! For example, you might consider:

- Herbal tea party

- Monthly potluck with dishes made from local plants

- Annual feast to celebrate the season

- Herbal remedy swap (share your elderflower cordial in exchange for a friend's dandelion root tea)

- Plant medicine–making skill share

- Community medicine–making event

- Gardening work party

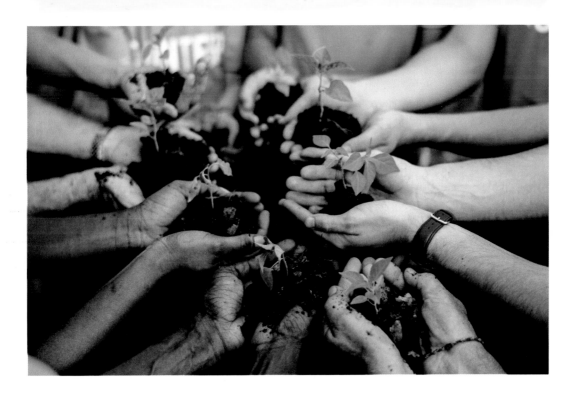

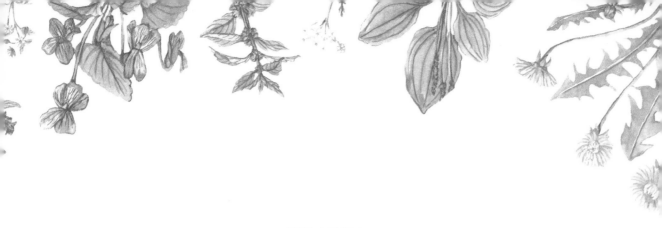

CHAPTER 7

THE JOY OF RECONNECTION: LIVING DEEPLY WITH THE SEASONS

Of all the phenomena of nature, none is as spectacular
or as subtle as that of the changing seasons.

— BERND HEINRICH

Our busy modern lives make it easy to live disconnected from the seasons. Indoor climate control means we can ignore outside weather with the click of a button. Supermarkets allow us to eat tomatoes in winter (even if they taste like mushy cardboard). Alarm clocks wake us up at the same time year-round, no matter how light or dark the sky is. This detachment sometimes begins when we are young. Many of us were taught about the seasons at school but rarely learned about the world around us.

Rosalee remembers her elementary school teacher decorating the classroom with a snow theme for the month of December—even though she lived in the Southwest desert where snow is absent. A life divorced from seasonal rhythms can be frustrating or simply mind-numbingly boring.

Immersing yourself in nature's rhythms provides simple yet profound delights such as taking pleasure in the tender greens of spring or sensing the first nip of autumn, tracking the sun from dawn to twilight or the cycle of the moon as it waxes and wanes. The seasons bring a flow of new insights as flowers and leaves unfurl, pollinators visit, fruits ripen, and then it all dies back to begin the cycle of growth all over again.

The plants in the following seasonal chapters are arranged according to general patterns of plant growth in temperate regions. For some readers, these correspondences will line up perfectly. For others, they may be off. The harvest time for many plants can also span more than one season. Although celestial paths define the official beginning and end of a season, the actual lived experience varies from place to place. The plants one person encounters in March may not show up for another person until July. Rather than equating certain months with each season,

look for the patterns of daylight hours, weather, and plant growth where you live.

It's not unusual for people new to wildcrafting or foraging to ask for a readymade harvesting calendar so they know when to gather plants. This is impossible! Not only do plants have widely different seasons depending on location, but they can also shift their growing seasons in response to changing climate. The following pages contain journal prompts and exercises designed to help you get to know *your* local seasons and plants. Keep in mind that you do not need to complete the exercises all at once. As each season progresses and you notice changes in yourself and the world around you, you can revisit the questions. It's okay not

journal:
REFLECTION

What are some seasonal patterns where you live? In what ways do you live with the seasons? In what ways is it a challenge? Do you have a favorite or least favorite season? What makes it so?

Here is Emily's reflection on this topic: *I grew up in the humid, subtropical climate of San Antonio, Texas, and now live in the Mediterranean climate of Los Angeles, so my experience of the year—and its rhythm of plants—has rarely matched the stereotypical four seasons. In L.A. we typically have hot, dry summers and temperate, wet winters. Winter rains awaken the growth of classic "springtime" plants, so while snow covers many parts of the country, my local hills are awash in the greens of chickweed, mallow, and mustard. After a busy winter and spring of gathering plants, I often slow down from midsummer to autumn, when annuals have died back and the land is dry and dusty.*

Adding complexity, we have many microclimates, and conditions can fluctuate from year to year and from one part of town to another. Plus, we have global climate change to contend with. Some years I'm gathering elderflowers in January, other years in May. All of this has taught me to continually engage my senses and experience the world as it unfolds, rather than remain attached to expectations. Instead of relying on someone else's calendar, I get to be an active observer and participant in the place where I live.

to have all the answers! Your sense of curiosity is what's important.

Tuning in to these natural rhythms roots your everyday experiences and reveals a never--ending spiral of wonder. Nature is constantly moving, teaching us to recognize the impermanence of life and therefore the joy of living in the moment. Taking time to appreciate the gifts of each season can fill our hearts with gratitude and give our lives meaning. We experience this every time we take in a brilliant sunset, notice the grace of falling snow, or listen to the trills of a favorite songbird.

SIT SPOT SENSES EXERCISE

Regularly visiting your sit spot (see page 14) is one of the most powerful ways to tune in to your local natural rhythms. Aim to visit at least once a week and do this exercise. As you become familiar with the prompts, you'll be able to do it without referring to the text, which will keep you more focused on your senses. Each of us has unique sensory abilities and sensitivities. So, as you move through this exercise, cultivate a practice that feels right to you.

To begin, take five slow, deep breaths, paying attention to the air flowing in and out of your lungs. Close your eyes if you feel comfortable and safe doing so.

- *Smell:* Turn your attention to your sense of smell. What scents do you notice?

- *Taste:* Our sense of smell and taste are closely related. As you breathe through your nose, what do you taste? Experiment with breathing through your mouth and detecting tastes and smells in the air.

- *Touch:* Now focus on your skin. Do you feel sunshine, wind, moisture, warmth, or cold on your face, arms, and other body parts?

- *Sound:* Listen to the world around you, giving yourself some time to let the variety of sounds unfold. What do you hear? Is each sound loud, quiet, near, far, from a certain direction?

- *Sight:* Open your eyes if you've had them closed. What shapes, colors, and movements do you see?

- *Touch (Texture):* Reach out and touch something nearby: feel the texture of a rock, the bark of a tree, or the petal of a flower (avoiding any poisonous plants, of course!).

With your senses engaged, enjoy being present where you are. You can do this for as long as you like.

journal:
SIT SPOT JOURNALING

After doing the Sit Spot Senses Exercise, record your observations and reflections in your journal. You might consider writing or sketching about:

- Date, time, weather

- Sense observations, including smell, taste, touch, sound, sight

- Plants, fungi, animals, and how they interact with one another

- Plants' life-cycle phases (e.g., leaf buds, leaves, flowers, seeds)

- Geology, soil, and slope observations

- Environmental disturbances (e.g., fires, windstorms, clear-cutting)

- Patterns or connections you notice

- Questions or things you are curious about

- Reflections on your experiences and feelings

SET SEASONAL INTENTIONS

At the beginning of each season, consider how you will put the Wild Remedies Ideals (and your own ideals) into practice. You might feel like setting one goal or ten; here are some ideas to get you started.

This season, I will . . .

- *Visit my sit spot on:* Sunday afternoons

- *Learn about where I live by:* observing birds outside my window

- *Practice gratitude by:* giving thanks when I pick chickweed

- *Give back to plants by:* cleaning up my neighborhood park

- *Learn about this plant:* chickweed

- *Make this food or remedy:* chickweed salve

- *Take care of myself by:* starting each day with a cup of herbal tea

- *Take care of the earth by:* building a native bee hotel

- *Cultivate community by:* listening to an elder's story

- *Share my love of nature by:* inviting friends over for a meal of seasonal ingredients

MAKE SEASONAL OBSERVATIONS

During each season, focus on the world both inside and outside your body. This will help you engage with the plant world and tune in to the foods, herbal remedies, and activities that best nourish and support you.

Looking outside . . .

- How would you describe the temperature and humidity?

- What time is sunrise and sunset? When are the full and new moons?

- What plants, fungi, animals do you notice?

- What local foods are in season?

- Do any colors catch your attention? You might notice the colors of the sky, insects, plants.

Looking inside . . .

- How would you describe your energy level and movement patterns?

- Are you craving any particular foods or drinks?

- What are your health joys and challenges?

- What makes you feel most alive?

- How can you best support your health and well-being this time of year?

REFLECT ON THE SEASON

As each season winds down and transitions into the next, take some time to reflect. Recording your observations from year to year can be a powerful way to become aware of seasonal rhythms.

- What plants and animals did you observe?

- What plants did you identify, harvest, and make food and remedies with?

- What seasonal activities or traditions did you enjoy?

- What sights, smells, colors, tastes, textures, and sounds caught your attention?

- How did you practice self-care?

- How did you take care of the earth around you?

- What were your joys? Challenges?

- What were you grateful for this season?

- What do you look forward to this time next year?

GET TO KNOW A PLANT

In each of the chapters that follow, you will read about a plant's gifts and ways to identify and work with it. But that is only an introduction. As you get to know each plant personally, your relationship will deepen. You'll learn more about what the plant offers you and how you can help tend the plant and its ecosystem.

In your journal, draw a simple sketch of each plant you study as you consider the following questions.

- Can you find this plant growing near you? What do you notice about where it likes to grow? What ecological connections do you observe?

- Where else might you be able to find this plant (e.g., botanical garden, grocery store)?

- Is it appropriate to harvest this plant in the wild where you live? Why or why not?

- How would you describe its shapes, colors, textures, scents? Do you associate any sounds with it?

- What does it taste like? Does it feel hot, cold, moist, or dry?

- What gifts does this plant offer in your life?

- In what ways can you give back to this plant?

- What foods or remedies would you like to make with this plant? With whom would you like to share them?

- Who could teach you more about this plant or where it lives?

You can use a blank journal to record your answers to the prompts in this chapter. To make it easier, we've also created a *Wild Remedies Journal* that you can download. Get your copy at: wildremediesbook.com/resources.

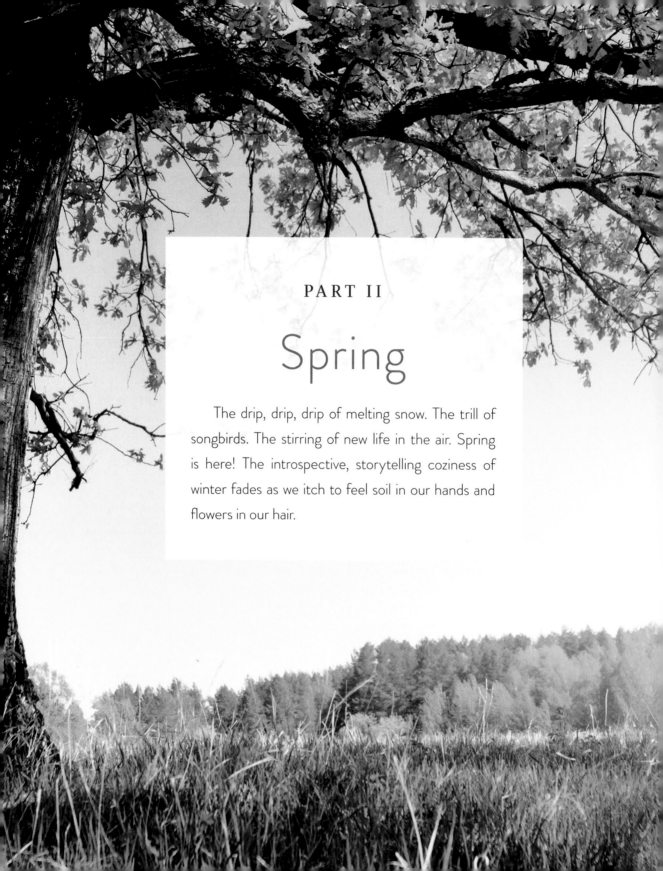

PART II

Spring

The drip, drip, drip of melting snow. The trill of songbirds. The stirring of new life in the air. Spring is here! The introspective, storytelling coziness of winter fades as we itch to feel soil in our hands and flowers in our hair.

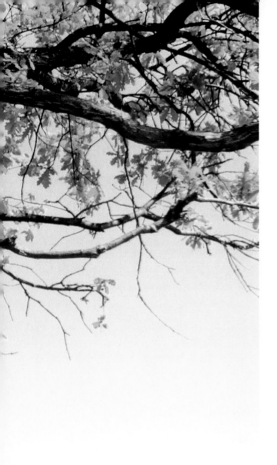

Plans are made: Which plants will you grow with this year? What will fill your baskets? In what ways will you give back?

The beginning of spring can test the plant lover's patience as you eagerly await your green friends' return. Slowly leaves unfurl, tree buds open as catkins give way to green canopies. The new growth of spring builds upon itself gradually, layer tumbling upon layer. Soon, however, it's hard to track every unfolding. Chickweed! Dandelions! Peach blossoms! Earthworms tunnel up through the soil beneath your feet. Insect wings flutter in the glistening light.

Spring teaches us how to slowly wake from a long slumber. It's a gentle push-pull. One morning you are harvesting violet flowers in sunshine; the next you are huddled inside to avoid freezing rain. Yet as the temperature rises and falls, as rains come and go, the sun graces the sky longer each day. Fresh spring greens fill your plate, and their slightly bitter tastes stoke your metabolic fires.

As the earth renews its gardens, we, too, can freshen our inner and outer worlds. Spring cleaning gives us the opportunity to assess our apothecaries. What herbs and remedies did you use? What simply collected dust? How can you use up last year's bounty in order to make room for this year's? Take this time to listen to the chorus of peepers and give thanks for all new life.

Spring Activities

- Smell the damp earth
- Eat a salad of tender greens
- Make a nature arrangement
- Listen to birds sing
- Look for new plant buds and shoots

- Play in the rain
- Clean your wildcrafting tools
- Draw a leaf as it unfurls
- Host a brunch for friends
- Keep a journal (see Chapter 7)

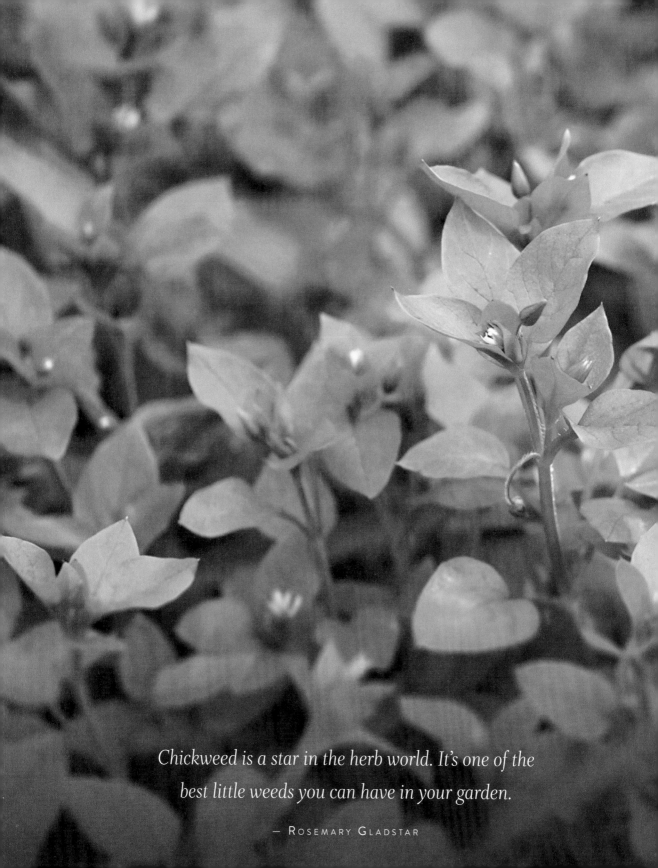

Chickweed is a star in the herb world. It's one of the best little weeds you can have in your garden.

— ROSEMARY GLADSTAR

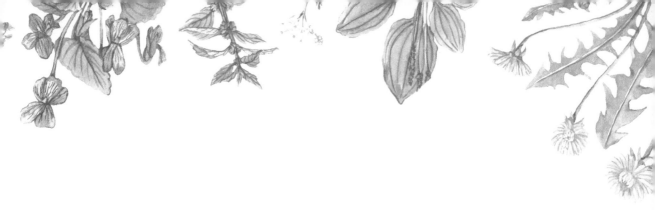

CHAPTER 8

CHICKWEED

A chickweed patch, whether it's found in a garden, a sunny forest, or a fallow field, is a sweet treasure, for this is a delicious food and wonderful healing remedy. Chickweed is best when fresh. You can eat bunches of it daily or preserve it as food or medicine. This starry delight will fade with warmer temperatures and bright, sunlit days.

Botanical name: *Stellaria media*

Family: Caryophyllaceae (pink/carnation)

Parts used: aerial portions (leaves, stems, flowers)

Energetics: cooling, moistening

Taste: salty

Properties: alterative, demulcent, diuretic, expectorant, febrifuge, inflammatory modulator, lymphagogue, nutritive, vulnerary

Uses: dry coughs, food, infections, inflammation, nutrient deficiencies, rashes, swollen lymph glands or stagnant lymph

Preparations: cream, food, oil, salve, succus (juice), tincture, vinegar

Native to Europe, chickweed is now one of the most common weeds in the world. It produces thousands of seeds, and a single plant can bear both seed heads and blooming flowers. It is sometimes used as a cover crop and is a favorite food of chickens.

MEDICINAL PROPERTIES AND ENERGETICS

Chickweed is a cooling and moistening herb for hot situations. It can soothe irritated eyes, dry coughs, an inflamed lymph system,

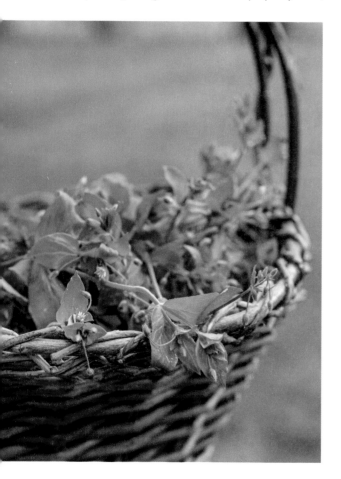

and skin conditions that are red, irritated, and itchy. Chickweed is high in saponins, soaplike constituents that act as an antimicrobial within the plant. In humans, saponins have a range of beneficial functions, including regulating blood sugar, supporting a healthy microbiome, and modulating inflammation.[1] We find many of these gifts in chickweed.

PLANT GIFTS

Provides Nutrient-Dense Food

Chickweed is a nutrient-dense plant, offering us deep nourishment in its fresh spring growth. This is especially valuable after the traditionally heavier foods of the fall and winter. Chickweed can be enjoyed by anyone and can also be used to support someone who may be chronically ill or recovering from a long-term illness. It contains many nutrients, including beta-carotene, calcium, fiber, iron, magnesium, niacin, phosphorus, potassium, vitamin C, and zinc.[2]

Quells Coughs

Not all coughs are the same, and therefore not all herbs that are "good for coughs" are the same. Sometimes coughs are thick and congested and you can support your lungs by thinning and expelling the mucus (see Chapter 10: Wild Mustard). At other times coughs come from irritation and dryness. In this latter case, chickweed excels at restoring moisture and decreasing irritation in the lungs. It can also gently support the fresh expectoration of mucus to help move stuck mucus out of the lungs. This may be due in part to the saponin content.

Soothes the Eyes

The moistening and cooling qualities of chickweed offer soothing relief to eyes that are irritated, red, or dry or have minor infections such as a sty or pink eye. For best results, apply the chickweed right to the problem area. You can easily do this by mashing up the fresh plant and then placing that juicy pulp on your closed eye for 10 to 20 minutes. If both eyes are affected, use separate poultices for each. This can be repeated multiple times and over the course of several days.

Heals Skin Conditions and Infections

Herbalists often reach for chickweed to address hot, inflamed, or itchy skin conditions such as eczema, blisters, scrapes, boils, diaper rash, and insect bites or stings. It can be used as a fresh poultice or as an infused oil or salve (see Chickweed Salve recipe on page 88). In addition to topical use, chickweed can support skin health when taken internally as a fresh green or as a vinegar or alcohol extract.

Herbalists have long used chickweed to address infections. In vitro studies have isolated various constituents in chickweed that show antiviral activity against herpes simplex 2 (HSV-2) and hepatitis B.[3]

Moves the Lymph

When the lymphatic system gets sluggish or swollen, there can also be associated signs of heat and swelling. Chickweed gently supports and moves the lymph. Consider it when lymph glands are swollen or when there is swelling and edema, indicating a stagnant interstitial fluid or lymphatic system. Many herbalists also use chickweed to address cysts.

HOW TO IDENTIFY

Chickweed typically likes cool weather and moist, somewhat shady spots, although it may be

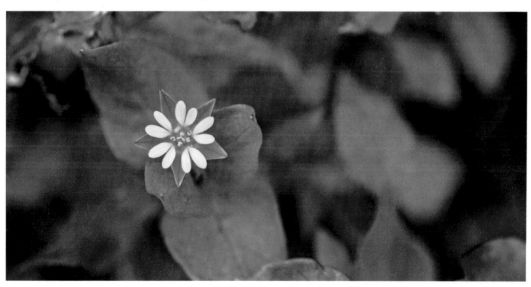

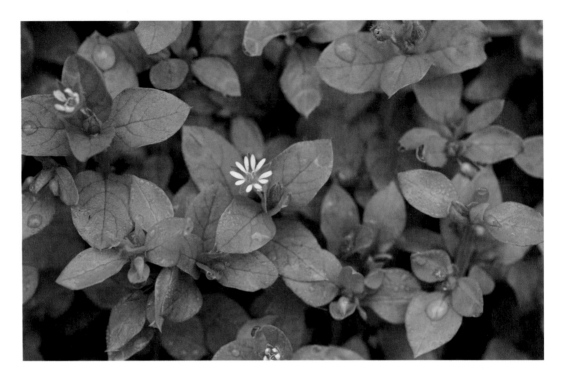

found in sunnier locations. Although often associated with early spring, it may also be found during autumn and winter in some places. It has a sprawling growth habit, its spindly stems often intertwining to form dense mats across the ground.

One of the plant's distinguishing characteristics is a line of fine hairs running down the side of the stem and changing sides at each node (the part of the stem where leaves are connected). The bright green ovate leaves have smooth margins and pointed tips, and are arranged in opposite pairs along the stem. The starlike white flowers are 2 to 5 millimeters in diameter. On first glance, each flower appears to have 10 petals, but a closer look reveals five deeply cleft petals. The color of the anthers ranges from yellow to green, brown, red, and purple. Egg-shaped fruits contain numerous tiny reddish-brown seeds.

ECOLOGICAL CONNECTIONS

Chickweed is a host to moth and butterfly larvae. The flowers attract small bees and flies, and occasionally butterflies and wasps, that feed on the nectar and pollen and help pollinate the plant. (Chickweed can also self-pollinate.) Small birds as well as mammals like rabbits, groundhogs, and deer browse on the foliage and seeds, helping to spread the seeds via their droppings. Seeds are also dispersed by ants.

HOW TO HARVEST

Harvest aerial portions of chickweed (leaves, stems, flowers) when the plants are young and tender. It may be harvested while flowering, but avoid harvesting it if it has gone

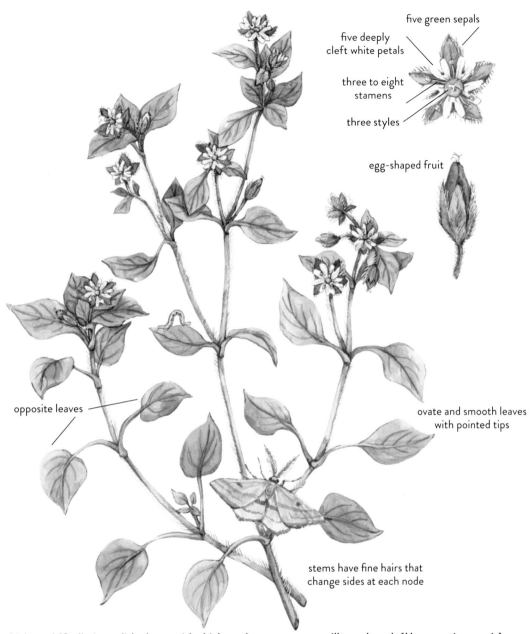

five green sepals

five deeply
cleft white petals

three to eight
stamens

three styles

egg-shaped fruit

opposite leaves

ovate and smooth leaves
with pointed tips

stems have fine hairs that
change sides at each node

chickweed (*Stellaria media*), shown with chickweed geometer caterpillar and moth (*Haematopis grataria*)

Life cycle: herbaceous annual or ephemeral
Reproduces by: seed
Growth habit: spreading, 2–12 inches tall
Habitat: disturbed areas, fields, gardens, lawns, meadows, orchards, roadsides, woodlands
Sun: full sun to partial shade
Soil: moist, fertile
USDA Hardiness Zones: 3–8

to seed, as it becomes tough and fibrous. Use scissors to snip the top portions of the plant, leaving several leaves behind. (If you try to pick chickweed with your hands, the elastic-like stems can be hard to break. You also risk pulling out the roots, something you should avoid unless you are trying to rid an area of the plant.) Regularly harvesting chickweed will cause it to branch and produce thick regrowth. Chickweed reproduces readily by seed, so leave enough flowers so it can produce them.

Harvesting Cautions

Chickweed has two poisonous look-alikes. When not in bloom, scarlet pimpernel (*Anagallis arvensis*) looks nearly identical to chickweed. However, it has hairless stems. The flowers are orange, red, or blue. The second look-alike to avoid is spurge (*Euphorbia* spp.). Spurge lacks chickweed's hairy stem and has different leaves, which grow opposite each other on the stem. When broken, spurge exudes a milky sap that can irritate the skin.

Chickweed also has two edible cousins: star chickweed (*Stellaria pubera*) and mouse-eared chickweed (*Cerastium vulgatum*).

GARDENING TIPS

A plant determined to reproduce, chickweed grows generously, easily seeds, and will continue to mature and set seed after being pulled. Before planting chickweed in your garden, be sure you want it—some relationships are for life! In early spring (or autumn in some places), directly sow seeds in rich garden soil, water well, and keep sponge-moist until you see many seedlings. Leave a small amount to reseed each year, or divide and replant divisions.

USING CHICKWEED IN YOUR LIFE

All tender, aerial parts of the plant can be used. Chickweed can be eaten as a raw salad green or prepared as a pesto. It makes a wonderful vinegar infusion, as the vinegar pulls out the plant's minerals.

Chickweed can also be made into a fresh plant alcohol extract. It can be infused into oil and made into a cream or salve. It can be dried for teas, but you'll notice its potency declines quickly over just a couple of weeks. If you want to dry it, use it up quickly.

Recommended Amounts

Chickweed is both medicine and food. As a result, the dosage can be quite high when eaten as a vegetable.

- *Tincture (fresh):* 1:2, 50% alcohol; 3 to 5 ml, 3 to 5 times daily

- *External:* Applications can be frequent and may need to be used consistently for several months to treat chronic skin irritation.

Special Considerations

Chickweed is a very safe herb. Because it is high in saponins, extremely large amounts may cause nausea or diarrhea in some people. As with any herb, start slowly until you see how your body reacts.

CHICKWEED VINEGAR

Apple cider vinegar is a wonderful medium for extracting all those wonderful minerals from chickweed. You can use this infused vinegar to make salad dressing or drizzle it on cooked greens.

Yield: 2 cups

---

2 cups minced chickweed

Up to 2 cups apple cider vinegar (at least 5% acidity)

1. Put the chickweed in a pint jar. Pour in enough vinegar to fill the jar and submerge the herbs completely. (You might not use the entire 2 cups.)

2. Cover the jar, preferably with a glass or plastic lid. If using a metal lid, place parchment paper between the lid and the jar (vinegar will corrode metal). Label the jar.

3. Let the jar sit at room temperature, out of direct sunlight, for about 4 weeks, shaking it every few days.

4. Strain the vinegar into a clean jar. Store in the refrigerator and use within 1 year.

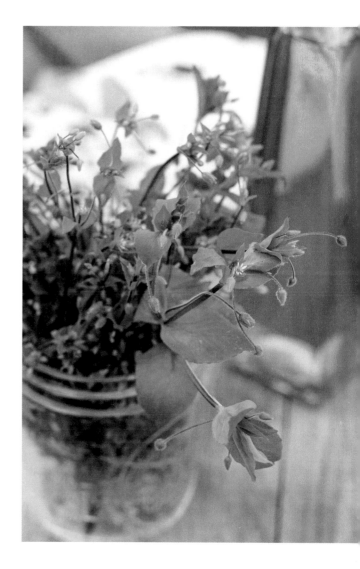

CHICKWEED PESTO

Slather chickweed pesto on pasta, sandwiches, eggs, rice, vegetables, or anywhere else you want the verdant taste of spring. If you're making this recipe with young, tender chickweed, you can use the whole stem, leaf, and flower. Older plants may have unpleasantly fibrous stems, so you'll have to pluck the leaves from the stems.

Yield: About 1 cup

¼ cup pine nuts

3 cups loosely packed fresh chickweed

2 garlic cloves

Kosher salt

½ cup extra-virgin olive oil

¼ cup grated Parmesan cheese

1. Toast the pine nuts in a dry skillet over medium-low heat, stirring frequently, until lightly toasted, about 2 minutes. Remove the nuts from the pan and let them cool.

2. Combine the pine nuts, chickweed, garlic, and ¼ teaspoon salt in a food processor. Pulse until finely chopped.

3. With the processor running, slowly pour in the olive oil and process until the mixture is smooth.

4. Add the cheese and pulse until just combined. Taste and adjust the ingredients and seasonings as desired.

5. Serve immediately, refrigerate for up to 3 days, or freeze for up to 3 months. To store in the refrigerator, transfer the pesto to an airtight container and pour a thin layer of olive oil on top to prevent oxidation. To store in the freezer, transfer the pesto to a freezer-safe container, or freeze in ice cube trays and then transfer the cubes to a freezer-safe container.

Variations: For a nut-free version, ½ cup shelled hemp seeds can be substituted for the pine nuts. For a dairy-free version, you can omit the Parmesan cheese and salt and add 1 tablespoon of chopped preserved lemon peel (see Preserved Lemons recipe on page 332).

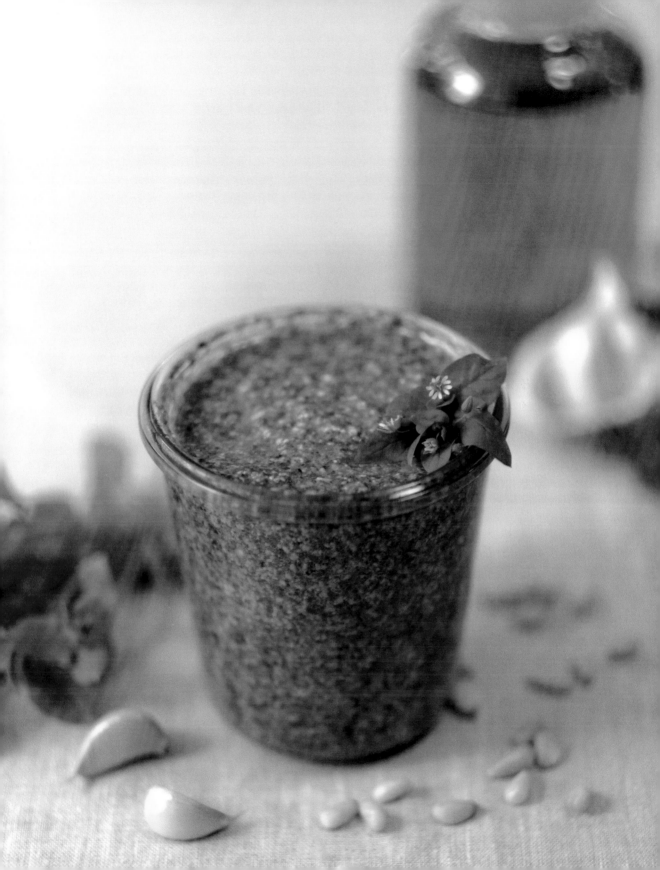

CHICKWEED SALVE

This salve brings soothing relief to hot and dry tissues. Rub it over bug bites, hot rashes, clean wounds, diaper rashes, or any itchy skin conditions. The optional lavender essential oil is also wonderful for the same conditions, provides a nice scent, and mildly helps the salve to last longer. This recipe makes a soft salve. If you anticipate storing it in a warm location, add more beeswax to help it solidify more. Up to 2 ounces (56 grams) of beeswax can be used in total.

Yield: 8 ounces

2 large handfuls fresh chickweed

1¼ cups olive oil

1 ounce (28 g) beeswax

30 to 50 drops (¼ to ½ teaspoon) lavender (*Lavandula angustifolia*) essential oil (optional)

1. *Prep the day before:* Chop the fresh chickweed finely and arrange it in a thin layer on a cutting board or cookie sheet. Allow to wilt for 12 to 24 hours.

2. *The next day:* Measure out the olive oil in a measuring cup. Add the wilted chickweed to the olive oil. You'll get the best results if there is roughly an equal amount of chickweed to olive oil, meaning there isn't a thick layer of oil or chickweed leaves at the top of the cup.

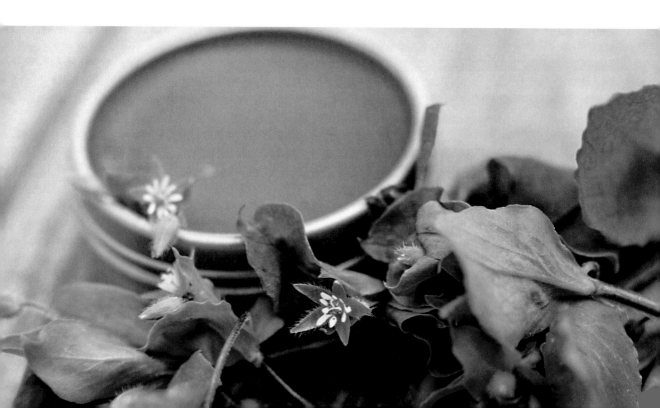

3. Place the chickweed and olive oil in a blender or food processor. Blend for 15 to 20 seconds or until the chickweed and olive oil are well blended. (This further breaks up the plant cell walls, helping the extraction process. However, this step can be skipped.)

4. Place the chickweed and olive oil mixture in the top part of a double boiler, or place a bowl on top of a pan that has 2 inches of water in it (the water should not touch the bottom of the bowl).

5. Bring the water to a boil, then reduce to a simmer. Stir the mixture occasionally and continue to heat until it is quite warm to the touch. Turn off the heat and allow the mixture to sit for several hours.

6. Repeat this process (reheating and allowing to cool) several times within a 24- to 48-hour period to fully extract the plant material into the oil. Throughout this process, do not let the oil get so hot that it smokes or begins to "fry" the plant material—you only need to get the oil warm to extract the goodness in the plant material.

7. After 24 to 48 hours, when the chickweed has infused well with the oil, the oil will have taken on green color. Strain off the chickweed through a double layer of cheesecloth.

8. Measure out 1 cup of the infused oil. (Extra oil can be used as a body moisturizer. If you don't have a cup of oil, add a little plain olive oil to make up the difference.)

9. Melt the beeswax in the top of a double boiler or a pan on very low heat. (*Tip:* The smaller your pieces of beeswax, the more easily they will melt.)

10. Once the beeswax has melted, add the chickweed oil. Stir well to combine, using as little heat as possible to keep the mixture liquid. (*Note:* It's normal for the beeswax to harden slightly when you add the oil. Allow it to melt again.)

11. Add the lavender essential oil, if using. Stir.

12. Immediately pour into tins or glass jars, and let the salve sit until it sets. Label and store in a cool place. This salve will last for a year, if not longer.

Cleanup tip: Use a paper towel to wipe out any container that held oil or the salve. Remove as much as possible, then wash with hot, soapy water.

Slow cooker method: Instead of using a double boiler for steps 4 to 6, you can use a slow cooker, yogurt incubator, or other low-temperature appliance that can maintain the oil temperature at 100°F.

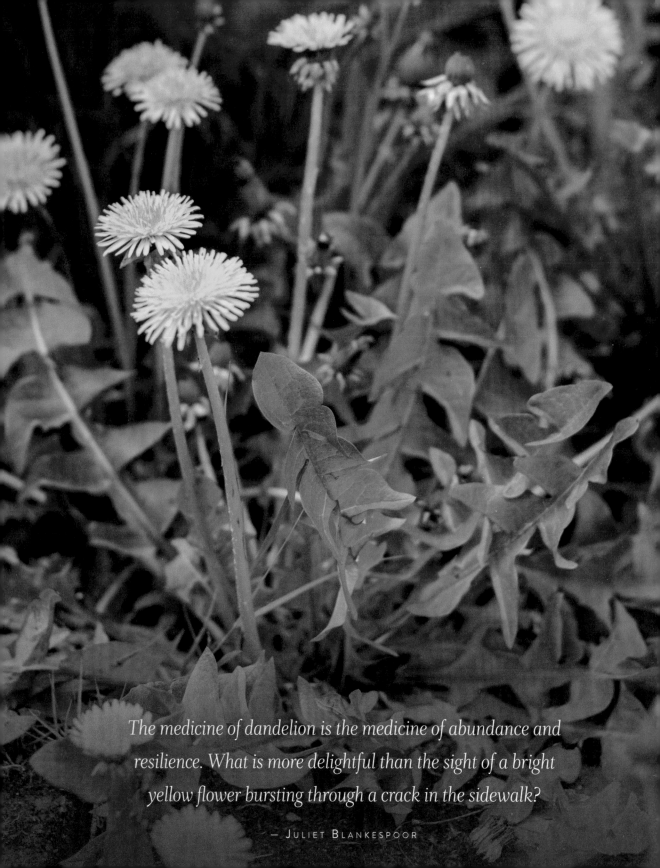

The medicine of dandelion is the medicine of abundance and resilience. What is more delightful than the sight of a bright yellow flower bursting through a crack in the sidewalk?

— Juliet Blankespoor

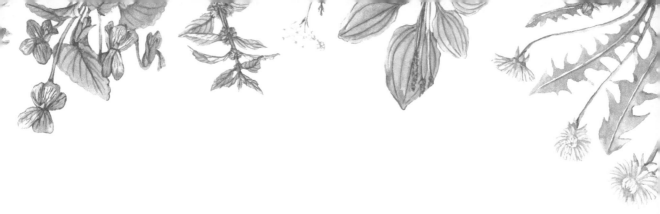

CHAPTER 9

DANDELION LEAF AND FLOWER

Dandelions tell us that spring is here! Often among the first flowers to emerge, especially in northern climates, dandelions bring important early nectar to honeybees and lift the hearts of all who anticipate longer days and warmer temperatures. The golden orbs fill lawns and meadows and even appear between the cracks in concrete. Dandelion is both tenacious and generous and is one of our most-needed plant medicines.

Botanical name: *Taraxacum officinale*
Family: Asteraceae (aster)
Parts used: leaves, flowers, sap, seeds, roots (see Chapter 26)
Energetics: cooling, drying
Taste: leaf is bitter, salty; flower is bitter, sweet
Properties: leaf is alterative, digestive stimulant, diuretic, nutritive; flower is anodyne, anti-oxidant, inflammatory modulator, nutritive
Uses: food, liver function, poor digestion, skin eruptions, water retention
Preparations: food, oil, tincture, vinegar

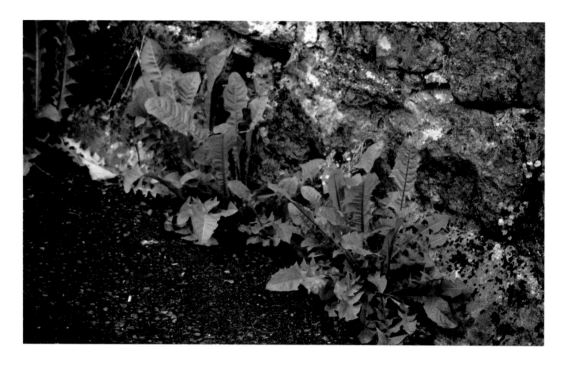

Dandelion is an opportunistic plant that originated in Eurasia and spread to all temperate climate zones of the world. Europeans have long loved the plant as both food and medicine and most likely intentionally (and unintentionally) brought the seeds with them to North America, where dandelion quickly spread. Anita Sanchez, author of *The Teeth of the Lion*, reports that a 1672 New England botanical survey listed dandelions as well established. Sanchez also says that the plants were introduced to Canada by the French and to the West Coast by the Spanish.[1]

It wasn't until the mid-19th century that the desire for the perfect lawn engendered a common disdain for this beautiful plant. Today consumers spend billions of dollars on ecologically harmful herbicides for their lawns, mostly to eradicate dandelions.

MEDICINAL PROPERTIES AND ENERGETICS

The energetic qualities of dandelion leaves and flowers are like spring itself: fresh, moving, and stimulating. The leaves are drying due to their digestive and diuretic effects. Both the leaves and the flowers are cooling in nature. Consider dandelion leaves and flowers for any type of sluggishness, whether it's the winter blues or stagnant fluids in the body such as edema or lymph.

PLANT GIFTS

Leaves Support Digestion

When dandelion leaves are young and tender, they have a slightly bitter taste, which stimulates many digestive functions and secretions.

For this reason the leaves are considered a spring tonic, something that is taken to enliven digestion after a winter of heavy meats and stored vegetables. Although we don't typically go without fresh foods for all of winter, dandelion leaves are still relevant today! They are some of our most nutrient-dense greens and can be considered a daily spark to maintaining healthy digestion. Dandelion leaves are filled with nutrients, including fiber, calcium, potassium, vitamin C, phosphorus, magnesium, beta-carotene, zinc, and manganese.[2]

The leaves also have high amounts of inulin. This starchy carbohydrate is broken down in the intestines and provides nutrients for healthy gut flora. While probiotics are currently popular, many surmise that increasing intake of prebiotics, like inulin, can help foster a healthy microbiome in the intestines. We are just beginning to understand how regularly eating inulin-rich foods could be helpful for a wide range of health issues. One study found that children with celiac disease who took inulin had a 31 percent increase in short-chain fatty acids and an improvement in their gut flora. Researchers are investigating whether inulin can help restore gut homeostasis in children with celiac disease.[3] Many studies have shown that a diet high in inulin can reduce blood glucose and insulin levels, indicating that it can be an important way to address insulin resistance and type 2 diabetes.[4]

Leaves Act as a Diuretic

Eating many dandelion leaves will make you urinate. A lot. This is such an obvious effect that the common name for dandelion in France is *pissenlit*, which translates to "pee the bed." Herbalists commonly use dandelion leaves to address edema, urinary stagnation, and symptoms of high blood pressure. Preliminary human clinical trials have confirmed the diuretic effect of dandelion tincture (alcohol and water extraction).[5]

Flowers Bring Joy and Nutrition

Spend a sunny morning picking bright yellow dandelion flowers and you'll undoubtedly experience one of their "side effects": they bring joy and laughter to those who spend time with them. This simple gift is perhaps the most profound that dandelion has to offer! What is more precious than joy? If that's not enough, then wait a while, and as the yellow blooms turn to seed heads, dandelions offer up another gift: free wishes!

Dandelion flowers are both food and medicine. As a food, they have a sweet, bland taste and are high in nutrients like lutein and beta-carotene, both known for the ability to support eye health. In addition to vitamins and minerals, dandelion flowers are high in flavonoids. One study looked at dandelion leaf and flower extracts and determined that the flowers have especially high flavonoid content. The study concluded they may be beneficial for diseases associated with oxidative stress (e.g., atherosclerosis, cancer, type 2 diabetes, rheumatoid arthritis, and cardiovascular diseases).[6]

Flowers Relieve Pain and Protect Skin

Freshly wilted dandelion flowers can be infused into oil and used to relieve muscle aches and pains. Consider pairing it with Cottonwood Oil (see recipe on page 342) or goldenrod oil, which are both great for pain relief. Herbalists also recommend dandelion flower–infused oil as a way to support healthy lymphatic tissues topically (see page 147 for a Spring Flowers Massage Oil recipe). The infused oil can be made into creams or serums to support skin health. One in vitro study found that dandelion leaf and flower extracts act as potent protective agents against UVB damage.[7]

HOW TO IDENTIFY

This plant is so well known that it may seem unnecessary to provide a description. However, people often mistake other yellow-flowered plants for dandelions, so it is useful to go over the details. Dandelions have a dense basal rosette of lanceolate or oblong leaves that are

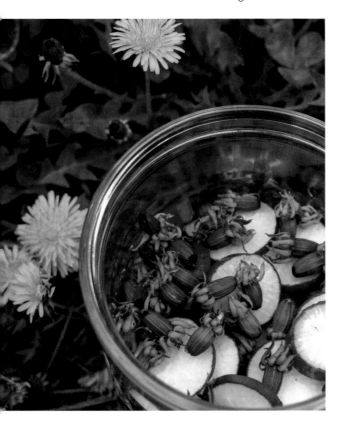

2 to 14 inches long and 0.5 to 3 inches wide. Each leaf has deeply lobed, irregular teeth and is generally broader at the tip. When broken, the leaves and stems exude a milky sap.

From the center of the rosette arises one or more flowering stalks. Each stalk is hollow and leafless and has a solitary yellow flower head. The composite flower head is 1 to 2 inches in diameter, cupped by pointy green bracts, and composed of numerous yellow ray florets. (It has no disk florets.) The fruit is a dry brown or gray seed with a tuft of silvery white hairs, which gives the mature flower head its round, furry appearance and helps disperse the seeds in the wind.

ECOLOGICAL CONNECTIONS

Many species of moth caterpillars eat the foliage of the dandelion, as do mammals, including rabbits, groundhogs, pocket gophers, deer, elk, and bears. The flowers provide nectar and pollen to insects such as honeybees, native bees, bee flies, and hoverflies. Small birds, including goldfinches and English sparrows, eat the seeds.

HOW TO HARVEST

Leaves and flowers can be gathered by hand or with scissors throughout the growing season. The leaves are best when young, as they become more bitter and tough as they age. There's no set rule as to when they are tasty and when they're not. Look for visibly young leaves then nibble some to let your palate decide.

Flowers and buds can be used whenever they are available. The flowers will readily go to seed, so it's best to harvest them and then use them immediately.

When harvesting flowers, keep in mind that they provide early spring food for bees and other insects. Dandelions tend to thrive on their own, but you can help keep a stand going by maintaining some of the roots (see How to Gather on page 295) or letting the flowers go to seed.

Harvesting Cautions

Every year billions of dollars are spent on herbicides attempting to eradicate the dandelion. Harvest dandelions in an area that hasn't been poisoned for at least three years and is free of heavy metals.

Potential look-alike plants include cat's ear (*Hypochaeris radicata*), hawkweed (*Hieracium pilosella*), sow thistle (*Sonchus* spp.), chicory (*Cichorium intybus*), and young wild lettuce (*Lactuca* spp.).

GARDENING TIPS

Dandelion is easy to grow in almost every type of soil. Establishing a garden bed or large containers with loose, friable soil will make root harvest easier. Direct sow seeds in early spring and keep moist until germinated. Seeds are distributed by the wind; remove flowers before they set seed to control their invasive generosity. There are numerous cultivars that produce thicker leaves and offer less bitterness.

USING DANDELION LEAF AND FLOWER IN YOUR LIFE

As we've said, dandelion leaves and flowers are a nutrient-dense and delicious food. The leaves can be added to salads, sautéed, or made into a pesto. Dandelion flowers can be eaten whole, added to salads, prepared as jam or wine, or added to baked goods.

Dandelion leaves can be used as a diuretic when fresh or dried. They can also be made into an alcohol extract (tincture). The flowers can be infused into oil when freshly wilted. Due to the high water content, a hot water bath infusing method is best; see the Spring Flowers Massage Oil recipe (page 147) for an example.

Recommended Amounts

- *Tea or powder (dried leaf):* 1 to 3 grams

- *Tincture (dried leaf):* 1:5, 30% alcohol; 3 to 5 ml, 3 times daily

- *Tincture (fresh leaf):* 1:2, 50% alcohol; 3 to 5 ml, 3 times daily

Special Considerations

Some people are sensitive to plants in the Asteraceae family, which can result in rare and usually mild reactions to dandelion.

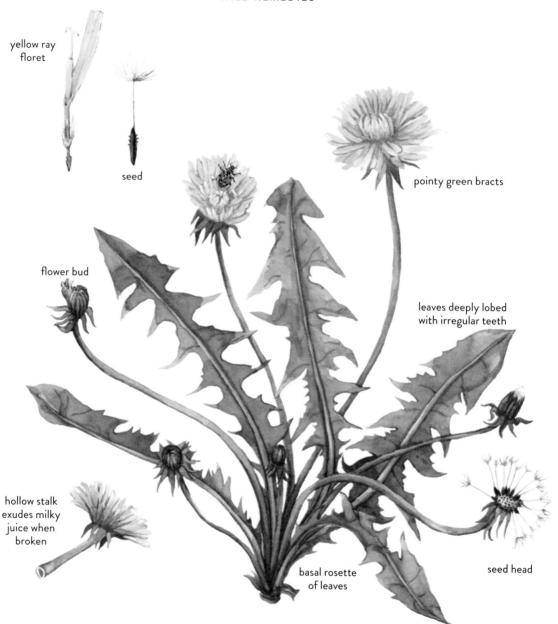

yellow ray
floret

seed

pointy green bracts

flower bud

leaves deeply lobed
with irregular teeth

hollow stalk
exudes milky
juice when
broken

basal rosette
of leaves

seed head

dandelion (*Taraxacum officinale*), shown with convergent lady beetle (*Hippodamia convergens*)

> **Life cycle:** herbaceous perennial
> **Reproduces by:** seed, root
> **Growth habit:** basal leaf rosette with upright stem, 2–12 inches tall
> **Habitat:** disturbed areas, fields, lawns, meadows, pastures, roadsides, sidewalk cracks
> **Sun:** full sun to partial shade
> **Soil:** prefers loamy, moist
> **USDA Hardiness Zones:** 5–9

FERMENTED DANDELION BUDS AND RADISHES

This recipe preserves the taste (and nutrients) of spring by transforming spicy radishes and bright dandelion buds into sour lacto-fermented pickles. These are filled with beneficial bacteria that aid digestion and support healthy immune function. Enjoy them on sandwiches, with a cheese snack, or in salads.

When harvesting dandelion buds, be sure they are unopened buds and not spent flowers. Unopened buds look like buttons, while spent flowers have their yellow petals peeking out the top. To process the dandelion buds, remove the stem entirely and then taste the bud. If it tastes good to you, use it as is. If it is too bitter, then remove the bracts before using.

This recipe uses a 3-cup fermentation jar but can be easily changed to fit your desired jar size. You can also use a quart canning jar with a fixed lid; however, you'll need to remove the lid daily to let pressure escape. You will also need a weight to keep the radishes below the brine. You can buy glass weights made for this purpose or use a rock that has been sanitized.

Yield: 3 cups

1½ tablespoons kosher or coarse sea salt

2 cups chlorine-free water (see note on water, page 67)

1 teaspoon mustard seeds

1 teaspoon whole black peppercorns

6 large radishes, sliced to ⅛ inch (approximately 2 cups sliced)

4 garlic cloves

½ cup dandelion buds

1. Begin by mixing the salt and water. Stir to dissolve and set aside.

2. Place the mustard seeds and black peppercorns in a 3-cup fermentation jar or 1-quart canning jar.

3. Place a layer of radishes over the spices. Add some of the dandelion buds and a clove of garlic. Continue layering with the radishes, dandelion buds, and garlic. End with a thick layer of radishes.

4. Pour the salt brine over the radishes and dandelions until they are completely covered. Leave at least 1 inch of space between the top of the brine and the lid. Discard any leftover salt brine. Use a weight to keep the radishes below the surface of the brine.

5. Let the jar sit at room temperature, out of direct sunlight . After 3 days, taste the radishes. If you like them as is, remove the weight and store in the refrigerator. They can be fermented for up to a week or even longer, depending on your desired taste.

SOCCA WITH DANDELION GREENS

Socca, or farinata, is a savory chickpea-flour pancake popular in the Mediterranean region. We love topping it with pesto (such as the Chickweed Pesto on page 86) or a salad made with dandelion leaves. In this recipe, lightly caramelized onions, sweet raisins, and toasted nuts complement and temper the bitterness of the dandelion greens. Serve this as an appetizer or a light meal.

Yield: One 10-inch flatbread, 2 main-dish servings or 4 to 6 appetizers

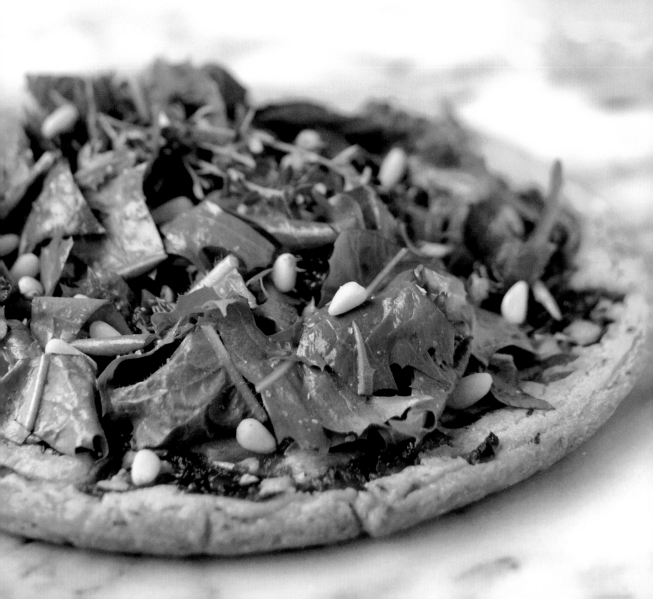

1. Place the chopped dandelion greens in a large bowl with enough water to cover. Set aside while preparing the socca. (Soaking the greens tames the bitterness; you may skip this step if you wish.)

For the socca:

1. Combine the chickpea flour, 1½ tablespoons of olive oil, garlic, thyme, salt, pepper, and 1 cup of water in a bowl and whisk to form a batter. Let stand for at least 30 minutes. (You can also leave it overnight at cool room temperature or in the refrigerator.)

2. Preheat the oven to 450°F with a rack in the center.

3. Heat 1 tablespoon of olive oil in a large saucepan over medium heat. Add the onion and cook, stirring occasionally, until it starts to brown, about 10 minutes. Reduce the heat to medium-low and cook, stirring every few minutes, until golden, about 10 more minutes. As the onion is cooking, add 1 or 2 tablespoons of water as necessary to prevent it from sticking to the pan. Remove from the heat and set aside.

4. Place a 10-inch cast-iron skillet or similar-size baking dish in the oven to preheat for 5 minutes. Carefully remove the skillet from the oven, add 1 tablespoon of olive oil, and swirl to coat the bottom. Stir the chickpea batter and pour it into the skillet. Sprinkle the onions on top and return the skillet to the oven.

5. Bake about 20 minutes, until the socca is cooked in the middle (yet still tender) and crisp around the edges. Halfway through baking, dab the top of the socca with the remaining ½ tablespoon of olive oil.

6. Remove the skillet from the oven. Use a spatula to lift the socca from the skillet and transfer it to a cutting board, then prepare the topping.

For the topping:

1. Drain and thoroughly dry the dandelion greens. Place them in a large bowl.

2. Combine olive oil, vinegar, mustard, honey, and pepper in a small saucepan over medium heat. Heat until warm, 1 to 2 minutes. Stir in the raisins and immediately pour the warm dressing over the dandelion greens. Toss to coat.

3. Pile the dandelion greens on top of the socca. Sprinkle some salt over the greens and scatter the pine nuts and goat cheese (if using) on top. Cut into wedges and serve.

Socca

1 cup (4 ounces) chickpea flour or garbanzo bean flour

¼ cup extra-virgin olive oil, divided

1 garlic clove, crushed or grated

2 teaspoons chopped fresh thyme, or ¾ teaspoon dried thyme

½ teaspoon salt

⅛ teaspoon freshly ground black pepper, divided

1 cup water

1 medium yellow onion, thinly sliced

Topping

3 ounces (about 4 cups) dandelion greens, tough stems discarded, and cut into 1½-inch pieces

Water for soaking the greens

3 tablespoons extra-virgin olive oil

2 tablespoons sherry vinegar

1 teaspoon Dijon mustard

½ teaspoon honey

⅛ teaspoon freshly ground black pepper

¼ cup golden or dark raisins

⅛ teaspoon salt

2 tablespoons pine nuts, toasted

2 ounces goat cheese, crumbled (optional)

DANDELION MAPLE SYRUP CAKE

Here's a delicious way to enjoy sunny dandelion blooms. Serve this cake as part of a brunch or as an after-dinner dessert. It pairs well with Roasted Roots Brew (page 298). To make this recipe, harvest about 2 cups of flower heads just before you begin to bake; otherwise, they may turn into puff balls on your counter. Process the flower heads by removing all the sepals and bracts, basically separating out the yellow flowers from all the green bits.

Yield: One 9-inch cake, about 8 medium servings

Cake

½ cup butter, softened

½ cup maple syrup

2 large eggs

1 teaspoon vanilla

¾ cup freshly picked dandelion flowers (sepals and bracts removed)

1 cup whole wheat pastry flour (or gluten-free all-purpose flour)

1 cup rolled oats

1 teaspoon ground cinnamon

½ teaspoon baking soda

½ teaspoon salt

¼ cup raisins, chopped (optional)

¼ cup walnuts, chopped (optional)

Frosting

8 ounces cream cheese, softened

¼ cup butter, softened

¼ cup maple syrup

¼ cup freshly picked dandelion flowers (sepals and bracts removed)

For the cake:

1. Preheat the oven to 375°F. Grease a 9 x 2-inch glass pie plate.

2. Mix the butter, maple syrup, eggs, and vanilla in a medium bowl. Add the dandelion flowers and mix well. Set aside.

3. Mix the flour, oats, cinnamon, baking soda, and salt in a medium bowl.

4. Add the dry mixture to the wet mixture and stir well. If using, mix in the raisins and/or walnuts.

5. Press the batter into the greased pie plate. Bake for 30 to 35 minutes or until a toothpick inserted into the center comes out clean. Let cool.

For the frosting:

1. Use a handheld mixer to combine the cream cheese, butter, and maple syrup. Taste and add more maple syrup if desired.

Assemble the cake: When cooled, invert the cake onto a sheet pan or large, flat plate. Frost the top and sides. Sprinkle the dandelion flowers on top.

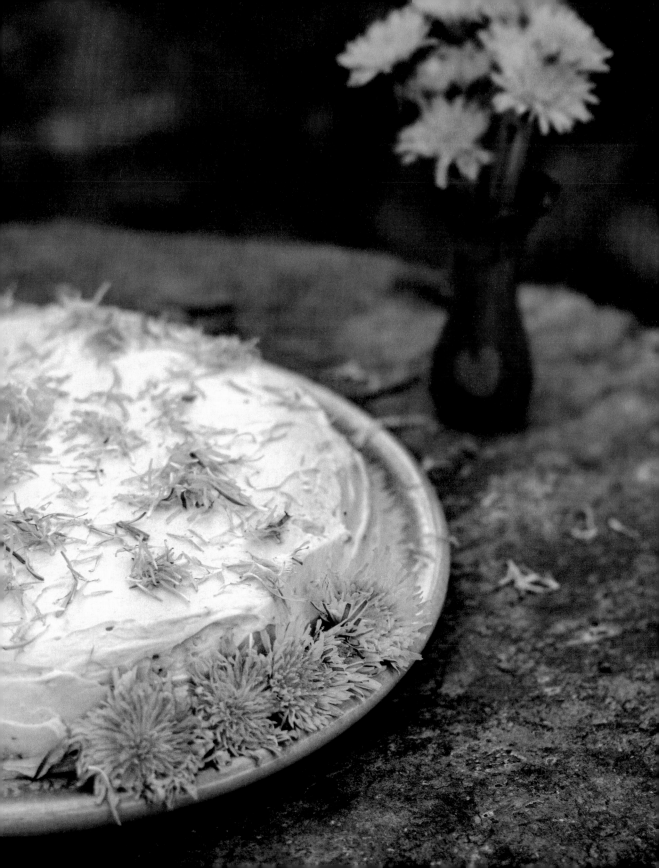

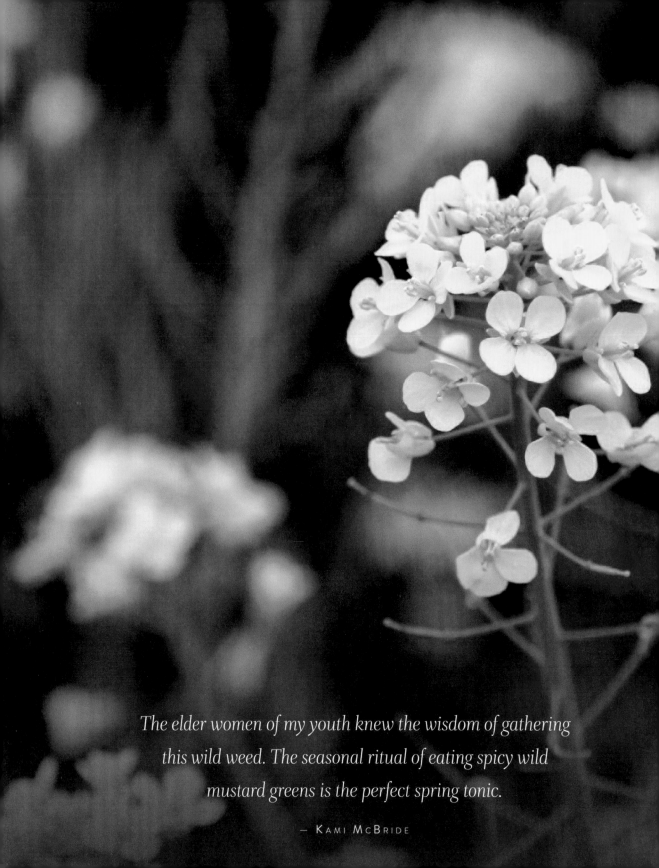

The elder women of my youth knew the wisdom of gathering this wild weed. The seasonal ritual of eating spicy wild mustard greens is the perfect spring tonic.

— Kami McBride

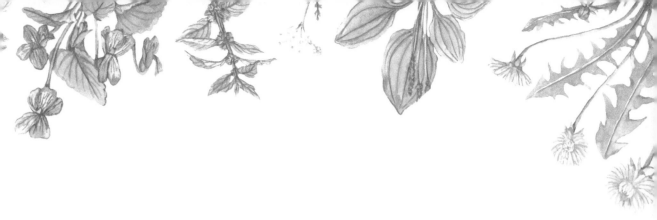

CHAPTER 10

WILD MUSTARD

Once you learn to recognize plants in the mustard family, you'll find friends wherever you may travel. With more than 4,000 recognized species growing in practically every corner of the world, mustards generously offer their gifts as food and medicine. They often flower in the spring, with some species erupting into displays of brilliant yellow blossoms along roadsides, in fields, and in disturbed areas. Many of our important food crops, like cabbage, kale, and broccoli, are in the mustard family. Countless species that grow wild can be used in similar ways for food and medicine.

Botanical names: *Alliaria petiolata, Brassica* spp., *Capsella bursa-pastoris, Lepidium* spp., *Sinapis* spp., *Sisymbrium* spp., *Thlaspi* spp., and many more
Family: Brassicaceae (mustard)
Parts used: leaves, flowers, seeds
Energetics: warming, drying
Taste: pungent, acrid
Properties: carminative, diaphoretic, digestive, expectorant, nutritive, stimulant
Uses: colds and flu, food, digestive, pain
Preparations: food, plaster, tea, vinegar

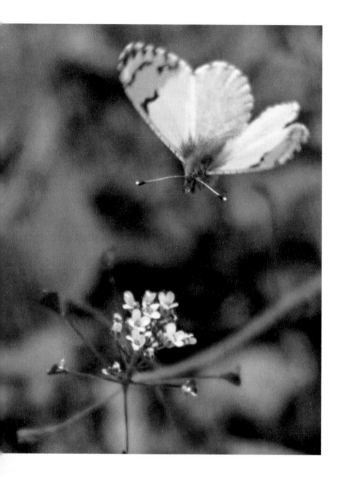

The mustard family is big and common! But while its members often share the same gifts, it's hard to lump them all together. For example, some mustards are endemic to certain parts of the world, meaning they are found only in that one area. Other mustards are notoriously free-wheeling and have voraciously spread into new homes around the world. Many mustards are cultivated and used as food or cover crops. The Chinese may have cultivated mustards more than 5,000 years ago.[1] And there's archaeological evidence that one mustard species was used as a spice more than 6,000 years ago in northern Europe.[2]

MEDICINAL PROPERTIES AND ENERGETICS

Most mustard family plants are, to some degree, spicy and hot in flavor. This quality, called pungency in herbal medicine, signifies something that can warm you up and stimulate movement. You've likely experienced this if you've ever eaten a bowl of spicy soup. The warmth often flows out from your middle to warm your entire body. In addition to stimulating circulation, it can also relieve mucus congestion.

PLANT GIFTS

Alleviates Cold and Flu Symptoms

Mustard's spicy nature can be used many ways to ease the symptoms of an upper respiratory infection, especially when you feel cold and have congestion. It can warm you when you are chilled and can be used to support the fever process (stimulating diaphoretic). A famous folklore remedy is to use mustard topically as a poultice or plaster to break up congestion in the lungs and ease coughing. Herbalists call a plant with this action a stimulating expectorant, meaning that it thins mucus and stimulates its release in order to get excessive amounts out of the body.

Relieves Pain

The spicy qualities of mustard can be a bit irritating when applied to the skin. This irritation can actually be therapeutic! Herbalists call plants with this action a rubefacient or counterirritant. Rubefacients, like mustard, increase blood flow to an area, which means your own body's natural healing abilities can work faster. Mustard plasters and poultices can be used topically to relieve arthritic pain, especially when the pain is worse with cold. Mustard is also prized for its ability to relieve pain associated with overused muscles. We recommend adding mustard powder to an Epsom salt bath to ease sore and tired muscles.

Stops Bleeding

While many mustards are used similarly, shepherd's purse (*Capsella bursa-pastoris*) has a unique use within herbal medicine. This plant is a strong styptic herb that can be used to stop excessive bleeding. It is particularly effective at stopping excessive internal bleeding such as menstrual flooding (menorrhagia) and post-partum hemorrhaging. Midwives commonly used it as a fresh tincture for this effect.

A recent study looked at the ability of shepherd's purse to stop postpartum hemor-rhaging. This study split 100 people into two groups. Fifty people received oxytocin and sublingual drops of shepherd's purse tincture, and the other 50 people received oxytocin and a placebo. Those taking the shepherd's purse saw significantly less bleeding than those who took the placebo.[3] Another clinical trial showed that shepherd's purse was effective as stopping heavy menstrual bleeding.[4] Herbalist Karta Purkh Singh Khalsa recommends 1 ounce of the dried herb made into a tea for menstrual flood-ing associated with perimenopause.

Adds Spice to Food

All plants in the mustard family are edible, but some are more tasty than others. Besides the spicy seeds, the young spring leaves and flowers can be eaten raw, made into a variety of condiments, used as a spice to flavor food, and cooked with foods such as vegetables, meats, and soups. As the plant matures, the spicy qualities intensify and, depending on the species, may render the leaves unpalatable. Try your local species of wild mustards to find your preferred edible, and note how the taste changes as the plant goes through its life cycle.

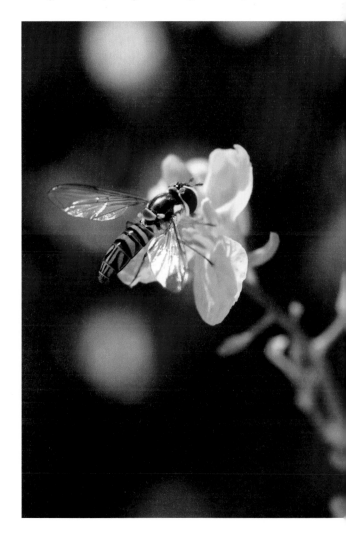

HOW TO IDENTIFY

Each mustard species has its own identifying characteristics, and you should consult a local guide for specific information. Fortunately, all species of mustard are edible (though not necessarily palatable), so if you learn how to identify Brassicaceae family plants, you're in a good position to forage.

Generally speaking, mustards can be easily identified by their flowers, which have four sepals, four petals (arranged in a cross or X shape), and six stamens (four tall, two short). The flowers are usually white, yellow, or lavender and grow in terminal clusters. The seeds are encased in pods called siliques or silicles, which grow in a radial pattern and vary in shape from long, narrow oblongs to short and flattened.

ECOLOGICAL CONNECTIONS

Mustard flowers provide nectar and pollen for bees, hoverflies, and other insects. Even if the mustards are not native to an area, they may be an important source in the absence of native wildflowers—even those they have crowded out themselves. The seeds may be eaten by birds and rodents.

Brassicaceae family plants can spread aggressively, and some of them are allelopathic, meaning they produce chemicals that inhibit the growth of other plants. Or, in the case of garlic mustard (*Alliaria petiolata*), the plant contains chemicals that are toxic to the native butterfly larvae that try to eat it. What is the solution? In some places it might be to eradicate the mustard and grow native plants. In others it might be to eliminate some mustard but leave enough for the bees, especially if human activity has damaged native plant habitats. The issue is complex and illustrates why foraging "rules" are not absolute.

Mustard plants may also be able to clean contaminated soil and water. For example, researchers have studied Indian mustard (*Brassica juncea*) and found that it has the potential to phytoremediate heavy metals, including cadmium, lead, and zinc, in water and soil.[5]

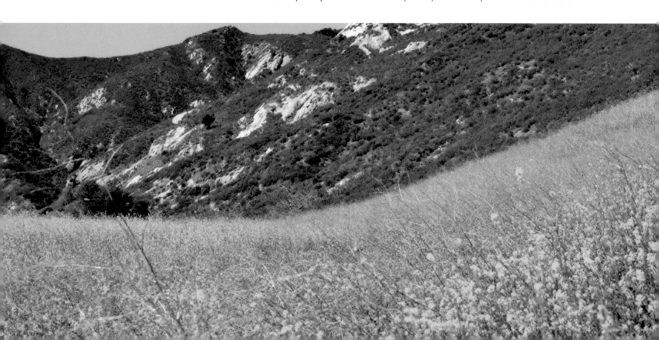

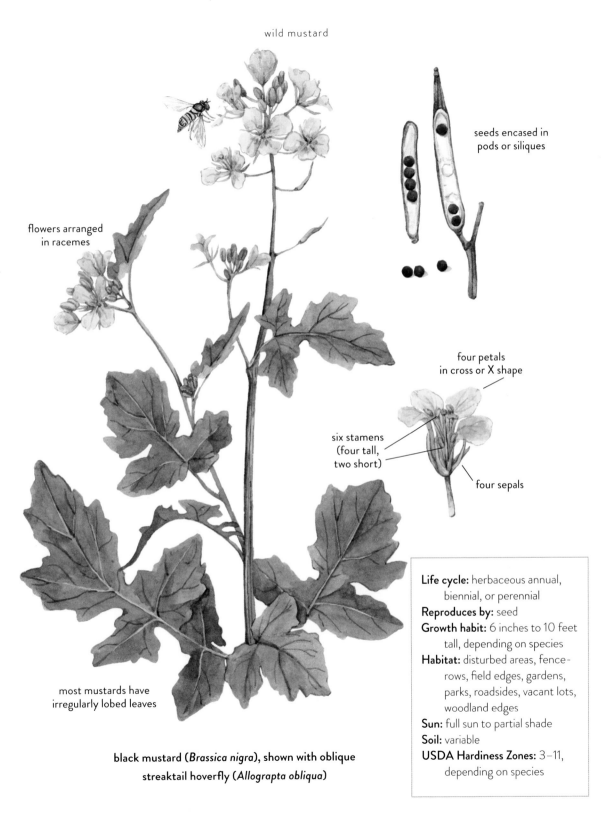

wild mustard

seeds encased in
pods or siliques

flowers arranged
in racemes

four petals
in cross or X shape

six stamens
(four tall,
two short)

four sepals

most mustards have
irregularly lobed leaves

black mustard (*Brassica nigra*), shown with oblique
streaktail hoverfly (*Allograpta obliqua*)

Life cycle: herbaceous annual,
biennial, or perennial
Reproduces by: seed
Growth habit: 6 inches to 10 feet
tall, depending on species
Habitat: disturbed areas, fencerows, field edges, gardens,
parks, roadsides, vacant lots,
woodland edges
Sun: full sun to partial shade
Soil: variable
USDA Hardiness Zones: 3–11,
depending on species

HOW TO HARVEST

Mustard greens are usually best gathered early in the growing season, when they are tender and not overly pungent; however, let your own taste buds guide you. Individual leaves, unopened flower buds, and open flowers can be plucked with your fingers or snipped with scissors.

To collect the seeds, gather the mature, dried pods and place them in a paper bag or pillowcase. You can then shake and rub the bag to separate the seeds from the pods.

There are usually plenty of mustard plants around, but do be aware that if you harvest too many flowers and seeds, the population can dwindle.

Harvesting Cautions

Farmers and park managers may be happy to have you remove invasive mustards; ask for permission, and make sure the area hasn't been sprayed with herbicides. Because mustard can pull up heavy metals from the soil, pay extra attention to your harvesting areas.

GARDENING TIPS

Many mustard species are easily grown by seed and do well with regular watering and garden soil. Propagation is by sowing seed onto weed-free soil, tamping in, and watering. Sow in early spring and late summer for cold-hardy species. Some species will become spicier with summer heat. If young leaves are preferred, stagger sowing every couple of weeks to keep a supply coming in. Note that certain species, like *Alliaria petiolata*, are classified as "noxious" and "invasive" weeds in some U.S. states.

USING MUSTARD IN YOUR LIFE

Mustards vary in taste and spice. Generally the young, tender greens are the most edible. For some species, cooking the mustard can lessen the sharp, hot flavor. The greens may be eaten fresh in salads or sautéed with olive oil, added to soups, fermented in kimchi, and more. The unopened flower buds of some species are delicious steamed, boiled, or stir-fried, and the open flowers make a good garnish for salads and sandwiches. Seed pods may be eaten when tender and green and can make a good trailside snack or pickle. The dried seeds from many species can be collected and used like a culinary mustard.

Mustards can be made into a tea (fresh or dried), extracted into vinegar, or made into an alcohol extract (tincture). They can also be mashed up into a poultice and used topically or dried and added to bathwater.

Recommended Amounts

Mustards are eaten as food, and sensitive individuals may find that too much can cause a mild stomachache.

Special Considerations

- Wild mustards vary considerably in taste and spice. When trying a new mustard, take it slow and experiment with amounts to find something that works for your purposes without overdoing it.

- In rare cases, mustards can cause a moderate to severe contact dermatitis in sensitive individuals. If using mustard topically, try it on a small area first.

FIVE-SPICE MUSTARD FLOWER BUDS

Because wild mustards vary in intensity, you'll need to do some tasting before you harvest. Use flower buds that are pleasantly bitter but not aggressively pungent; they should taste similar to rapini (broccoli rabe). Gather the flower buds before they open, picking the top 2 to 6 inches of the plant, including the buds and perhaps some tender leaves and stalks. Chinese five-spice powder can be purchased, or you can make your own—see Rosalee's book *Alchemy of Herbs* for a recipe. This dish is adapted from a recipe for Chinese broccoli by Victoria Granof in *Cookie* magazine.

Yield: 4 servings

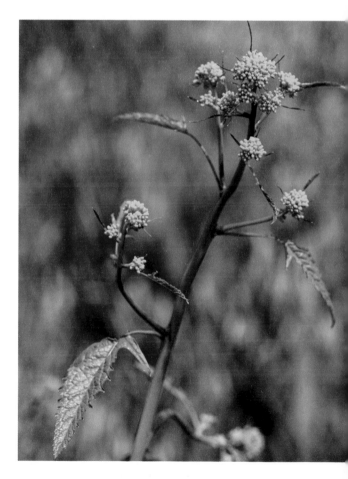

1 pound mustard flower buds

3 tablespoons unsalted butter or peanut oil

2 garlic cloves, minced

1 tablespoon soy sauce

½ teaspoon Chinese five-spice powder

¼ cup roasted peanuts or almonds, coarsely chopped

1. Bring a large pot of salted water to a boil. Cook the mustard flower buds until they are just tender, about 2 minutes. Drain well.

2. Melt the butter in a large skillet over medium heat. Add the garlic and cook until softened and fragrant, about 1 minute. Stir in the soy sauce, five-spice powder, and 1 tablespoon of water. Add the mustard flower buds to the pan, toss to coat, and cook until heated through.

3. Transfer to a serving dish and sprinkle the peanuts on top.

MUSTARD GREENS CHERMOULA

Chermoula is an herby, earthy North African sauce that traditionally accompanies grilled fish. This recipe gives it a pungent kick with the addition of mustard greens, and we don't stop at using it on seafood. This versatile sauce brings fantastic flavor to grain bowls, roasted cauliflower, eggs, grilled chicken or tempeh, sandwiches, and more. Like all recipes with wild mustard, you'll probably want to use younger and more mild-tasting leaves rather than leaves with an intensely bitter or spicy flavor.

Yield: About 1 cup

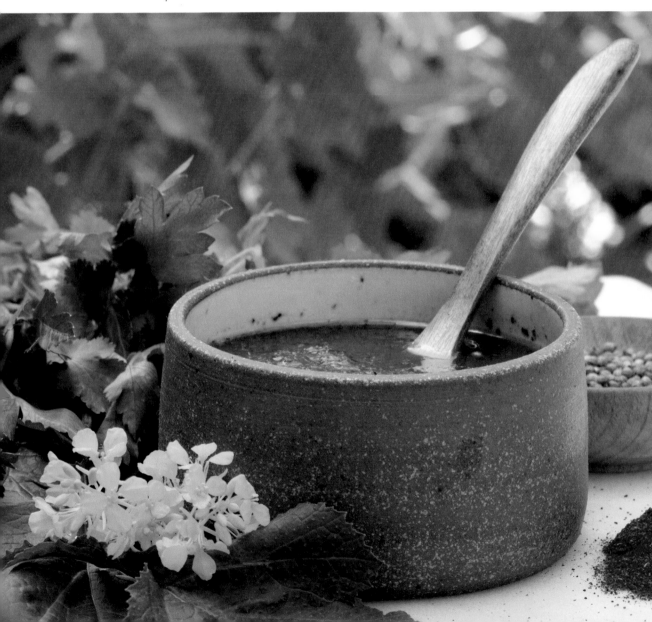

1 cup packed mustard leaves

½ cup packed cilantro

½ cup packed flat-leaf parsley

1 teaspoon grated lemon zest
(from about ½ lemon)

1 tablespoon fresh lemon juice
(from about ½ lemon)

2 garlic cloves

1 teaspoon whole coriander
seeds, toasted

1 teaspoon whole cumin seeds,
toasted

1 teaspoon paprika

½ teaspoon kosher salt

¼ teaspoon ground cayenne
pepper

½ cup extra-virgin olive oil

1. Combine the mustard leaves, cilantro, parsley, lemon zest, lemon juice, garlic, coriander, cumin, paprika, salt, and cayenne in a food processor. Pulse until finely chopped.

2. Keep the processor running and slowly pour in the olive oil. Process until the mixture is smooth.

3. Taste and adjust the ingredients and seasonings as desired.

4. Serve immediately or refrigerate for up to 3 days. To store in the refrigerator, transfer to an airtight container and pour a thin layer of olive oil on top to prevent oxidation.

Variation: Preserved lemon (see recipe on page 332) can be substituted for the fresh lemon zest and juice. Start with 1 teaspoon of minced preserved lemon and add more as desired. You may also want to reduce the amount of added salt.

AVOCADO TOAST WITH MUSTARD FLOWERS

Milder than the leaves but still packing a punch, mustard flowers are fabulous garnishes for salads, eggs, and sandwiches. Their peppery bite pairs nicely with creamy avocado, and naturally that includes avocado toast! Think of this recipe as a guide and feel free to add a pinch of this or that; chickweed, fennel pollen, and wild radish flowers often make their way onto our toasts, too. For a vegan version, you could use smashed cooked chickpeas instead of eggs.

Yield: 2 servings

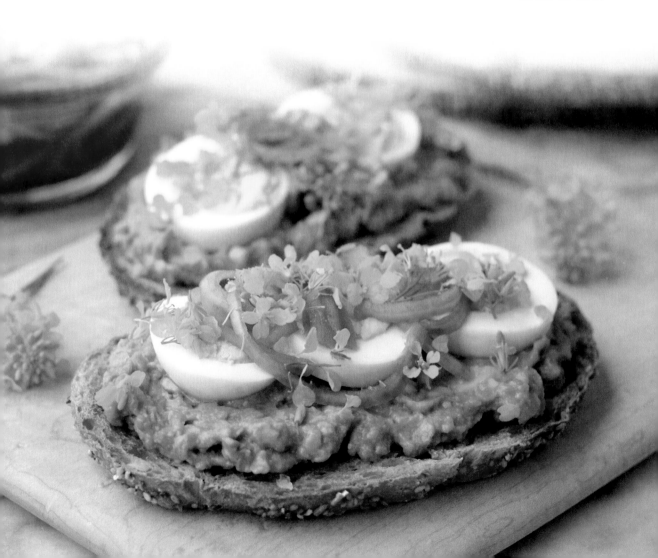

2 slices bread (any kind)

1 ripe avocado, pitted and peeled

2 teaspoons extra-virgin olive oil

2 to 3 teaspoons fresh lemon juice, to taste

Salt and freshly ground black pepper

2 hard-boiled eggs (below)

2 tablespoons pickled red onions (below)

Handful of mustard flowers

Flaky sea salt, for serving

1. Toast the bread.

2. Meanwhile, combine the avocado, olive oil, lemon juice, and salt and pepper to taste in a small bowl. Lightly mash with a fork.

3. Peel the hard-boiled eggs and cut each egg cross-wise into 4 slices.

4. Spread the avocado mixture on the slices of toast and arrange the eggs on top. Garnish with the pickled onions, mustard flowers, and a sprinkle of sea salt. Serve immediately.

To make hard-boiled eggs: Place eggs in a single layer in a saucepan and add cool water to cover the eggs by 1 inch. Bring to a boil over high heat. Turn off the heat, cover the pan, and let stand for 10 minutes (or 15 to 20 minutes at high altitude). Transfer the eggs to a bowl of ice water and let cool. You can make these ahead and refrigerate for up to 1 week.

To make pickled red onions: Place thinly sliced red onions in a glass jar and cover with red wine vinegar or apple cider vinegar. Let stand for at least 15 minutes and up to 1 hour. Drain just before using. You can make these ahead and store in the refrigerator for up to 2 weeks.

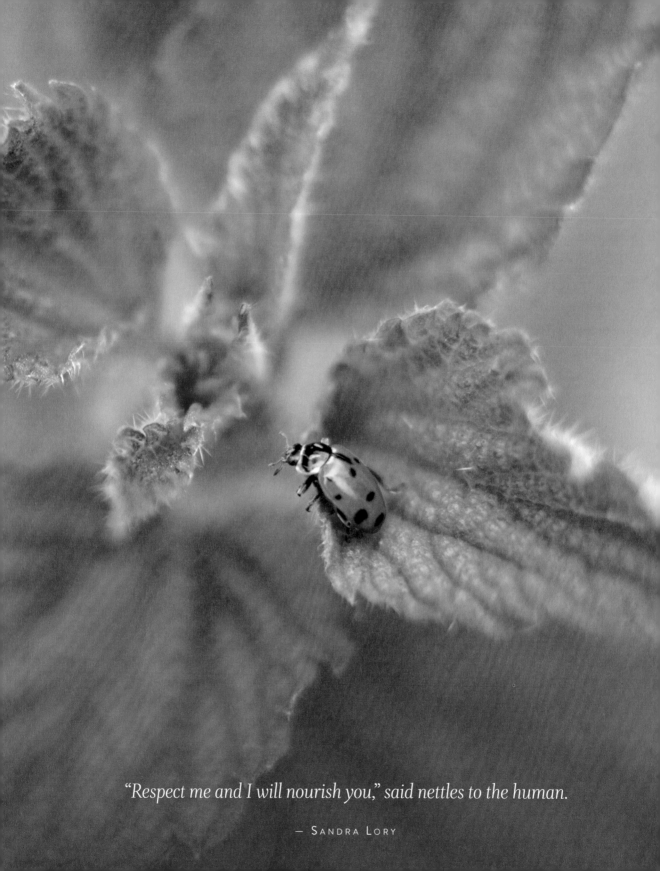

"Respect me and I will nourish you," said nettles to the human.

— SANDRA LORY

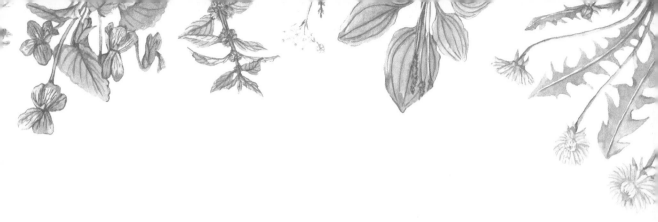

CHAPTER 11

NETTLE

Do you know that many of our modern-day fruits and vegetables are missing nutrients? Perhaps we bred these nutrients out while making our fruits sweeter and tastier (as with apples and tomatoes, for instance). Or maybe they were lost as an unintentional consequence of monoculture and nutrient-depleted soils. In any case, our foods don't contain the vitamins, minerals, and phytonutrients they once did.[1] The good news is that eating nettle is a powerful way to replace those nutrients, naturally!

Other common name: stinging nettle
Botanical names: *Urtica dioica, U. dioica* ssp. *dioica, U. dioica* ssp. *gracilis, U. dioica* ssp. *holosericea, U. chamaedryoides, U. urens*
Family: Urticaceae (nettle)
Parts used: young leaves, roots, seeds
Energetics: cooling, drying
Taste: salty
Properties: astringent, diuretic, kidney/adrenal trophorestorative, nutritive, styptic
Uses: arthritis, asthma, building blood, eczema, fatigue, food, hypothyroid, insulin resistance, low lactation, low metabolism, menstrual cramps, seasonal allergies, type 2 diabetes, urinary tract infections, weak hair/teeth/bones
Preparations: food, freeze-dried product, nourishing herbal infusion, tea, tincture

Native to Africa, Asia, Europe, and North America, nettle grows all over the Northern Hemisphere, and wherever it stands, humans take notice! The plant is covered in tiny hairs that are like hollow needles. Casually brushing up against the leaves or stems releases a slew of irritating chemicals into the surface of your skin, which results in a mild but uncomfortable rash. Who knows how many tens of thousands of years ago our ancestors figured out how to cook or dry the leaves to avoid the sting. At any rate, we've been enjoying the many gifts of nettles ever since.

In addition to food and medicine, humans have long used nettle in fiber arts. Native American peoples have traditions of making nettle clothing, rope, and fishing nets. In Denmark, researchers found a Bronze Age burial shroud made from nettle. Nettle textiles were widely produced in Europe until the 19th century and are still made today.

MEDICINAL PROPERTIES AND ENERGETICS

This plant embodies food as medicine. Nettle's many gifts are often attributed to its wide-ranging nutrients—and most people could benefit from all those nutrients—but nettle isn't for everyone. Especially when first drinking it as a tea or eating it in meals, it can be a strong diuretic (the diuretic effect can lessen over time). As a result, nettle is very drying, and those who tend to already be dry (dry hair, skin) can easily experience an unwelcome increase of dry symptoms when using nettle. Sometimes adding moistening herbs like mallow or violets to nettle formulations can help offset this, but sometimes it's simply too drying. Nettle is also cooling in nature. For people who tend to be warm and moist, nettle is a nourishing and building plant with countless benefits.

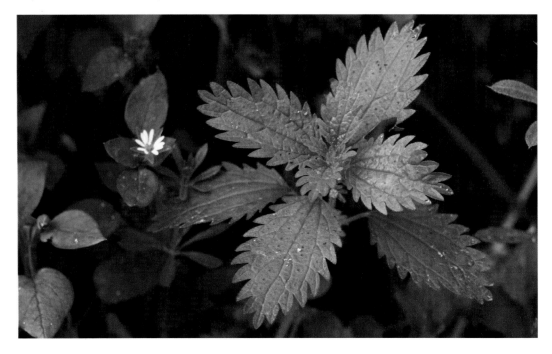

PLANT GIFTS

Leaves Provide Deep Nourishment

Nettle leaves are high in nutrients, including calcium, fiber, protein, potassium, flavonoids like rutin, ascorbic acid, glucosamine, beta-carotene, vitamin K, and many more.[2] Few plants boast the nutrient content of nettle, and few plants have benefits as dramatic when enjoyed frequently. Eating nettle or drinking its strong tea regularly often results in healthier bones, stronger teeth, and more vibrant hair. Nettle can also improve skin health and is frequently used to reduce eczema and acne.

Time and again we've heard from people who start drinking strong nettle teas daily that they are amazed at how much better they feel: their minds are sharper and their energy is higher and is sustained all day. A good candidate for nettles is someone who wants to do more but doesn't have the energy to do much.

Leaves Build Blood and Promote Lactation

Nettle leaves contain iron and are also believed to help the body better assimilate it. Herbalists commonly recommend nettle to help pregnant people maintain healthy iron levels. Nettle is also used for excessive menstruation (menorrhagia) leading to anemia.

Herbalists have long recommended nettle tea to help nursing parents create an abundant supply of milk for their newborns. A study in 2017 showed that nettle tea increases milk in nursing parents with premature babies without any adverse effect.[3]

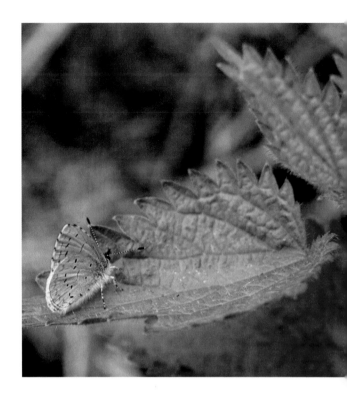

Leaves Reduce Inflammation

Nettle can modulate inflammation, which can be beneficial in a variety of ways. Seasonal allergy sufferers can find relief from their symptoms by drinking a strong nettle tea starting a couple of months before the allergy season starts. Freeze-dried nettle can be taken for immediate relief of acute seasonal allergy symptoms.[4]

Several studies have shown that a fresh alcohol extract of nettle leaves can reduce inflammation and blood glucose levels in people with type 2 diabetes and insulin resistance.[5] One recent study showed that nettle "may decrease risk factors of cardiovascular incidence and other complications in patients with diabetes mellitus."[6]

Nettle can also reduce pain associated with inflammation. Some of its nutrients, like magnesium, can help relieve musculoskeletal pain. Researchers have shown that a combination of nettle, rose hips, and devil's claw was effective at addressing knee pain.[7] Even the uncomfortable sting of fresh nettle can be used to bring blood flow to an area and decrease pain. If that last example sounds strange, you don't have to take our word for it. Researchers have done two studies showing that fresh nettle brushed against the thumb and knees can reduce pain and inflammation.[8] Those must have been some interesting studies to sign up for!

Seeds Increase Energy and Support the Kidneys

It is not recommended to eat nettle leaves after the plant matures, flowers, and goes to seed. But its seeds, hanging in small clusters from the leaf axils, are another potent herbal remedy. Nettle seeds can be eaten or extracted in alcohol and used to increase energy. Some herbalists think the increased energy is due to its supporting action for the adrenals.

Herbalist David Winston had the insight that nettle seeds could be used to help people with severe kidney disease. Since then, many herbalists have used nettle seeds to help people with failing kidneys.[9]

Roots Support Prostate Health

Herbalists often reach for nettle root to support prostate health and to alleviate the symptoms of benign prostatic hyperplasia (BPH), a noncancerous enlargement of the prostate.[10] It is often combined with saw palmetto. In one study using nettle root and saw palmetto, researchers concluded that the herbs were more effective and safer than the conventional drugs prescribed for BPH.[11]

HOW TO IDENTIFY

Nettle loves damp, nutrient-rich soils and can spread to form dense colonies. It has erect, occasionally branched stems that are covered with bristly hairs and somewhat square in cross-section. The oppositely arranged leaves are ovate to lanceolate with a pointed tip and sharply serrated margins. The leaves may be smooth or hairy. Leaf veins are noticeably sunken on the upper surface. In most species, long clusters of spike-like flowers droop from the leaf axils and have small greenish-white or pinkish-white flowers. These mature into tiny, flattened, egg-shaped seeds.

You may want to consult a local field guide to distinguish among the different species and subspecies. *Urtica urens* differs the most as it is an annual, not rhizomatous, and shorter with a sharper sting.

ECOLOGICAL CONNECTIONS

Nettle is a host plant for many insect young, including butterfly and moth caterpillars, beetle larvae, and midge larvae. Two butterflies associated with nettle include the red admiral (*Vanessa atalanta*) and question mark butterfly (*Polygonia interrogationis*). Tall and dense stands of nettle also provide shelter for insects, birds, reptiles, amphibians, and small mammals.

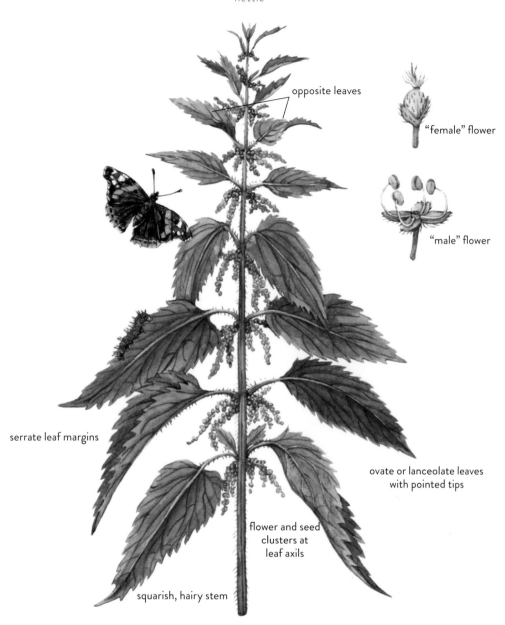

opposite leaves

"female" flower

"male" flower

serrate leaf margins

ovate or lanceolate leaves
with pointed tips

flower and seed
clusters at
leaf axils

squarish, hairy stem

nettle (*Urtica dioica*), shown with red admiral caterpillar and butterfly (*Vanessa atalanta*)

Life cycle: herbaceous perennial
Reproduces by: seed, rhizome
Growth habit: dense rhizomatous clumps; upright, leafy stems 1–9 feet tall
Habitat: disturbed areas, ditches, fields, floodplains, marshes, meadows, riparian areas,
riverbanks, seeps, thickets, woodlands
Sun: sun to shade
Soil: moist, rich, well drained
USDA Hardiness Zones: 3–10

HOW TO HARVEST

Harvest the leaves before the plant flowers and goes to seed. Using your (gloved) fingers or scissors, pinch off the top few inches of fresh growth. Picking the tops of established plants can encourage them to grow more leaves, and you can continue to harvest from established plants one or more times during a season. However, take care not to harvest too many tops too often, so that plants in the stand can flower and go to seed.

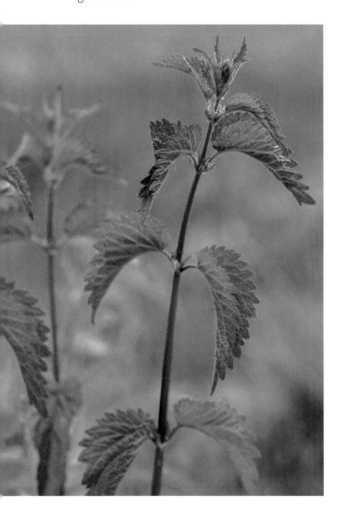

Gather the seeds when they are mature and green. (Some species of *Urtica* have separate "male" and "female" plants, so make sure you're harvesting from the "female" plants that have seeds.) Cut the flowering stalks, bundle them together, and hang them to dry with a paper bag around the bundle. The bag will catch any seeds that fall as they dry, and you can use gloved fingers to pull off the rest.

Dig the roots from a large, established patch after the plants have died back, using a garden fork to loosen the soil.

Nettle can be propagated by seed or rhizome transplanting.

Harvesting Cautions

Collect nettles carefully to avoid getting stung; we suggest wearing gloves and long sleeves. Because nettles can concentrate heavy metals and inorganic nitrates, pay extra attention to your harvesting areas. Look-alike plants include wood nettle (*Laportea canadensis*), which is edible; false nettle (*Boehmeria cylindrica*); and clearweed (*Pilea pumila*).

GARDENING TIPS

Nettle prefers nutrient-dense and humus-rich soils. Water regularly to maintain moist soil, or plant near a pond or stream. Nettle earns its invasive weed reputation because of its dual propagation strategies—windblown seeds and creeping underground rhizomes—so contain it with barriers and harvest seeds before they ripen. Propagation by seed is easy, with about a 50 percent germination rate. Propagation by division of established plants should be done in early spring.

USING NETTLE IN YOUR LIFE

Nettle leaves are nourishing greens and can be consumed in larger quantities like spinach or kale. They must be cooked or dried prior to eating to eliminate their stinging hairs. Use gloves while handling them to avoid the sting. We like to blanch the young leaves quickly in boiling water before using them in stir-fries, pestos, and other dishes. Consider using nettles anywhere you might use spinach—soups, lasagna, spanakopita, saag paneer, etc. The leaves can also be blanched and frozen for later use. Dried and powdered leaves can be added to smoothies and other foods.

Nettle leaves have a wide range of medicinal applications. The benefits you are looking for will determine how best to use them. For their nutrient content and support of general health and vitality, you can eat them fresh or use them as a strong tea or decoction. Research showing benefits for people with insulin resistance used the fresh leaf alcohol extract.

Nettle seeds can be eaten fresh, extracted into alcohol, or dried to sprinkle on food. See the dosage recommendation below, and keep in mind that some herbalists prefer to use even smaller amounts.

Nettle roots are generally dried and taken as a tea, tincture, or capsule.

Recommended Amounts

For nettle leaf:

- *Tea (dried):* 28 grams or 1 ounce (approximately 2 cups of finely crumbled leaves) daily

- *Tincture (fresh):* 1:2, 75 to 95% alcohol; 3 to 5 ml, 3 to 5 times daily

For nettle seed:

- *Seed (fresh):* 1 to 3 teaspoons

- *Tincture (dried):* 1:5, 30% alcohol, 3 to 5 ml, 3 times daily

For nettle root:

- *Decoction (dried):* 1 to 5 grams

- *Tincture (dried):* 1:5, 30% alcohol; 2 to 3 ml, 3 times daily[12]

Special Considerations

- It is not recommended to eat nettle leaves after the plant has gone to flower/seed.

- Use nettle with caution in people with dry constitutions.

- For some, nettle can be a strong diuretic.

- Very occasionally people report that nettle gives them a headache.

NETTLE FRITTATA

This recipe was inspired by kuku sabzi, a Persian frittata made with an abundance of greens. The result is a light and delicious way to enjoy the gifts of spring. This is a very forgiving recipe that is open to many variations. Use whatever greens may be lurking in your refrigerator or growing strong in the garden. This can be served warm or at room temperature.

Yield: 4 to 6 servings

6 tablespoons olive oil, divided

7 large scallions, sliced (including the green parts)

3 garlic cloves, minced

1 teaspoon ground black pepper

1 teaspoon dried rosemary

1 teaspoon dried thyme

1 teaspoon dried mustard powder

6 large eggs

1½ teaspoons salt

1 teaspoon baking powder

3 cups finely chopped nettle leaves (use gloves when chopping)

1 cup finely chopped dill leaves

1½ cups finely chopped parsley

1. Preheat your oven broiler on high. Heat 3 tablespoons of the olive oil in an 8-inch broiler-safe skillet on medium-high heat. Add the scallions and sauté for 3 to 5 minutes or until they are softened and the white parts are becoming translucent. Add the minced garlic, black pepper, rosemary, thyme, and mustard and sauté for 1 minute more. Remove from heat.

2. Mix the eggs, salt, and baking powder in a medium bowl. Whisk until well combined and a bit frothy. Gently stir in the nettle, dill, parsley, and scallion mixture to the eggs.

3. Heat the remaining 3 tablespoons of olive oil in the skillet. Pour the egg mixture into the skillet and spread evenly. Cook on medium heat, covered, for 8 to 10 minutes or until the bottom is set.

4. Uncover the skillet and place it under the broiler for 1 to 2 minutes or until it is cooked through. It can quickly burn, so don't leave it unattended—keep checking it until the egg mixture is set.

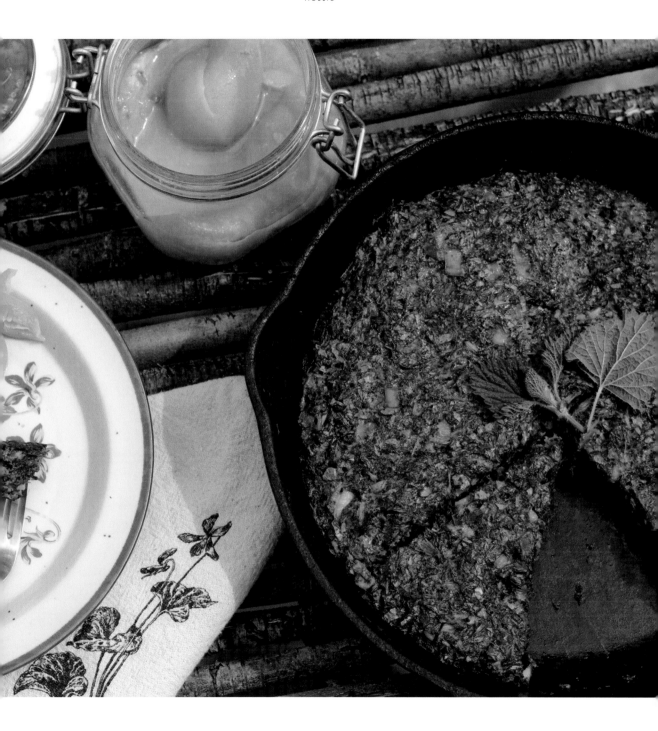

NETTLE AND ASPARAGUS SOUP

Serve a taste of spring with this savory and delicious soup! Perfect for a Sunday brunch or a cozy evening meal, this recipe is a synergistic combination of two favorite seasonal plants.

Yield: 3 quarts

5 tablespoons olive oil, divided

1 medium onion, diced (about ½ cup)

7 garlic cloves, minced (about 2 tablespoons)

1 tablespoon dried rosemary

2 teaspoons dried thyme

1 teaspoon freshly ground black pepper

1½ teaspoons salt

5 cups broth (bone broth or vegetable broth) or water

2 medium potatoes, diced (about 1 ½ cups)

1 bunch asparagus (about 10 ounces), cut into 1-inch pieces

5 cups chopped fresh young nettle leaves (use gloves when chopping)

1 tablespoon lemon juice

Dash of cream (optional)

1. Heat 3 tablespoons of the olive oil in a large saucepan over medium heat. When hot, add the onion and sauté until translucent.

2. Add the remaining 2 tablespoons of olive oil and wait a few moments for it to heat. Add the garlic, rosemary, thyme, black pepper, and salt. Sauté for 1 minute or until aromatic.

3. Add the broth, cover, and bring to a boil.

4. Add the potatoes and simmer for 5 minutes.

5. Add the asparagus and nettle leaves and simmer for 5 to 7 minutes or until the asparagus pieces are fairly soft.

6. Once the asparagus are soft, turn off the heat. Add the lemon juice.

7. Using a blender (immersion or upright), blend the soup on high until thoroughly creamed. (If using an upright blender, be sure to allow steam to escape while blending to avoid a big, hot mess.)

8. Add salt and pepper to taste. Serve in bowls with a dash of cream (optional).

Variation: A simple mushroom topping works wonderfully with this soup. You can make it while the soup is simmering. Heat 1 tablespoon butter in a small saucepan. Add 1 minced garlic clove and sauté for 30 seconds or until fragrant. Add a handful of minced mushrooms (morels, shiitakes, chanterelles, buttons, or whatever you like), and cook until tender. Top each serving of soup with a few spoonfuls.

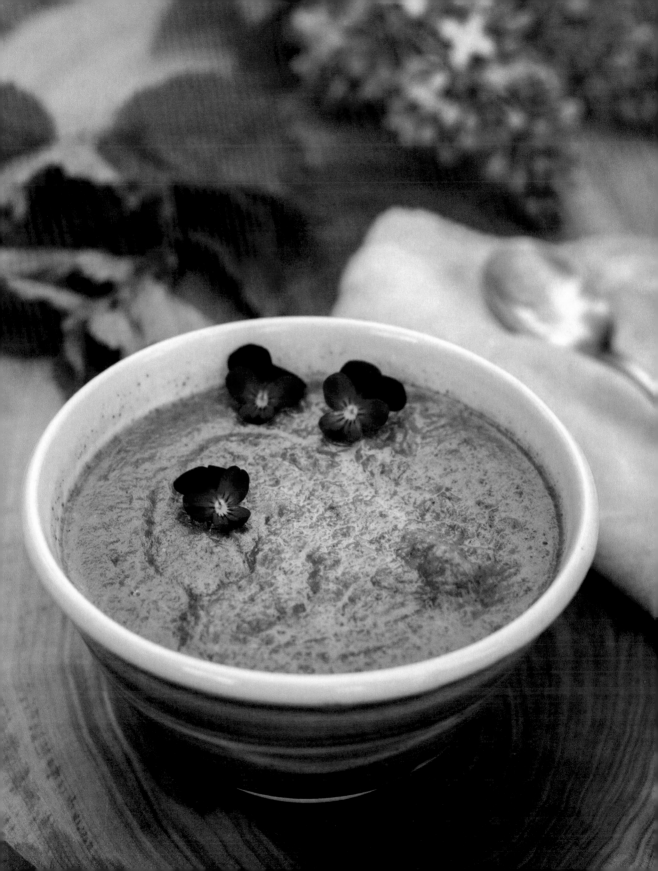

POTATO PANCAKES WITH NETTLE

Potato pancakes get a boost of nutritious nettle in this recipe, which makes a tasty appetizer, side dish, or snack. Inspired by Korean gamjajeon, these pancakes are crisp on the outside and chewy in the middle. A soy and vinegar dipping sauce provides a nice balance to the starchy potatoes and earthy nettles. Or you can serve these latke-style with sour cream or applesauce.

Yield: 16 to 20 3-inch pancakes

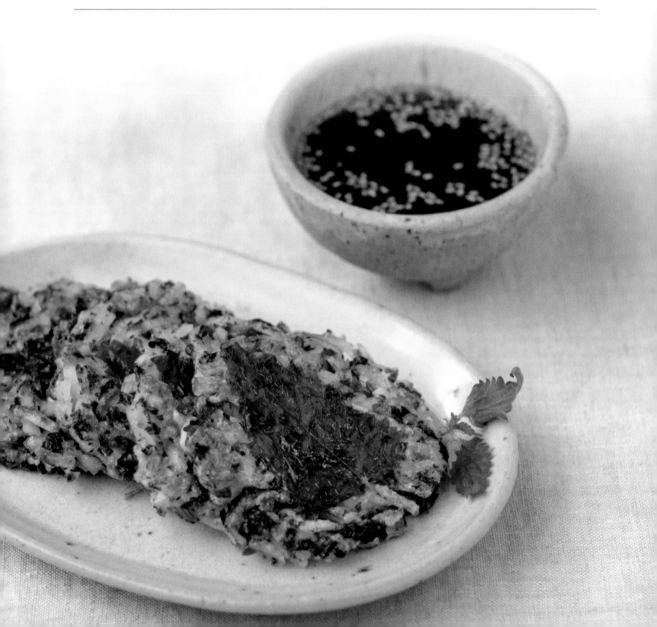

For the dipping sauce:

1. Combine all the ingredients in a small bowl. Set aside until ready to serve.

For the pancakes:

1. Set aside 16 to 20 nice-looking nettle leaves, which will be used to decorate the pancakes.

2. Bring a large pot of water to a boil. Add the remaining nettle leaves to the pot and cook, stirring frequently, for 2 minutes. Drain and squeeze out excess water. (You can reserve the nettle cooking water to drink as tea or to feed when cooled to plants.) Finely chop the cooked nettles.

3. Grate the potatoes using a box grater or the grater insert in a food processor. Place the potatoes in a fine-mesh strainer over a bowl and use the back of a spoon to press out as much liquid as possible. After a couple of minutes, a starchy paste will settle at the bottom of the bowl. Carefully pour off the liquid. Combine the starch with the grated potatoes, nettles, green garlic or scallions, jalapeño (if using), and salt and mix well.

4. Heat 1 tablespoon of oil in a large skillet over medium-high heat. Drop a heaping tablespoon of the potato mixture into the pan, using the back of a spoon to flatten and shape it into a 3-inch pancake. Gently press a reserved nettle leaf onto the top of the pancake. (We like handling the leaves with chopsticks, but you can also use gloves.)

5. Repeat this process to fill the pan and cook the pancakes until they are crisp and golden on the bottom, about 3 minutes. Turn the pancakes over and cook until crisp and golden on the other side, about 3 more minutes. Remove from the pan and drain on paper towels.

6. Repeat with the remaining pancake mixture, adding more oil to the pan as needed.

7. Serve warm with dipping sauce on the side.

Dipping sauce (optional)

3 tablespoons soy sauce

1 tablespoon rice vinegar

½ teaspoon sugar or honey

½ teaspoon toasted sesame seeds

Pancakes

2 cups packed fresh nettle leaves (use gloves when handling)

1 pound russet potatoes (about 2 medium), peeled

2 stalks green garlic or scallions, finely chopped (about ¼ cup)

1 jalapeño, seeded and finely chopped (optional)

½ teaspoon kosher salt

Vegetable oil, for frying

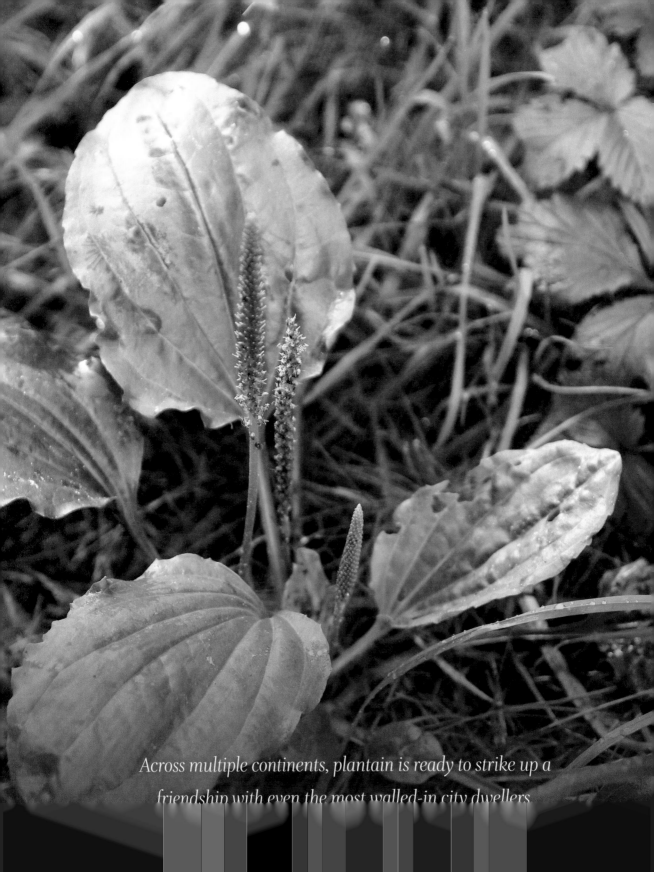

Across multiple continents, plantain is ready to strike up a
friendship with even the most walled-in city dwellers.

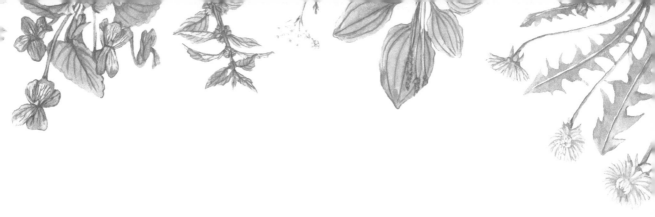

CHAPTER 12

PLANTAIN

Growing everywhere from sidewalk cracks to seaside rocks, the humble plantain
has many virtues, its utility ranging from acute first-aid situations to chronic
conditions. Best of all, if you know how to spot it, you can most likely find
this plant whenever you need it. (By the way, *Plantago* is completely unrelated
to the plantain of the banana family, which is part of the *Musa* genus!)

Other common names: fleawort, ribwort, white man's footprint
Botanical names: *Plantago major, P. lanceolata, P. rugelii, P. rhodosperma, P. virginica*, and
    other species
Family: Plantaginaceae (plantain)
Parts used: leaves, seeds
Energetics: cooling, moistening
Taste: salty, bitter
Properties: antimicrobial, demulcent, diuretic, expectorant, inflammatory modulator,
    nutritive, slightly astringent, vulnerary
Uses: dry coughs, food, healing of tissues, insect and spider bites, splinters/drawing out,
    ulcers and other gastrointestinal inflammation, urinary infections, wounds
Preparations: food, oil, poultice, salve, tea, tincture, vinegar

Various species of plantain are native to Africa, Asia, Europe, and the Americas. In North America, the most commonly found species came from Europe. Plantain loves disturbed soils and can even grow in hard-packed earth with lots of foot traffic. When European settlers brought the seeds to North America, they spread so readily via horses' hooves and wagon wheels headed west that plantain was commonly called "white man's footprint."

MEDICINAL PROPERTIES AND ENERGETICS

You could spend a lot of time trying to memorize plantain's medicinal applications, but you will have a deeper understanding of its abilities when you view it through the lens of its energetic properties. Plantain is energetically cooling and excels when used to counteract hot conditions such as redness (sometimes yellowness), sharp pain, swelling, inflammation, or simply feeling overheated. Burns are an obvious example of a hot condition as the burned area feels warm to the touch and turns red. A red, hot, itchy rash is another example. A fresh plantain poultice can soothe burns and rashes by both pulling out the heat and healing the damaged tissue.

PLANT GIFTS

Heals Bites, Stings, and Wounds

Plantain may be most famous for its ability to soothe painful insect bites and stings. It's used to treat bee stings and even to counteract the venom from spider bites. We've seen this work again and again on many types of bites and stings. For best results, apply a plantain leaf poultice as quickly as possible after the sting and change the poultice every 20 minutes or when it feels warm to the touch. A plantain salve will also work well, especially on common itchy insect bites, like those from flies and mosquitoes.

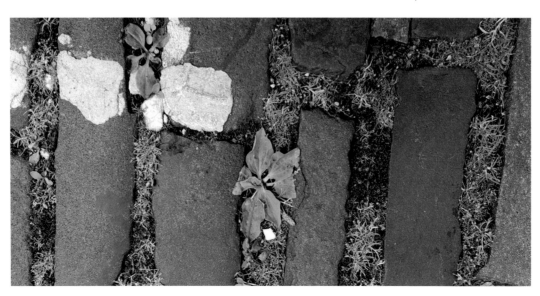

Plantain can promote skin healing after minor wounds such a cuts, scrapes, burns, and blisters. Because it has the ability to draw things out, plantain is perfect for treating splinters or boils. Plantain also is antimicrobial, so it helps to prevent infections in wounds as they heal. We like to combine it with echinacea when an infection is suspected or already present.

Soothes Gastrointestinal Inflammation

Plantain leaf can heal the mucous membranes of the digestive tract. A strong plantain leaf infusion (tea) can be one of the most dramatic healers for inflammatory digestive problems, including intestinal permeability (leaky gut), ulcers, and inflammatory bowel diseases (see Healing Digestive Tea on page 135). In this situation, plantain soothes the inflamed tissues, helps to heal the tissues (vulnerary), prevents bacterial overgrowth (antimicrobial), and can seemingly knit those tissues back together (astringent).

It can also heal the upper digestive tract. For example, it can relieve the pain of canker sores and speed up the healing of the affected tissues. It's also a nice tea for people who have acid reflux, as it can soothe and heal the tissues of the esophagus.

The seeds are mucilaginous and high in fiber. Seeds from *Plantago ovatum* and *P. psyllium* are sold as "psyllium" seed and husk, which are used to maintain bowel regularity. Psyllium is the basis for the Metamucil brand name. The seeds from *Plantago major, P. rugelii,* and *P. lanceolata* can be used similarly, but the process of harvesting enough of those tiny seeds is time-consuming.

Relieves Coughs

You know that type of dry, hacking cough that seems endless and oh so painful? The one you typically get at the end of a cold or flu or from inhaling small particles such as dust or smoke? Plantain soothes hot, dry, and spasmodic coughs. It moistens the lungs and cools the heat, thus relieving the irritation causing the cough. (See page 262 for a Healthy Lungs Tea recipe.)

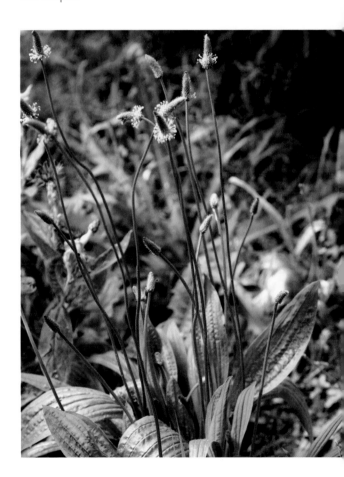

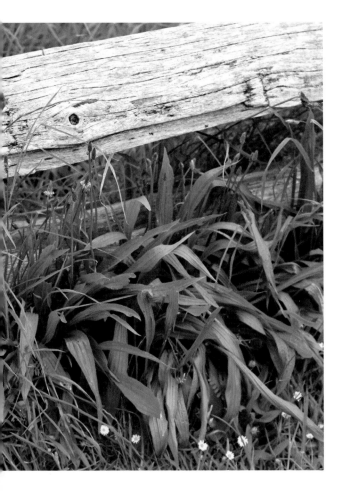

green, or yellow flowers. The flowers mature into tiny, egg-shaped capsules that contain the seeds.

ECOLOGICAL CONNECTIONS

Insects that feed on the leaves, buds, and flowers include grasshoppers, flea beetles, and moth and butterfly caterpillars. Mammals such as squirrels, rabbits, groundhogs, and deer eat the flower spikes. The seeds are eaten by birds and small mammals like mice and squirrels. Animals (including people) help disperse the seeds, which can stick to feet and fur.

Plantain also has potential for phytoremediation. For example, researchers have studied the ability of *Plantago major* to accumulate lead as well as pesticides in contaminated soil and water, with promising results.[1]

HOW TO HARVEST

The leaves may be gathered at any time during the growing season. If you plan to eat them, they are most palatable when young. If using them for medicine, they are likely to be more potent before the plant has flowered and gone to seed. You can use your fingers to pluck the leaves at the base, although the stringy veins can sometimes be hard to break, so scissors are preferable.

Harvest the seeds after they have turned brown or black. Cut off the stalk and shake the seeds into a bag.

Plantain is pollinated by wind and generally doesn't need our help to thrive. As long as you let the plant develop flowers and seeds, it should reproduce easily.

HOW TO IDENTIFY

Plantain thrives in areas with human disturbance, from hiking trails to parking lots. Each species has its own identifying characteristics, and you should consult a field guide for specific information.

Generally speaking, plantain has basal leaves that are simple with conspicuous parallel veins. If you tear a leaf, you'll see that the veins look like white strings, similar to celery. Arising from the leafy base are slender, leafless stalks with a cylindrical spike of inconspicuous white,

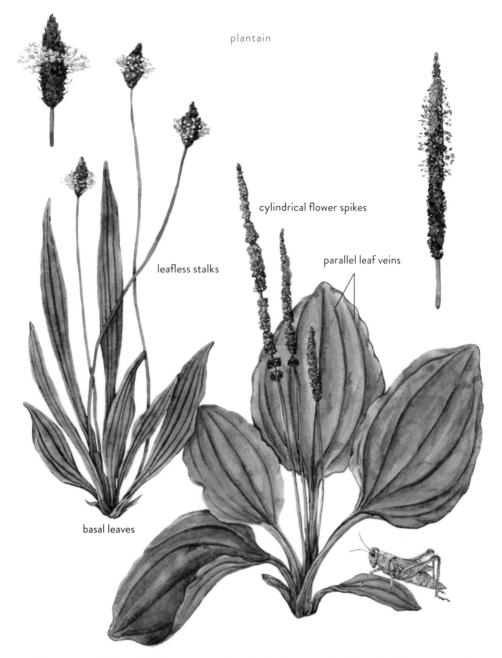

cylindrical flower spikes

leafless stalks

parallel leaf veins

basal leaves

left: narrowleaf plantain (*Plantago lanceolata*) and right: broadleaf plantain (*Plantago major*), shown with two-striped grasshopper (*Melanoplus bivittatus*)

Life cycle: herbaceous perennial, sometimes annual
Reproduces by: seed
Growth habit: basal leaves with flowering stalk up to 1 foot tall
Habitat: disturbed areas, fields, footpaths, lawns, parks, roadsides, stream banks and riverbanks, vacant lots, woodlands
Sun: full sun to partial shade
Soil: varied, dry or moist, often compacted
USDA Hardiness Zones: 3–9

Harvesting Cautions

Because plantain pulls up heavy metals from the soil, pay extra attention to your harvesting areas.

GARDENING TIPS

There are more than 200 species of plantain, and they adapt to all types of soil and conditions. Propagation is by seed, abundantly provided by existing plants. Sow seeds on the surface of soil and tamp down lightly to keep seed in place, then let spring's cool temperatures and moisture activate germination. Plantain is drought tolerant, but regular watering will produce lush growth. Remove flower heads to prevent seed dispersion. Plantain is suitable for containers.

USING PLANTAIN IN YOUR LIFE

Young plantain leaves are nutrient dense and considered edible, but they admittedly aren't always palatable. Depending on the plant, they can be quite bitter. We've chopped them up finely and added them to salads and stir-fries. They can also be blanched first to remove some of the bitterness. Young leaves are best.

As the leaves get older, the strings within them get tougher and more difficult to eat.

The seeds are also edible and don't have a lot of flavor. They can be eaten raw or added to cooked foods, or whole plantain seed stalks can be steamed and eaten if you find it too tedious to collect the seeds.

Fresh plantain is best for addressing wounds, burns, bites, and stings. A poultice can be made by mashing the fresh leaves in a mortar and pestle or simply chewing up a wad of leaves to make a "spit poultice." To make an oil infusion, let the leaves wilt overnight before infusing them. We prefer fresh leaves when making an alcohol extract. Dried plantain works well for teas and sitz baths.

Recommended Amounts

- *Tincture (fresh leaf):* 1:2, 75 to 95% alcohol; 3 to 5 ml, 3 to 5 times daily

- *Tea (dried leaf):* Up to 30 grams daily

Special Considerations

Plantain is regarded as safe, and there are no common allergies or adverse effects associated with its use.

HEALING DIGESTIVE TEA

Strong herbal teas are a powerful way to support digestive system healing. They are easy for your body to break down and absorb and are also a direct topical aid. This tea is carefully formulated to restore gut integrity and help heal damaged tissues. Rosalee has recommended this for people with ulcers or symptoms of intestinal permeability. To learn more about calendula and rose, download the bonus chapters at wildremediesbook.com/adventures.

One caution: this tea is slightly bitter—don't expect it to taste like a lovely afternoon beverage! If it's too bitter for you, try adding a pinch of salt or a bit of honey. A teaspoon of mint could be used in place of the fennel seeds.

Yield: 3 cups

½ cup (8 grams) finely crumbled dried plantain leaves

½ cup (8 grams) dried calendula flowers

¼ cup (3 grams) dried rose petals

1 tablespoon (2 grams) finely crumbled dried mallow or marshmallow leaves

1 teaspoon fennel seeds

3 cups water

1. Place all of the herbs in a quart jar (or quart-size tea press).

2. Bring 3 cups of water to a boil. Pour the water over the herbs, stir well, and cover. Infuse for 30 minutes.

3. Strain well and drink within 24 hours.

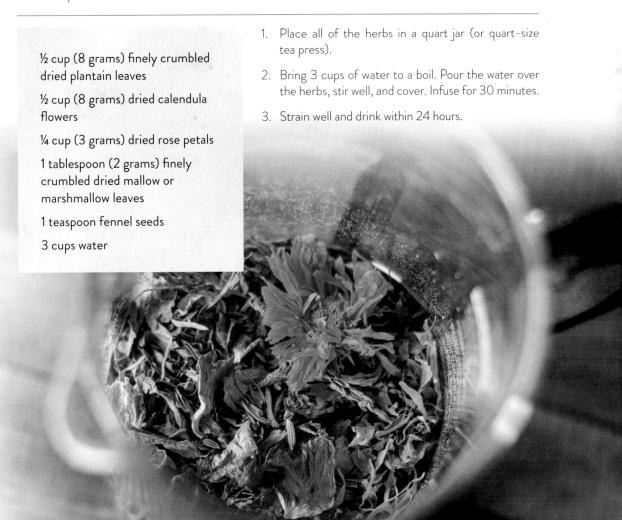

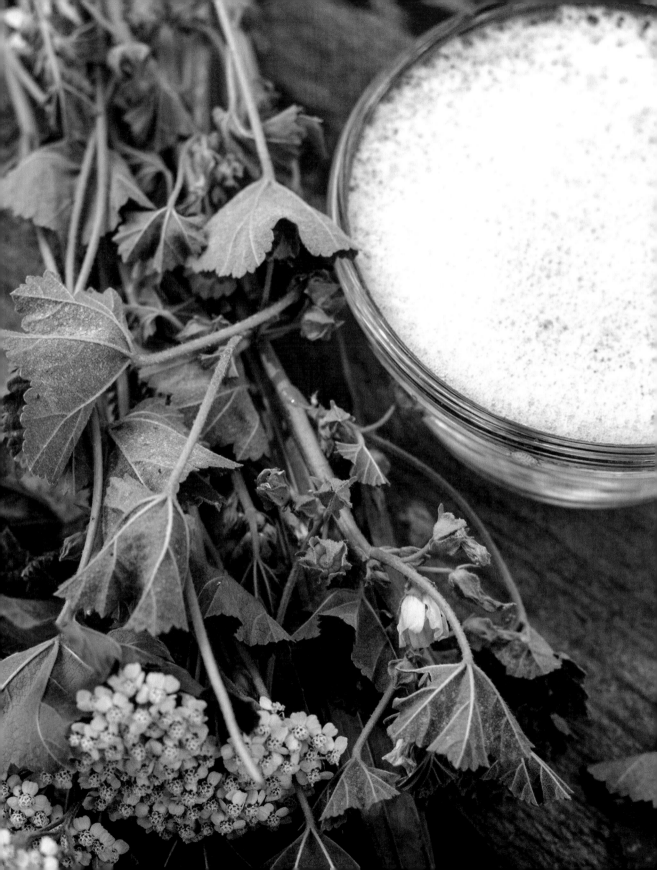

WILD AND WEEDY SHAMPOO AND BODY WASH

Making your own herb-infused shampoo is easy. It's also cheaper than store-bought shampoos and can cut down on plastic waste. Look for bulk castile soap at health food stores. You'll notice this shampoo has a much thinner consistency than commercial shampoos; it will lather up nicely all the same! We like to put it in a squirt bottle and apply it directly to the scalp. It also works well as a body wash.

This recipe is not ideal for color-treated hair. If you have light-colored hair, substitute goldenrod flowers or chamomile flowers for the plantain leaves to prevent accidental discoloration.

Yield: 1¼ cups

1. Place the distilled water in a small saucepan and bring to a boil. Remove from the heat. Add the plantain, mallow, and yarrow. Stir well, then cover. Infuse for 10 minutes.

2. Strain and let the infusion cool to room temperature. Add the castile soap, aloe vera gel, rosemary antioxidant extract, and lavender essential oil, if using. Stir well.

3. Pour into a shampoo container. Shake well before each use. Use within 2 weeks; discard if you see signs of mold growth.

1 cup distilled water

1 tablespoon dried plantain leaves

1 tablespoon dried mallow leaves

1 tablespoon dried yarrow flowers

⅓ cup castile soap

3 tablespoons aloe vera gel

1 tablespoon rosemary antioxidant extract (or other herb-infused oil of your choice)

30 drops (¼ teaspoon) lavender (*Lavandula angustifolia*) essential oil (optional)

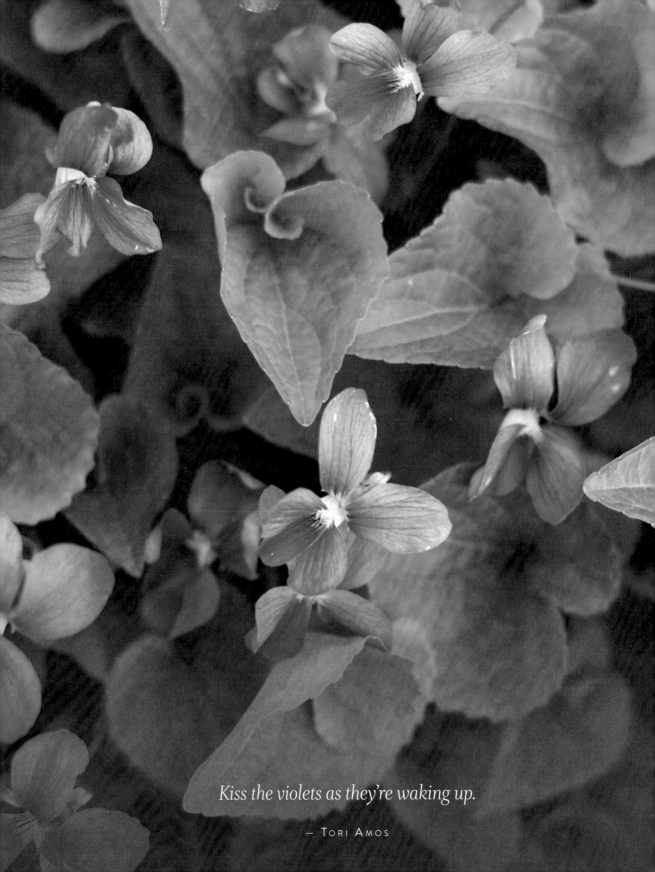

Kiss the violets as they're waking up.

— TORI AMOS

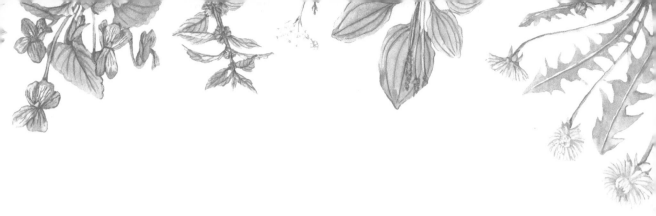

CHAPTER 13

VIOLET

Violets are the harbingers of spring. Their smiling, colorful blooms gladden our hearts and brighten our faces as they pop up in lawns, line stream banks, and fill feral meadows. These small and delicate plants offer us so much: food, medicine, and a balm to our hearts.

Other common name: Johnny-jump-up
Botanical names: *Viola odorata, V. sororia,* and other species
Family: Violaceae (violet)
Parts used: flowers, leaves
Energetics: cooling, moistening
Taste: salty, sweet
Properties: alterative, demulcent, inflammatory modulator, lymphagogue
Uses: breast health, cysts, food, hot inflamed tissues, sore throats, swollen lymph glands
Preparations: cream, food, oil, poultice, salve, syrup, tea, tincture

For at least a thousand years, herbalists have recommended violets for their cooling and moistening qualities, including for dry coughs, hot headaches, hot fevers, and hot skin conditions.[1] Many species of violets grow in temperate climates. The sweet violet, *Viola odorata*, is native to Europe and Asia but has spread to North America and parts of Australia. In ancient Greece, sweet violets were the emblem of Aphrodite and the flower of Athens.[2]

MEDICINAL PROPERTIES AND ENERGETICS

Violet's energetics mirror where it thrives, a beautiful example of how place is reflected in plants' gifts. To best understand its virtues, find a patch of violets and then get down on their level. You can kneel, but lying down and curling up close is best. You'll notice the air is cooler here and feel how the dampness of the earth seeps into you. Hello, violet.

As you touch those soft, delicate flowers and cup those heart-shaped leaves, you'll probably notice something else. Happiness. Relaxation. Contentment. By spending intimate time with violet, you've absorbed everything you need to know to understand how this medicine works. Violet is cooling and moistening. It brings calming and soothing relief, especially to dry and tense tissues.

PLANT GIFTS

Supports the Lymphatic System and Skin

Your lymphatic system is like a great waterway running throughout your body. And, just as rivers and streams can run smoothly or become stagnant and swollen, so it is with your lymphatic vessels. Violet loves to grow near clear running water, and it can be used to keep your

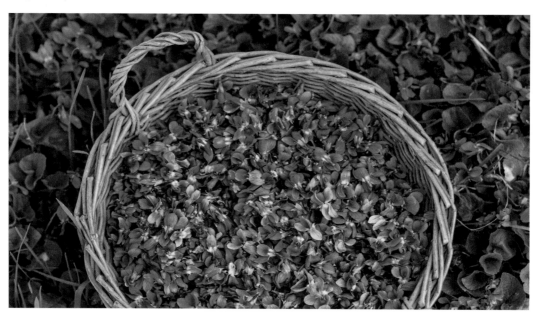

internal rivers running smoothly as well. Violet is revered for being able to break down hardened cysts, especially chronic ones. It is commonly used as a topical aid for fibrocystic breasts or other cysts below the skin's surface.

Violet is one of our best remedies for hot and dry skin. While it undoubtedly works in many ways, its cooling and moistening qualities combine with its ability to modulate inflammation to relieve hot, dry, and inflamed skin.

Several historical texts mention using violet for cancer. To date we do not have any clinical trials to confirm this; however, there have been some interesting in vitro studies.[3] One of these found certain constituents of *Viola odorata* "with robust cytotoxicity that may be promising chemosensitizing agents against drug resistant breast cancer."[4] We look forward to human clinical trials to further illuminate violet's possible benefits against cancer.

Quells Dry Coughs

Nibble on a fresh violet leaf and you'll find out why it is the perfect remedy for dryness. Those sweet, demulcent leaves are soothing and moistening. Irritated spasmodic coughs are often caused by dryness, and a violet tea restores moisture and relieves irritation. One double-blind randomized clinical trial with children aged 2 to 12 years found that violet syrup could help the coughs of children with intermittent asthma.[5]

Relieves Dryness and Inflammation

Violet leaves are a wonderful addition to your life if you tend to have a lot of dryness and inflammation in general. Regularly drinking violet tea can relieve dryness and soothe systemic inflammation. Herbalists commonly use it for dry, inflamed skin rashes as well as dry, painful joints such as arthritis.

Soothes the Nervous System

Violet's ability to soften and soothe hot and inflamed tissues also applies to your moods! Herbalist jim mcdonald recommends violet for people who react to stress by screaming until they are red in the face or for those who are overly rigid. "Violet softens," he explains. "It inspires flexibility."[6] Hildegard von Bingen, the German Benedictine abbess born in 1098, used violets extensively and recommended them in wine for "anyone oppressed by melancholy with a discontented mind, which then harms his lungs."[7]

Improves Insomnia

Using violet for sleep is not common practice in Western herbalism, but there was an interesting study of this traditional Iranian remedy. Researchers gave 50 patients with chronic insomnia two drops of a *Viola odorata* oil in each nostril nightly before sleeping. After a month, patients showed improvements in sleep.[8]

Provides Delicious Food

Violet flowers and leaves are sweet and demulcent and are a tasty addition to salads. In addition to their fresh flavor, violets are high in rutin, an antioxidant known to support heart health by strengthening and increasing flexibility in blood vessels, reducing cholesterol, and preventing and dissolving blood clots. Violet flowers can also add lovely color to a variety of preparations.

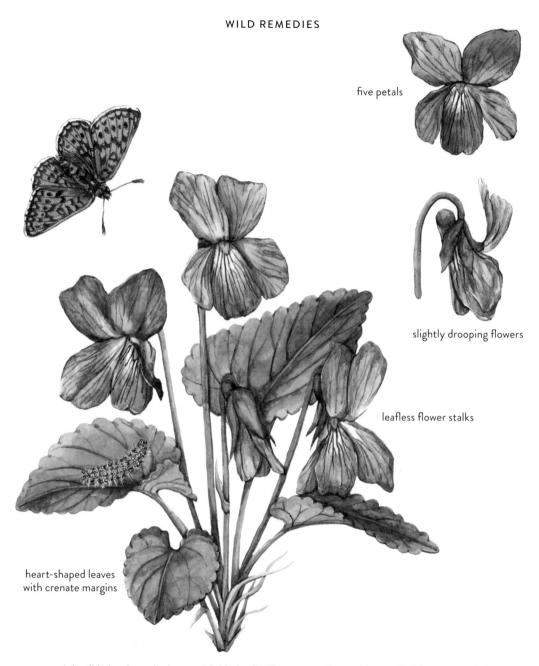

five petals

slightly drooping flowers

leafless flower stalks

heart-shaped leaves
with crenate margins

violet (*Viola odorata*), shown with Niobe fritillary caterpillar and butterfly (*Argynnis niobe*)

Life cycle: herbaceous perennial
Reproduces by: seed, rhizome
Growth habit: low-growing, 1–12 inches tall
Habitat: fields, forests, hedgerows, lawns, meadows, riverbanks, woodlands
Sun: partial shade, sometimes full sun
Soil: moist, rich, well drained
USDA Hardiness Zones: 2–11, depending on species

HOW TO IDENTIFY

Violets typically prefer cool, moist places, and they grow close to the ground with alternate or basal leaves. Leaves may be shaped like a heart or kidney with crenate margins. The slightly irregular flowers grow on upright, leafless stalks; are slightly drooping; and have five petals that are purple, blue, white, or yellow. Except for *Viola odorata*, most violet flowers don't have a strong fragrance. In some species, the showy flower is sterile and the plant produces a tiny, inconspicuous flower near the base, called a cleistogamous flower. This self-pollinated flower is where the seeds are formed.

ECOLOGICAL CONNECTIONS

For violet species that rely on pollinators for fertilization, the bright flowers attract insects like carpenter bees, mining bees, sweat bees, hoverflies, skippers, and small butterflies. Violets can also serve as host plants for butterflies and moths. Similar to the way that monarch butterflies depend on milkweed plants, several species of fritillary butterflies (tribe Argynnini) will lay their eggs only where there are violets for the larvae to eat. The seeds of some violets are coated with a sugary gel that attracts ants. These ants then carry the seeds, aiding in their dispersal.

HOW TO HARVEST

There is a lot of poor-quality dried violet on the market, so harvesting and growing your own can give you the best quality. While the leaves and flowers may be gathered at any time during the growing season, tender young leaves are best and are found early in the season. Older leaves may be too stringy to eat but are fine for infusions. If you plan to dry the flowers, pick them on a dry day without dew or rain. Wild violets should be picked judiciously, if at all. Use scissors or your fingers to pick individual leaves and flowers—just a few from each plant—and take care not to disturb the roots.

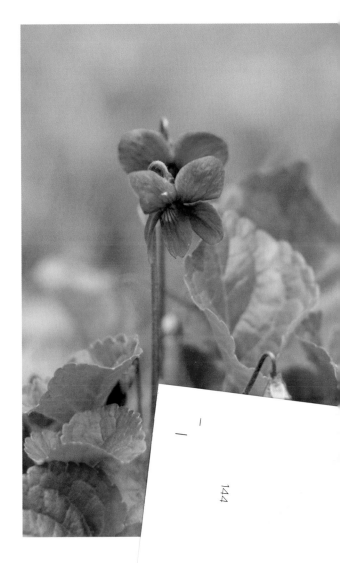

In some locations, violets may be a scarce native wildflower. Harvest only from abundant, well-established patches. Violets spread by rhizomes, and it's important not to uproot an entire plant.

Harvesting Cautions

Violets, especially before flowering, have many look-alikes, including edible plants as well as poisonous ones like monkshood (*Aconitum* spp.) and lesser celandine (*Ficaria verna*). Be certain you can identify the plant before harvesting.

GARDENING TIPS

Violets prefer cool and need extra attention during periods of excessive heat. Seeds benefit from a 90-day stratification before being sown indoors and are sporadic sprouters with a low germination rate. Transplant in spring, and water heavily to maintain production. Violets are reliable self-sowers, sometimes to the point of invasiveness, but can also be divided and replanted. Their small size makes them ideal for containers filled with soil high in organic matter.

USING VIOLET IN YOUR LIFE

Violet flowers can be used in teas, infused vinegars, syrups, and jellies. Fresh or candied flowers make lovely garnishes for salads and desserts. The leaves can be eaten fresh in salads, steamed, or sautéed. Different violet species have varying degrees of saponins in the leaves. This soapy constituent has medicinal benefits but can cause nausea if consumed in large amounts. Taste your leaves first to make sure they are palatable.

Dried violet leaves or flowers can be made into a hot or cold tea. The cold tea may be more mucilaginous. For best results drink the tea regularly. Fresh violets can be made into an alcohol extract or tincture. Topical applications for violet range from a simple fresh poultice to an oil infusion, salve, or cream.

For the sinuses and eyes, herbalist jim mcdonald recommends an eye or nasal wash: "A mild tea of fresh or dried violet leaves can be made into a nasal rinse by adding ¼ teaspoon of salt per 8-ounce cup of well-strained tea, and it is wonderfully soothing when dryness accompanies inflammation of the sinuses. This same preparation can be used as an eyewash and is really quite impressive; use it when the eyes are dry and blinking feels like someone's scratching sandpaper over your cornea."[9]

Recommended Amounts

Violet leaves and flowers can be used therapeutically in large, foodlike amounts.

- *Tea (dried leaves/flowers):* 5 to 28 grams daily

- *Tincture (fresh leaves/flowers):* 1:2, 40% alcohol; 3 to 5 ml, 3 times daily

Special Considerations

Violet is regarded as a safe herb, and there are no known contraindications.

VIOLET VINEGAR

You can use any species of edible *Viola* for this recipe, but those with deep purple blossoms will make the most exquisite jewel-colored vinegar. Drizzle violet vinegar over fruit and salad greens, or drink it in the form of an oxymel or cocktail.

Yield: 2 cups

1 cup fresh violet flowers

Up to 2 cups champagne vinegar or white wine vinegar (at least 5% acidity)

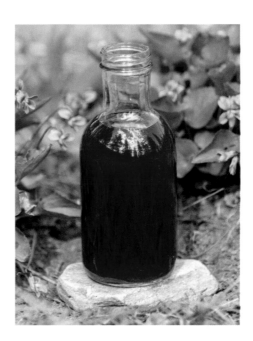

1. Put the violets in a pint jar. Pour in enough vinegar to fill the jar and submerge the flowers completely. (You might not use the entire 2 cups.)

2. Cover the jar, preferably with a glass or plastic lid (vinegar will corrode metal). If using a metal lid, place parchment paper between the lid and the jar. Label the jar.

3. Let the jar sit at room temperature, out of direct sunlight, for 1 to 2 weeks, shaking it daily. The longer you let it infuse, the stronger the flavor will be.

4. Strain the vinegar into a clean jar with a nonreactive lid. Store in the refrigerator for up to 1 year.

VIOLET OXYMEL

When you combine violet vinegar with honey, you get an oxymel that can be sipped by the spoonful to soothe a dry cough, mixed with sparkling water, or used in a cocktail (see recipes on page 146). Use a mild honey, such as light clover or wildflower, so you don't overpower the flavor of the violets. You can make any amount you like; just be sure to use equal parts vinegar and honey.

Yield: 1 cup

½ cup Violet Vinegar (recipe above)

½ cup honey

1. Combine vinegar and honey in a bowl and whisk to combine.

2. Pour the oxymel into a clean jar and cover with a nonreactive lid. Store in the refrigerator for up to 1 year.

SIMPLE VIOLET COCKTAIL

Here's a simple cocktail featuring violet oxymel, followed by one that's a bit more fancy. Use London dry or Old Tom gin, or a new-school international gin if you think it would pair well with the violet.

Yield: 1 cocktail

2 ounces gin

1 ounce Violet Oxymel (see page 145)

¼ ounce fresh lime juice

Chilled club soda, to taste

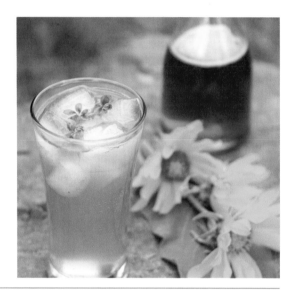

1. Fill a glass with ice. Add the gin, violet oxymel, and lime juice and stir to combine. Top off with club soda.

VIOLET GIN FIZZ

Yield: 1 cocktail

¼ ounce fresh lime juice

1 ounce Violet Oxymel (see page 145)

2 ounces gin

1 medium egg white or ¾ ounce aquafaba (drained chickpea liquid)

Chilled club soda, to taste

Violet flowers for garnish (optional)

1. Combine the lime juice, violet oxymel, gin, and egg white in a cocktail shaker. Shake vigorously until frothy, about 1 minute.

2. Fill the shaker with cracked ice and shake again until chilled. Double-strain into a glass. Top off with club soda. Garnish with violet flowers, if desired.

SPRING FLOWERS MASSAGE OIL

Violet and dandelion flowers combine to provide a gentle and nourishing oil. This can be rubbed into bellies, breasts, armpits, or wherever there are lymphatic glands. Use this as a daily ritual of preventive care to maintain healthy lymphatic flow.

Yield: About 2 cups

1 cup fresh violet flowers

1 cup fresh dandelion flowers

2 cups carrier oil (e.g., olive oil, apricot kernel oil, sweet almond oil)

30 to 50 drops (¼ to ½ teaspoon) lavender (*Lavandula angustifolia*) essential oil (optional)

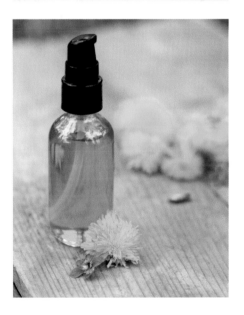

1. Place the flowers and oil in the top part of a double boiler, or place a bowl on top of a saucepan that has 2 inches of water in it (the water should not touch the bottom of the bowl).

2. Bring the water to a boil and then reduce to a simmer. Stir the oil occasionally and continue to heat until the oil is quite warm to the touch. Turn off the heat and allow the mixture to sit for several hours.

3. Repeat this process (reheating and allowing to cool) several times within a 48- to 72-hour period to fully extract the plant material into the oil. Throughout this process, do not let the oil get so hot that it smokes or begins to "fry" the plant material—you only need to get the oil warm to extract the goodness in the plant material.

4. When ready, strain off the flowers through a double layer of cheesecloth. If using, add the essential oil and stir well.

5. Label and store in a cool, dark place. Use within 1 year.

Slow cooker method: Instead of using a double boiler for steps 2 and 3, you can use a slow cooker, yogurt incubator, or other low-temperature appliance that can maintain the oil temperature at 100°F.

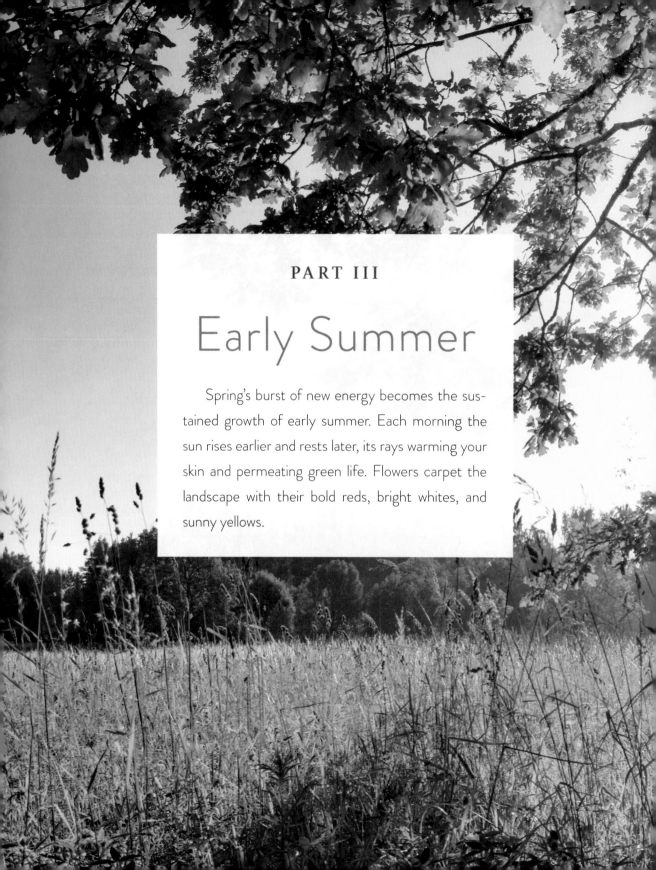

PART III

Early Summer

Spring's burst of new energy becomes the sustained growth of early summer. Each morning the sun rises earlier and rests later, its rays warming your skin and permeating green life. Flowers carpet the landscape with their bold reds, bright whites, and sunny yellows.

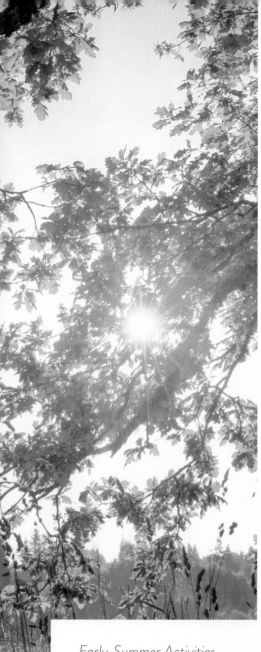

With long days comes renewed energy. Hands grow busy with tending plants, cultivating growth, and harvesting. Kitchen counters meet a procession of herbs, flowers, and berries as they are made into foods and remedies. Jars of dried plants and herbal potions fill your shelves. Animals are busy now, too, from caterpillars munching on green leaves to hummingbirds sipping nectar to mammals raising their young.

Even as summer is filled with energy, it is also a time to relax and relish life's joys. Rest sustains movement, and we can balance outer energy expenditure with inner nourishment. Caress the ground with your bare feet, doze in a hammock, quench your thirst with a cool glass of iced mint tea. Have a picnic or potluck and enjoy laughter with family and friends.

Summer can feel endless as you bask in the warmth, growth, and contentment of days spent outside. Your body may feel weary from the succession of long, busy days. But in many places, late-summer and autumn harvests lie just ahead. Before the next big push of the growing season, sink into the grass and feel the sun on your face.

Early-Summer Activities

- Check out a new hiking trail
- Make a nature arrangement
- Draw a flower
- Soak up the sunshine while daydreaming
- Go swimming

- Make a plant press
- Pick a plant bouquet
- Celebrate the summer solstice
- Have a picnic or barbecue
- Keep a journal (see Chapter 7)

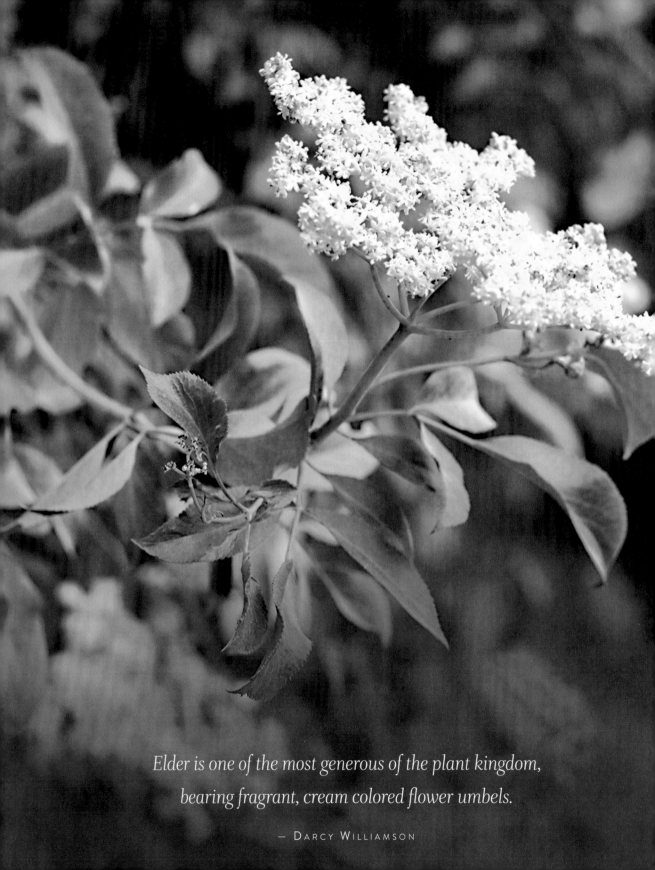

Elder is one of the most generous of the plant kingdom,

bearing fragrant, cream colored flower umbels.

— Darcy Williamson

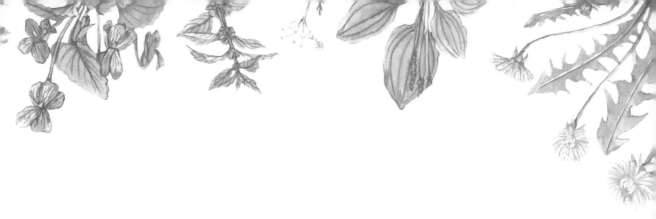

CHAPTER 14

ELDERFLOWER

Elderflowers erupt as a wave of white blooms, and shrubs that previously
were camouflaged in their anonymous green now jump out of the landscape. Those
sweet-smelling blossoms are a sure sign that warm weather has arrived. Attracted by its
evocative scent, pollinators spend their days sipping the nectar within. Meanwhile, two-
legged creatures dreaming of afternoon cordials and a well-stocked medicine
chest grab their baskets and pruners to head for the elder patches.

Botanical names: *Sambucus nigra, S. nigra* ssp. *canadensis, S. nigra* ssp. *caerulea, S. ebulus*
Family: Adoxaceae (moschatel)
Parts used: flowers, berries (see Chapter 22)
Energetics: cooling, drying
Taste: bitter, sweet
Properties: antioxidant rich, antiviral, diuretic, relaxing diaphoretic, relaxing nervine
Uses: colds and flu, ear infections, fevers, food, skin health
Preparations: cordial, cream, food, liqueur, oil, salve, syrup, tea, tincture

The elder shrub is native to many temperate and subtropical areas in both the Northern and Southern Hemispheres. People have long used it in food and medicine and for making musical instruments and tools, and many Indigenous peoples of North America continue to do so. Describing the importance of elder in her people's tradition, Chumash healer Cecilia Garza calls it "the music tree, our heartbeat. It helps restore the normal flow."[1] Elder also has an important role in European folklore, which often associates the plant with death, rebirth, and healing.

MEDICINAL PROPERTIES AND ENERGETICS

You know that experience of walking out of a stuffy room and into the cool, fresh air outside? Suddenly everything is brighter and your breaths become gratefully deeper. This is what elderflower does for you. It clears out stagnations, cools, brightens, and freshens.

PLANT GIFTS

Supports the Fever Process

Elderflower is one of our best herbal medicines to support the fever process. While fevers are commonly feared, they are actually among the body's most powerful immune system responses. As your body temperature rises, invading pathogens become increasingly uncomfortable. Stopping a healthy fever is like putting your guard dogs on a leash.

However, that's not to say that having a fever is a pleasant experience. First, you may get chills as your body shivers to generate muscle metabolism to heat you up. Then you can get uncomfortably hot, feel restless or lethargic, and have aches and pains. Elderflowers can be used for any stage of a cold or flu, but they especially shine when you feel hot and restless. Drinking a warm cup of elderflower tea opens your capillaries, stimulates sweating, and allows some heat to escape. Herbalist jim mcdonald equates this to opening the window in a hot room. Ahh, relief! Herbs that are used when someone with a fever feels hot and restless are called relaxing diaphoretics.

Herbalist Maude Grieve wrote in the 1930s that elderflowers are an "almost infallible cure for an attack of influenza in its first stage."[2] Today the traditional Western herbal formula of elderflowers, peppermint, and yarrow is still commonly used both to support fevers and to shorten the duration of a cold or flu (see Yarrow and Elderflower Tea recipe on page 214).

Nourishes the Skin

Herbalists often use relaxing diaphoretic herbs to support skin health. That same action of stimulating the capillaries to induce sweating during a fever can be called on to gently nourish and detox your skin. Historically, people often used elderflowers as external preparations—as a tea wash or infused in oil for a cream or salve. Elderflower washes or lotions can soothe red and inflamed skin conditions, such as rashes and sunburn. Elderflower water used to be a very common beauty regimen. Recent in vitro research has shown that topical elderflower preparations have the potential to deliver broad-spectrum UV protection.[3]

Modulates Inflammation

Elderflowers can be enjoyed as a tea, syrup, and food. They are high in antioxidants and have the ability to modulate excess and chronic inflammation. In vitro studies have shown elderflower tea used as a mouthwash to be an effective anti-inflammatory against periodontal pathogens like gingivitis.[4]

Elderflowers are also used against ear infections. They may be effective by soothing inflammation, addressing the infection, or stimulating the immune system.

HOW TO IDENTIFY

Each *Sambucus* species or subspecies has its own identifying characteristics, and you should consult a local guide for specific information. (It's also not uncommon for them to hybridize.) Generally speaking, elders are shrubs or small trees. Some have a single trunk, while others have multiple stems and can develop an arching or scraggly appearance. They have gray-brown bark, brittle wood, and pithy branches. The leaves are pinnately compound with an odd number (usually three to nine) of oppositely arranged leaflets. Each leaflet is lanceolate or ovate with serrated margins.

Flat-topped or slightly rounded inflorescences (cymose corymbs) measure from 3 to 10 inches across and have numerous white or cream-colored flowers. These are fragrant, their smell a combination of sweet and musty. Each tiny flower is about 1 centimeter wide and has five petals and five stamens arranged in a star shape. For a description of the berries, see page 247.

Many herbalists use the flowers of red elder (*Sambucus racemosa*) in a way that's similar to how they use *S. nigra*. Red elder can be distinguished from other species by its cone-shaped (instead of flat) flower clusters and its red berries.

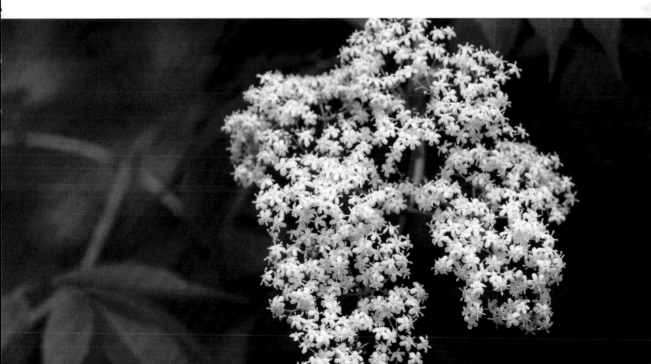

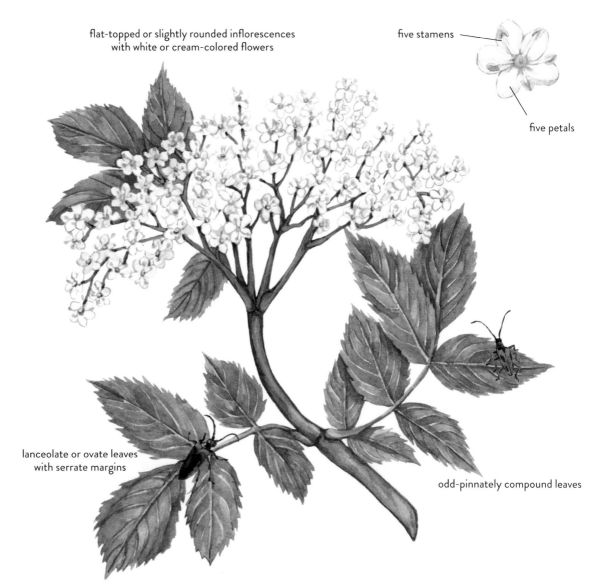

flat-topped or slightly rounded inflorescences
with white or cream-colored flowers

five stamens

five petals

lanceolate or ovate leaves
with serrate margins

odd-pinnately compound leaves

elder (*Sambucus nigra*), shown with valley elderberry longhorn beetles
(*Desmocerus californicus* ssp. *dimorphus*)

Life cycle: deciduous woody perennial
Reproduces by: seed, root
Growth habit: shrub or small tree, 5–30 feet tall
Habitat: ditches, fencerows, fields, forest edges, hedgerows, hillsides, low-lying areas, meadows, riparian areas, roadsides, stream banks, thickets, wetland margins
Sun: full sun to partial shade
Soil: moist and well drained; can tolerate some drought or wet sites
USDA Hardiness Zones: 3–9

ECOLOGICAL CONNECTIONS

Elders provide erosion control, nesting places for birds, and cover for small mammals, birds, and reptiles. The flowers attract a variety of bees, hoverflies, butterflies, and beetles. Carpenter bees and mason bees tunnel into broken stems to lay their eggs. Animals such as deer and elk browse the foliage, while birds, squirrels, mice, and other animals eat the berries.

Elderberry longhorn beetles (*Desmocerus* spp.) have an especially close relationship with this plant. These colorful beetles lay their eggs on the bark. When the larvae hatch, they burrow into and eat the stems, living within and eating the wood in their larval stage for one or two years. As adults, they feed on the leaves and flowers, helping with pollination in the process. Sadly, these beetles have declined in numbers, likely due to habitat destruction. One subspecies endemic to California, the valley elderberry longhorn beetle (*Desmocerus californicus dimorphus*), is listed as federally threatened.

HOW TO HARVEST

Collect the flowers when they are open, using your fingers or pruning shears to cut the entire cluster at the base. We find that flowers harvested in midmorning smell less musty than those harvested later in the day. You'll notice there are lots of little creatures enjoying the flowers. We recommend gently shaking the flower heads at your gathering spot to remove as many insects as possible. Once home, let the flowers sit for a couple of hours to allow any other insects to escape. You can also gently drop a cluster of flowers into a box or basket to jostle them out.

Any flowers you pick will not turn into berries, so keep in mind your future harvest, wildlife's needs, and the plant's reproduction. Elders reproduce by seed and spread by root suckers. They can also be propagated by cuttings.

Before using the flowers in food or medicine, completely separate them from the stems and leaves, which contain cyanogenic glycosides and can make you sick. They will be easier to remove when slightly or completely dry.

Harvesting Cautions

People have been known to confuse the flowers of the deadly poison hemlock (*Conium maculatum*), water hemlock (*Cicuta* spp.), and devil's walking stick (*Aralia spinosa*) for elderflowers. However, it is not difficult to differentiate them with careful observation of the flowers along with other characteristics.

GARDENING TIPS

Elder is easy to grow but requires space. There are several regional subspecies as well as ornamental varieties that have been cultivated for smaller size and beautifully colored foliage. They can be grown in a large container but require severe pruning each year. Purchase starter plants and plant in rich soil, watering regularly. They benefit from composted manure as fertilizer. Propagation by seed can be challenging, but propagation by softwood cuttings is easy and inexpensive. Do not harvest or prune a new elder for the first two years.

USING ELDERFLOWER IN YOUR LIFE

Fresh elderflowers can be made into a variety of foods and beverages, including elderflower fritters, jellies, infused vinegars, cordials, syrups, and liqueurs. Syrups and liqueurs can then be used in beverages and desserts from cake to sorbet. Dried elderflowers can often be used in recipes as well.

To support fevers, elderflowers are most commonly used as a warm tea made from the dried blossoms. If using a tincture, mix drops into hot water before drinking. A cool tea will have more of a diuretic effect. The flowers can also be infused into oil and made into creams or salves.

Recommended Amounts

- *Tea (dried):* 15 to 30 grams daily

- *Tincture (fresh):* 1:2, 40% alcohol; 30 to 90 drops (¼ to 1 teaspoon) per hour during acute phase

Special Considerations

The bark, stems, and leaves of elder contain toxic substances that can cause nausea and vomiting if ingested. (No precautions are necessary, however, for simply touching the elder plant.)

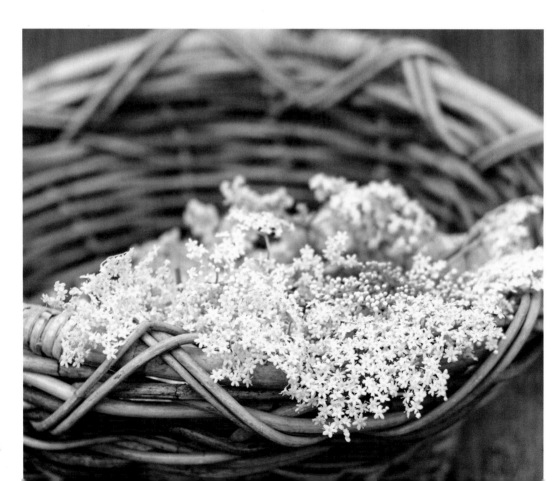

ELDERFLOWER AND ROSE PETAL TONER

Infusing elderflowers and rose petals in witch hazel magnifies their skin-toning gifts, making this a wonderful facial treatment. It also makes a soothing spray for sunburns. For both applications, it's handy to store this in a small spray bottle.

To learn more about rose, download the bonus chapter at wildremediesbook.com/adventures.

Yield: 2 cups

½ cup dried elderflowers

1 cup dried rose petals

Up to 2 cups witch hazel distillate

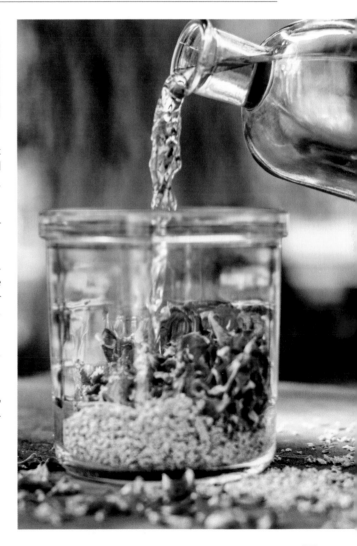

1. Place the elderflowers and rose petals in a pint jar. Pour in enough witch hazel distillate to fill the jar and submerge the flowers completely. (You might not use the entire 2 cups.)

2. Stir to release any air bubbles. Tightly cover the jar and label it.

3. Store the jar in a cool, dark place for 4 weeks. Shake the jar daily for the first week, and make sure the plant material stays submerged under the witch hazel for the remainder of the macerating time.

4. Strain the mixture through cheesecloth, squeezing it well to extract all the liquid.

5. Use a funnel to pour the toner into small, clean spray bottles. Store in a cool, dark place. Use within 1 year.

ELDERFLOWER CORDIAL

Elderflower cordial is a classic, and rightly so. A splash of this floral nectar brings the essence of sunny days to a glass of sparkling water, tonic, or wine. The cordial is also lovely drizzled over berries, cakes, and ices. We often double or triple this batch to make sure we have enough to last the year. Traditional recipes call for sugar, but this one uses honey. Use a mild honey so it doesn't overpower the delicate elder flavor.

Yield: About 2½ cups

---

1 cup packed elderflower heads (about 10 large)

Grated zest of 1 lemon (about 1 tablespoon)

Juice of 1 lemon (about 2 tablespoons)

1 cup mild-flavored honey

1½ cups water

1. Shake any insects out of the elderflower heads and separate the flowers from the stems (see How to Harvest on page 155). Place the flowers in a medium bowl along with the lemon zest and lemon juice.

2. Combine the honey and water in a small saucepan. Warm it over low-medium heat just to dissolve the honey; do not let it boil. Remove from heat and let it cool to room temperature.

3. Pour the syrup over the elderflower mixture. Cover the bowl with a clean dish towel and let it stand in a cool, dark place for 2 days.

4. Strain the cordial into a clean jar or bottle. Store in the refrigerator for 1 week or in the freezer for up to 1 year. If freezing, leave 1 inch of space at the top of the container to allow for expansion.

Variation: Sugar can be substituted for the honey. In the second step, use 2 cups of sugar and 2 cups of water. Bring to a boil, stirring to dissolve the sugar. Remove from heat, let cool to room temperature, and then proceed with step 3.

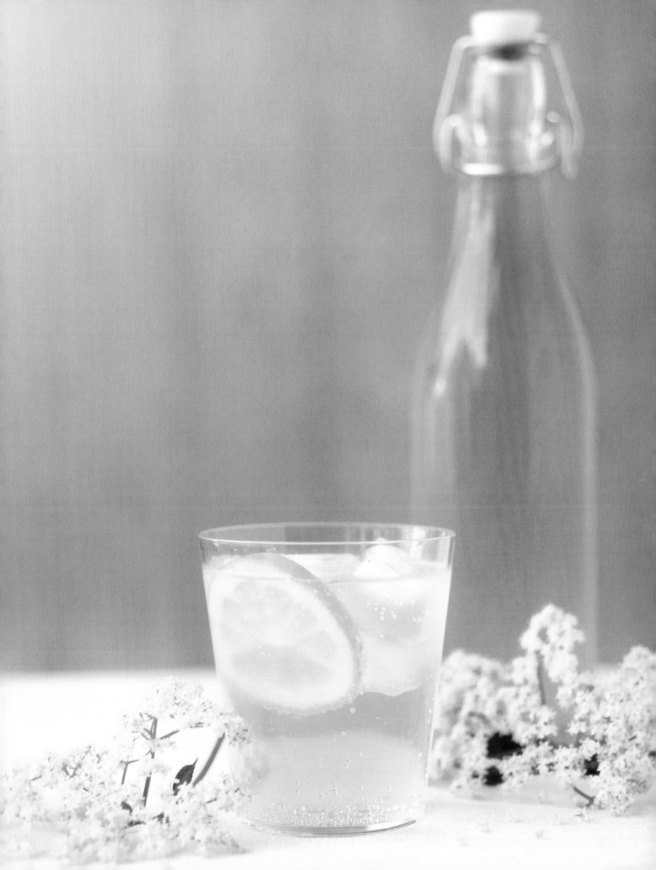

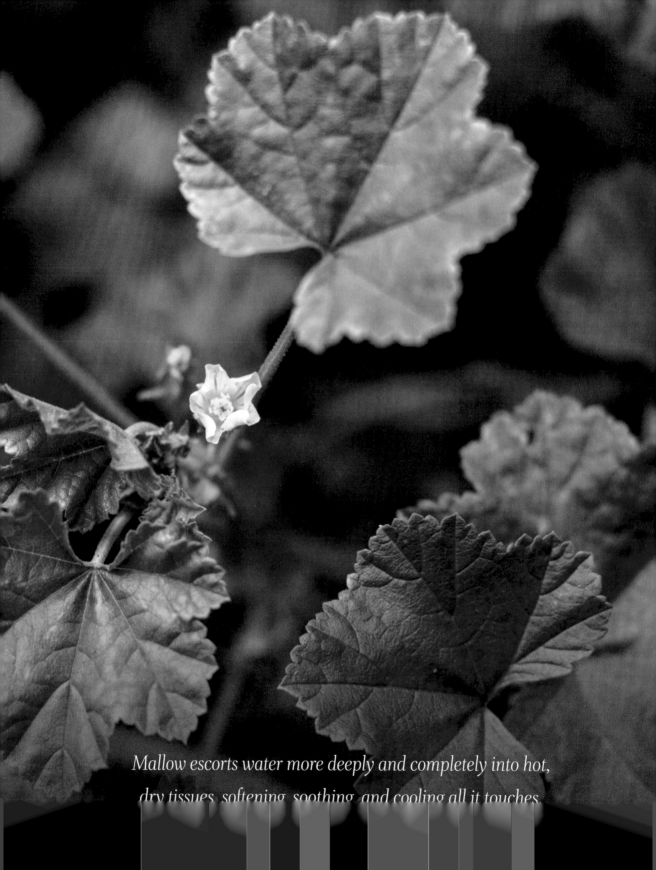

Mallow escorts water more deeply and completely into hot, dry tissues, softening, soothing, and cooling all it touches.

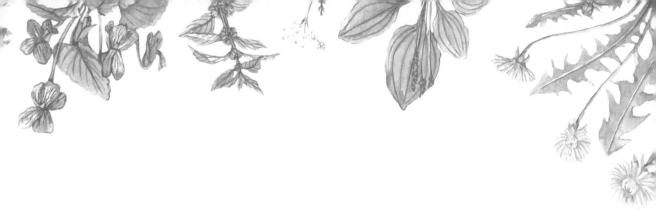

CHAPTER 15

MALLOW

Highly revered in times past, mallow is now frequently disdained as an invasive weed—an uninvited guest in gardens and disturbed soils. It's rare to encounter a whoop of gratitude when someone has an abundant amount of mallow; more commonly, people seek out ways to eradicate it. If you do not already love mallow, once you begin to rely on its many special gifts, you'll forever consider it a generous friend that offers its medicine freely.

Other common name: cheeseweed

Botanical names: *Malva neglecta, M. nicaeensis, M. parviflora, M. pusilla, M. sylvestris,* and other species

Family: Malvaceae (mallow)

Parts used: roots, leaves, flowers, fruits (seed pods), seeds

Energetics: cooling, moistening

Taste: sweet, salty

Properties: demulcent, emollient, expectorant, immunomodulator, nutritive, vulnerary

Uses: burns, digestive inflammation, dry and itchy skin, dry spasmodic coughs, food, sore and dry mouth and throat, urinary inflammation, wounds

Preparations: cold infusion (used internally and externally), decoction, food, low-alcohol tincture, powder, tea

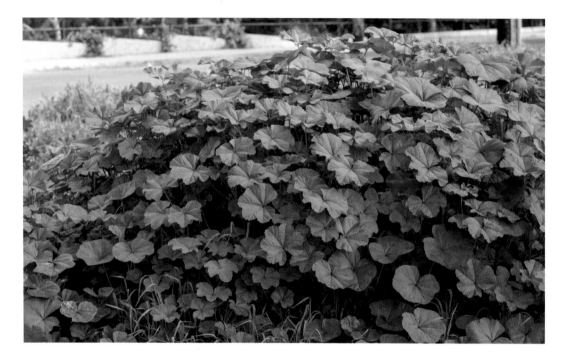

Many species of mallow have been used as both food and medicine for thousands of years. Experts believe that *Malva neglecta* originated in North Africa and Eurasia; *M. sylvestris* is common in Europe. *Althaea officinalis*, a close cousin to mallow commonly known as marshmallow, can be easily grown in the garden.

MEDICINAL PROPERTIES AND ENERGETICS

The core gifts of mallow lie in its slippery, slimy, and gooey qualities. We call these plants mucilaginous or demulcent. The gel-like nature of mallow is soothing and cooling, offering relief to hot and dry tissues. Mallow reminds us that plants work in mysterious ways. When we consume mucilage, it not only affects the tissues it comes into contact with but also promotes moisture systemically, reaching organs like the lungs and kidneys.

PLANT GIFTS

Soothes Irritated, Hot, and Dry Lungs

Your lungs work tirelessly to oxygenate your blood while exhaling carbon dioxide, making them a bridge between the external and internal. Ancient Chinese medical texts refer to the lungs as the delicate organ because they are very sensitive to imbalance and yet constantly under pressure to react to the quality of the inhaled air. Hot, dry, dusty, or smoky air can be an instant irritant. Humid air can feel heavy in the lungs. Inhaled pollutants and small particles are an increasingly common hazard in this modern age. Respiratory infections often invade the lungs, creating a myriad of symptoms such as congestion and coughing. What's a lung to do?

Mallow's mucilage wonderfully soothes hot, dry, and irritated lungs. It brings moisture and relief, easing pain and tightness in the chest while quelling spasmodic coughing. Mallow can be easily added to teas or eaten as a nutritious food. You can rely on mallow when there is wildfire smoke in the air, during the dryness of winter, or in the parched, hot months of summer.

Alleviates Cold and Flu Symptoms

Mallow's demulcent and potentially immune modulating qualities can address a variety of cold and flu symptoms. The thick, viscous fluid of the tea can ease a hot, swollen sore throat. The polysaccharides in mallow species have shown immunomodulating activity, helping the body to ward off an infection.[1] As mentioned above, mallow is also wonderful for easing a dry, spasmodic cough, although it is often combined with antispasmodics for best effects.

Relieves Urinary Symptoms

Mallow and its closely related cousin marshmallow (Althaea officinalis) are regularly used in herbal formulas for urinary tract infections and kidney stones. For the burning pain associated with these conditions, the systemically moisturizing effect of mallow brings soothing relief. For urinary infections, mallow is often combined with other herbs like goldenrod and yarrow.

Heals Wounds and Inflammation

Mallow can be used both internally and externally to heal wounds and soothe irritations like minor burns. Herbalists often recommend it for digestive inflammation such as ulcers or intestinal permeability (leaky gut). (See the Healing Digestive Tea on page 135.) It is also used to address constipation with dry stools. Topically it can be used to heal wounds and prevent infection. Preliminary tests have shown that mallow may be able to inhibit bacterial growth.[2] Another interesting in vitro test showed that mallow was able to address inflammation associated with osteoarthritis.[3]

Provides Food

Archaeologists have found evidence in dental calculi that suggests mallow was used as food (or medicine) at least 8,600 years ago in the Balkans.[4] In historical texts, Pliny (23–79 C.E.), Cicero (106–43 B.C.E.), and Diphilus of Siphne (3rd century B.C.E.) all mention eating mallow.[5] It remains a favorite wild edible among foraging enthusiasts today.

HOW TO IDENTIFY

Mallow tends to thrive in dry, disturbed soils. Some species spread close to the ground, while others grow up to six feet tall. The stems are somewhat hairy and have long-stalked, alternately arranged leaves. The leaves are rounded or kidney-shaped and shallowly lobed with dentate or crenate margins. They feel slightly hairy or velvety. Near the middle of the

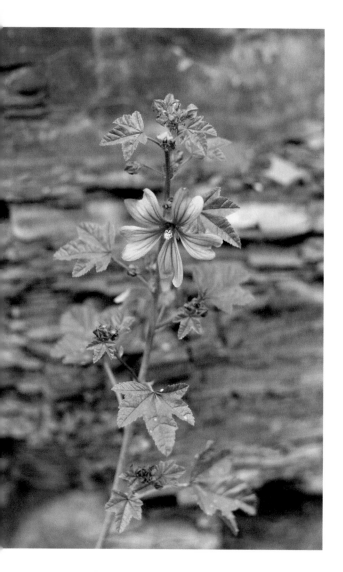

ECOLOGICAL CONNECTIONS

Mallow may be self-pollinating or pollinated by insects like bees and flies. Certain species are host plants for insects, including the painted lady butterfly (*Vanessa cardui*) and common checkered skipper (*Pyrgus communis*). When harvesting, keep an eye out for caterpillars feeding on the leaves.

HOW TO HARVEST

To gather the leaves, use your fingers, scissors, or pruning shears to snip the leaves close to where they attach to the stalk. Harvest the fruits when they are tender and green and the seeds when they are mature and dry; the latter can be gently plucked by hand. Harvest the taproot before the plant flowers; as it matures, the root becomes woody and harder to pull. To harvest roots, use a small shovel or digging tool.

Mallow reproduces by seed and often grows as an annual, so leave enough flowering plants and seeds to ensure future generations. Also consider sowing seeds in places with disturbed soil.

Harvesting Cautions

Because mallow absorbs minerals from the soil, pay extra attention to your harvesting areas.

leaf is a cleft where the stem is attached; there may be a little purple or red spot at this junction.

The flowers grow in clusters at the base of leaf stalks. They each have five petals and range in color from white to pink to purple, often with darker stripes. Mallow fruits or seed pods are round and flat, resembling a button. When dry, they look like a wheel of cheese with tiny wedged sections. The root is a long, woody taproot.

GARDENING TIPS

Stratify seeds for two to three weeks and plant in a loamy and moist soil. Mallow's germination rate is high, and it grows quickly once sprouted. Mallow can easily be grown in a container.

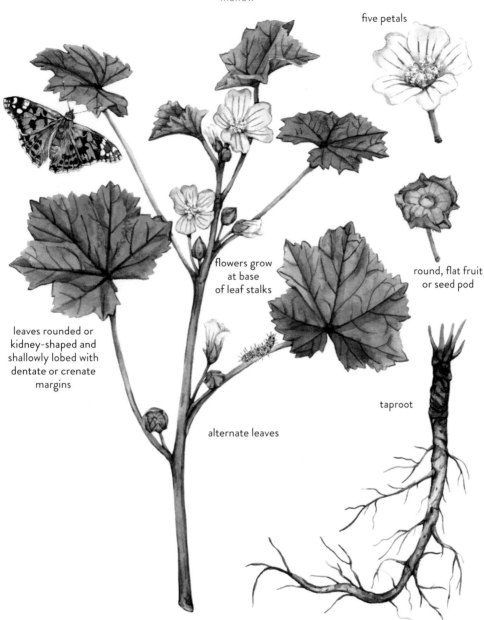

five petals

flowers grow
at base
of leaf stalks

round, flat fruit
or seed pod

leaves rounded or
kidney-shaped and
shallowly lobed with
dentate or crenate
margins

taproot

alternate leaves

mallow (*Malva* spp.), shown with painted lady caterpillar and butterfly (*Vanessa cardui*)

Life cycle: herbaceous annual, biennial, or short-lived perennial
Reproduces by: seed
Growth habit: low-growing and spreading to upright, with branching stems 1–6 feet tall
Habitat: agricultural fields, disturbed areas, gardens, lawns, parking lots, roadsides, sidewalk cracks, vacant lots
Sun: full sun to partial shade
Soil: variable; prefers dry, or moist and well drained
USDA Hardiness Zones: 5–8

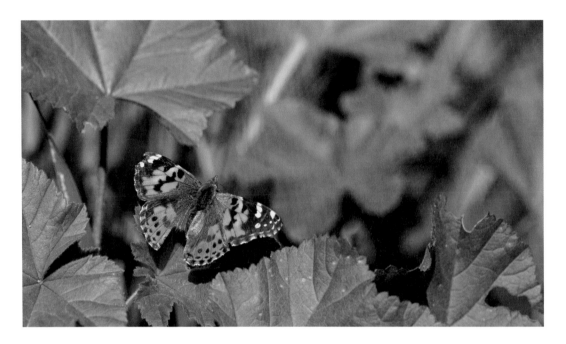

USING MALLOW IN YOUR LIFE

Mallow leaves and immature fruits can be eaten raw or cooked in a variety of ways. The mucilage of the leaves can be used to thicken soups and smoothies. The leaves can also be cooked like spinach or other greens, although they do have a slimier texture. Raw leaves, flowers, and fruits can be eaten in salads. Large leaves can be used as wraps and stuffed like grape leaves. Mallow leaves wilt very quickly; if using fresh ones, harvest them just before consuming.

The raw fruits, although somewhat tedious to harvest, can be pickled and eaten like capers. The fruits are especially nutritious, being a reported 21 percent protein and 15 percent fat.[6] The dried seeds can be ground and used as a thickening agent or binder similar to flax or chia seeds. The roots are also edible, but not as palatable as the leaves and fruits.

The entire plant, including the leaves, roots, flowers, and fruits, can be used either fresh or dried. Making a cool tea is often considered the best way to extract the mucilage from the plant. Mallow can be used as a simple herb or combined with other herbs to add moisture-enhancing qualities to a formula.

Recommended Amounts

- *Root:* 5 grams or as needed

- *Leaves:* 2 grams or as needed

Special Considerations

Mallow is considered a safe herb that can be consumed in large amounts as food or medicine.

MALLOW COLD INFUSION

There's no better way to extract mallow's soothing qualities than by making a cold infusion. If you use the roots, you will get a viscous drink that can relieve hot, inflamed conditions like dry sore throats, canker sores, urinary tract infections, and respiratory systems affected by dry winds or the airborne soot of wildfires. If you use the leaves, the result will be less goopy than a root-based tea—more like a simple, refreshing herbal water. (We often add mint and lemon.)

Yield: 2 cups

½ cup finely chopped dried mallow root (about 1 ounce), or ⅔ cup packed fresh mallow leaves, torn or chopped

Up to 2 cups cool water

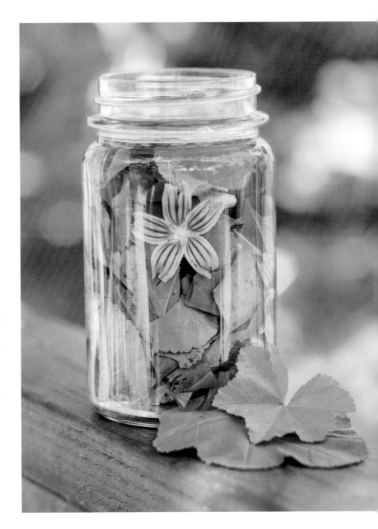

1. Place the mallow in a pint jar. Pour in enough water to fill the jar and submerge the herbs completely. (You might not use the entire 2 cups.)

2. Stir to moisten the herbs. Cover the jar and let it sit for a few hours or overnight in the refrigerator. The longer it infuses, the more viscous it will be.

3. Strain through a fine-mesh strainer. If you used roots, press down on them with the back of a spoon to extract as much of the gooey mucilage as possible.

4. Drink within 24 hours, sipping throughout the day as needed.

MALLOW AND QUINOA PATTIES

Though abundant and nutritious, mallow can be tricky to cook. When heated, the leaves turn slimy, so we typically eat them raw. However, in this vibrant recipe, mallow provides a fresh, green element to quinoa patties without any textural difficulties. Serve these as an appetizer, a component of a grain bowl or salad, or an on-the-go snack.

Yield: 14 patties

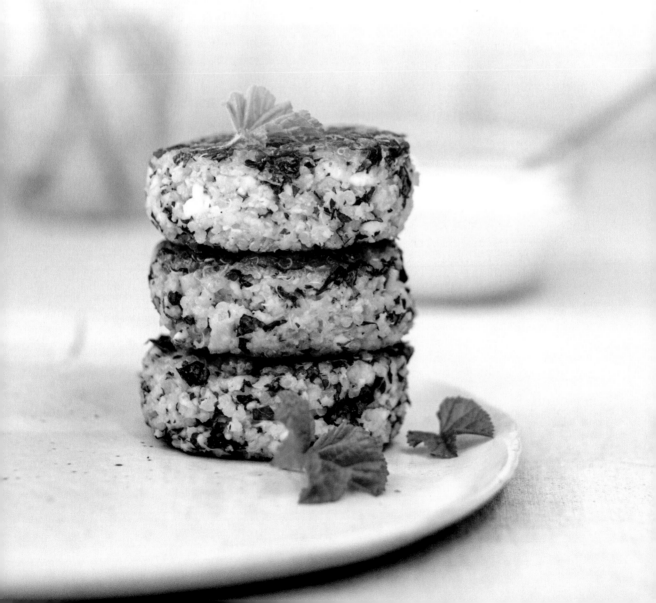

1. Cook the quinoa: Put the raw quinoa in a fine-mesh strainer and rinse with cool water. Drain. Combine the quinoa and 2 cups of water in a medium sauce-pan. Bring to a boil, then cover and turn down the heat to low. Simmer until the quinoa is tender and liquid is absorbed, about 15 minutes. Turn off the heat and let stand for 10 minutes. Transfer the quinoa to a large bowl, fluff it with a fork, and let it cool.

2. Lightly beat the eggs in a large bowl. Stir in the cooked quinoa, feta cheese, mallow leaves, onion, parsley, lemon zest, lemon juice, panko, salt, and pepper. Let the mixture stand for 5 minutes. Pick up a handful of the mixture; you should be able to shape it into a patty. If the mixture is too crumbly, stir in a little water (or more egg) until it holds together.

3. Line a baking sheet with parchment paper. Divide and shape the mixture into 14 patties, placing them on the baking sheet as you go.

4. Heat 1 tablespoon of oil in a skillet over medium heat. Gently place 4 of the cakes in the pan (or as many as will fit) and cook until golden brown on the bottom, about 4 minutes. Carefully turn the patties over and cook until golden brown on the other side, about 4 more minutes. Remove from the pan and drain on paper towels. Cook the rest of the patties, adding more oil to the pan as needed.

5. Serve topped with crème fraîche, yogurt, or other toppings of your choice, if desired.

---

1 cup uncooked white quinoa, or 3 cups cooked quinoa

2 cups water

4 large eggs

6 ounces feta cheese, crumbled (about 1½ cups)

2 cups mallow leaves, finely chopped

½ cup finely chopped yellow onion (about 1 medium)

¼ cup finely chopped flat-leaf parsley

Grated zest of 1 lemon (about 1 tablespoon)

4 teaspoons fresh lemon juice

1 cup panko (Japanese-style breadcrumbs)

½ teaspoon kosher salt

¼ teaspoon freshly ground black pepper

Olive oil, for frying

Crème fraîche or plain Greek-style yogurt, for serving (optional)

Variations: To make this recipe without gluten, use gluten-free panko or breadcrumbs. To make it without dairy, homemade tofu feta can be substituted for the cheese.

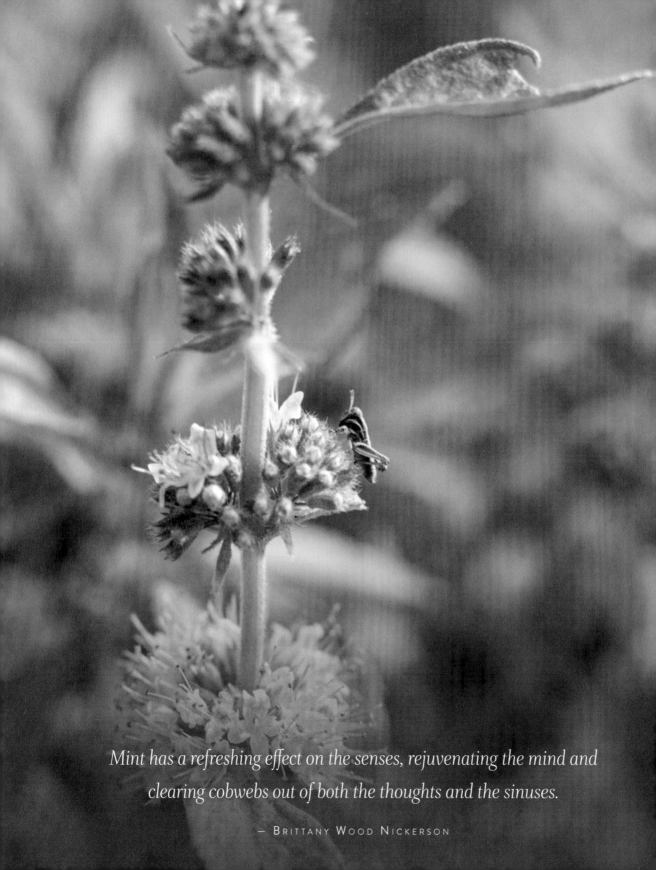

Mint has a refreshing effect on the senses, rejuvenating the mind and clearing cobwebs out of both the thoughts and the sinuses.

— Brittany Wood Nickerson

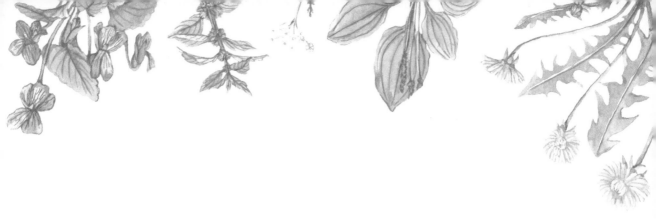

CHAPTER 16

MINT

Whether you find mint growing wild in a wet meadow, occupying a patch of your garden, or sold in bunches at your local farmers market, this aromatic plant has a cheery, fresh flavor that brightens teas, invigorates meals, and is now standard for breath mints, mouthwashes, and toothpastes. As with many plants, the exact chemical composition of mints changes depending on the exact species (they hybridize easily) and their growing conditions. Smelling and tasting mints reveal their complex nature. Can you detect the peppery sensation found in peppermint? Or the sweetness of spearmint? How strong is a feral mint compared with garden mint? This is just the beginning of mint's many secrets.

Botanical names: *Mentha aquatica, M. arvensis* (syn. *M. canadensis*), *M. x piperita, M. spicata, M. suaveolens,* and other species
Family: Lamiaceae (mint)
Parts used: aerial portions (mainly leaves, flowers)
Energetics: variable: warming to cooling, drying
Taste: pungent
Properties: analgesic, antispasmodic, aromatic, carminative, stimulating diaphoretic, stimulating nervine
Uses: bad breath, colds, fever, flu, food, gas, headaches, hiccups, itching and inflammation of the skin, nausea, sinus congestion, spasms, stomach upset
Preparations: essential oil, food, tea, tincture, wash

The fresh aromatics of mints have appealed to humans for thousands of years. Native to Africa, Australia, Eurasia, and North America, mints have historically been used across the world. While native species still exist today, their ability to easily hybridize has created a multitude of different mints. Wild mint (*Mentha arvensis*, syn. *M. canadensis*) grows wild in North America and Europe, where it loves moist meadows or stream banks. Peppermint (*M. x piperita*) is a commonly used hybridized mint that was first recognized in the 1600s, a cross between European spearmint (*M. spicata*) and a water mint (*M. aquatica*). Peppermint and spearmint are now widely cultivated and distilled for use in gums, candies, and breath mints, as well as mouthwashes, toothpastes, and other oral health products. Plant nurseries often carry many different mint cultivars.

MEDICINAL PROPERTIES AND ENERGETICS

Wild mint and peppermint are high in menthol, an aromatic chemical that imparts both a warming and a cooling sensation. Drinking a hot mint tea is an interesting experience of these differing energetics. Spearmint, though notably similar in flavor, doesn't contain menthol. Comparing the tastes of wild mint and spearmint shows you just how similar and different these plants can be. While all the mints offer unique gifts, for most purposes they can be readily interchanged.

PLANT GIFTS

Reduces Nausea, Stimulates Appetite, and Promotes Digestion

Plants repeatedly show us that they can be both gentle and strong. Mint is the perfect herb for addressing many digestive complaints or simply for promoting and maintaining healthy digestion. Its pleasing taste makes a comforting cup of tea, ideal for an after-meal brew and safe for all ages at the table. Yet, as pleasant and gentle as the tea can be, mint can also be used as powerful medicine. Researchers have shown mint to be effective for reducing nausea caused by chemotherapy.[1] It also is great for appetite loss due to the queasy feelings of anxiety. As an aromatic carminative herb, mint relieves flatulence. Enteric coated capsules of peppermint oil have been repeatedly shown to relieve irritable bowel syndrome (IBS) symptoms.[2] And one of mint's most handy uses is to quell stubborn hiccups.

Acts as an Antimicrobial

Mint species have been shown to have antimicrobial properties, which could be useful for both oral and digestive health. In vitro studies have shown various mints to be effective against the following bacteria and fungi pathogens: *Escherichia coli*, *Staphylococcus aureus*, *Streptococcus mutans*, *Aggregatibacter actinomycetem-comitans*, *Candida albicans*, *Fusarium graminearum*, *F. moniliforme*, and *Penicillium expansum*.[3]

Relieves Pain

Mint can relieve many types of pain, from headaches to osteoarthritis to menstrual cramps. Headaches related to stress and tension can be soothed with mint tea and a mint compress across the forehead and back of the neck. Researchers found that mint tea "improved stiffness and physical disability scores in adults with knee osteoarthritis."[4] Peppermint has been shown to decrease menstrual cramps in two clinical trials.[5] Mint tea as a wash or added to bathwater relieves minor skin irritations like insect bites, rashes, sunburn, and hives.

Soothes Cold and Flu Symptoms

Mint tea brings welcome relief to cold and flu symptoms. Hot tea can support the healthy fever process while also relieving tension and mild aches and pains. Mint-infused honey can soothe a sore throat and promote expectoration to relieve congestion in the lungs. A traditional Western herbal formula for soothing many cold and flu symptoms is a blend of elderflower, yarrow, and mint (see page 214 for a tea recipe).

HOW TO IDENTIFY

Although many species of mint grow in the wild and in gardens, they share some basic characteristics. All mints have square stems, which you can feel by rolling a stem between your fingers. The simple leaves are oppositely arranged on the stem. They are also aromatic—if you crush a leaf, it should smell like mint! Depending on the species, the plant's small tubular flowers may grow in terminal spikes or in whorls at the leaf axils. Each flower has five fused petals (typically an upper lip with two lobes and a lower lip with three lobes) and four stamens.

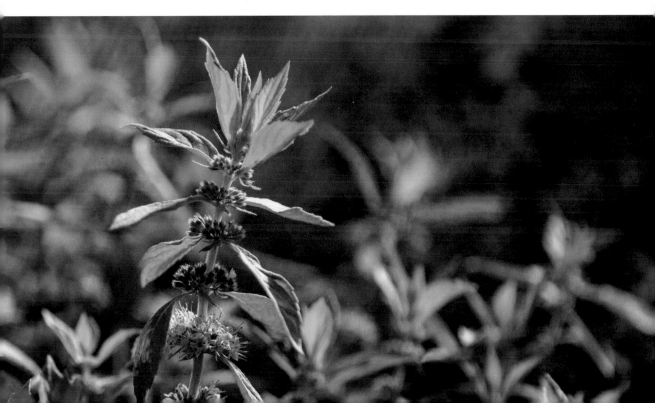

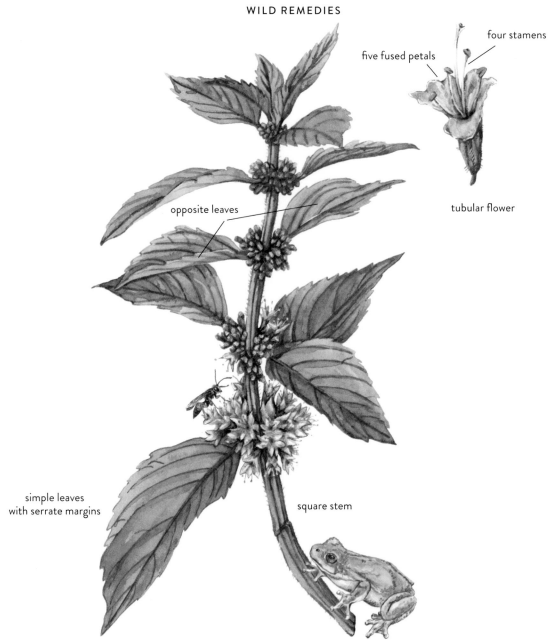

five fused petals

four stamens

tubular flower

opposite leaves

simple leaves
with serrate margins

square stem

wild mint (*Mentha arvensis*), shown with great golden digger wasp
(*Sphex ichneumoneus*) and Cope's gray tree frog (*Hyla chrysoscelis*)

Life cycle: herbaceous perennial
Reproduces by: rhizome
Growth habit: rhizomatous with stems 1–4 feet tall
Habitat: ditches, lakeshores, marshes, moist fields, riparian areas, riverbanks, streams
Sun: full sun to partial shade
Soil: moist, rich
USDA Hardiness Zones: 4–9, depending on species

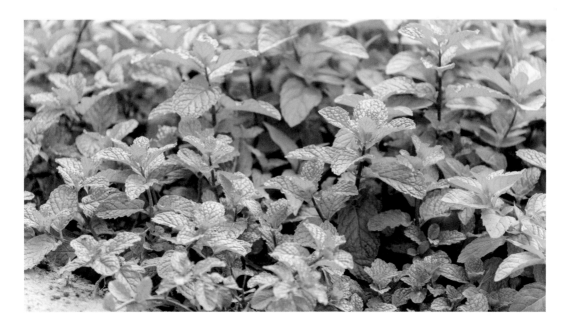

ECOLOGICAL CONNECTIONS

Mints attract insects such as honeybees, bumblebees, small native bees, flies, wasps, and butterflies. The plants can also help stabilize the soil along streams and riverbanks, preventing erosion.

HOW TO HARVEST

Harvest mint throughout the growing season, preferably before it flowers. Use your fingers or clippers to pinch off the top few inches of growth, and take care not to pull the roots. Frequently cutting mint encourages bushy growth, but do make sure you leave enough stems and leaves so the plant stays healthy.

Mint can spread prolifically by underground rhizomes. It can be propagated by stem or root cuttings from mature plants.

Harvesting Cautions

Be cautious with pennyroyal (*Mentha pulegium*), which has medicinal uses but can also be toxic; consult an experienced practitioner first. Potential look-alike plants include nettle (*Urtica dioica*), which you'll know by its sting, and anise hyssop (*Agastache foeniculum*), which smells like licorice.

GARDENING TIPS

The unruly behavior of mints often gets bad press in the gardening world. Fast-growing mints are strong producers, like to spread their joy via runners, and can be aggressive bullies in a small herb garden. Give them their own bed, but avoid planting different species close together; they will naturally hybridize, weakening both taste and medicinal properties. Propagation is best done by division and cuttings.

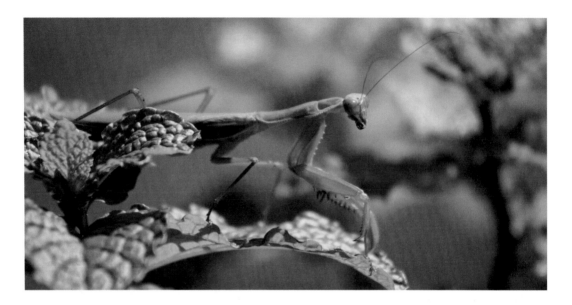

Seed for most mints is unreliable. Many mints benefit from well-drained, moist soil and partial shade. Gardeners intent on controlling mint by planting it in containers soon learn that mint doesn't care much about barriers!

USING MINT IN YOUR LIFE

Mint's fresh flavor has made it an important ingredient in many global cuisines, including Africa, Asia, the Mediterranean, and the Americas. Both dried and fresh mint are used for culinary purposes, depending on the recipe.

Mint can be used fresh or dried in teas and in hot or cold infusions. We often prefer a cold infusion for the fresh leaves; it makes a refreshing drink in hot weather. A hot infusion works well for the dried leaves and can be a comforting cup of tea and an after-meal treat. Mint can also be used externally as a poultice or compress. Mint extracts well into alcohol and glycerin. Peppermint and spearmint are readily found as essential oils.

Recommended Amounts

- *Tea (dried):* 1 to 3 teaspoons, 3 to 5 times daily

- *Tea (fresh):* 2 to 6 teaspoons, 3 to 5 times daily

- *Tincture (dried):* 1:5, 30% alcohol; 3 to 6 ml, 3 to 5 times daily

Special Considerations

- Avoid mints if you are susceptible to heartburn.

- Taken in excess, mint can dry up breast milk.

- Avoid excessive amounts when pregnant.

MINT CHIMICHURRI

Inspired by the zesty green sauce from Argentina and Uruguay, this mint chimichurri is endlessly versatile. Try spooning it over grilled meats and vegetables, tossing it into a grain bowl, and serving it as a dip for crudités. We especially love mint chimichurri slathered on cauliflower steaks and roasted potatoes. And it's a fast and flavorful way to perk up boring leftovers. We typically make this with spearmint. If you're using a stronger-flavored mint, you might want to adjust the recipe by using less mint or more parsley. Let your taste buds guide you.

Yield: About ⅔ cup

1 cup firmly packed fresh mint leaves

1 cup firmly packed fresh flat-leaf parsley leaves

2 garlic cloves

½ teaspoon salt

½ teaspoon red pepper flakes

1½ tablespoons red wine vinegar or apple cider vinegar

½ cup extra-virgin olive oil

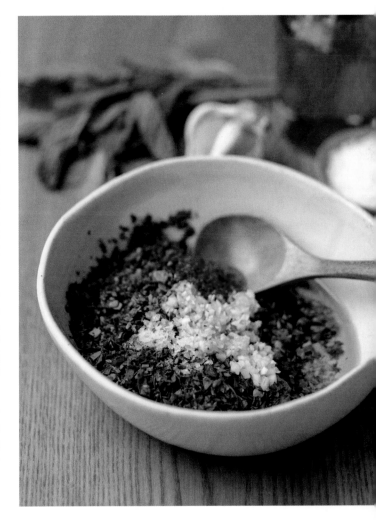

1. Finely chop the mint, parsley, and garlic. Place them in a small bowl. Using a fork, stir in the salt, red pepper flakes, vinegar, and olive oil. (Alternatively, you can pulse the ingredients in a food processor, being careful not to puree the mixture; it should have some texture.)

2. Although it can be used immediately, for best flavor let the sauce sit for 1 hour at room temperature before serving. Store in an airtight container in the refrigerator for up to 1 week.

FRESH SUMMER ROLLS

We love wrapping mint leaves and edible flowers into refreshing Vietnamese-style summer rolls, or goi cuon. Rolling these takes a little practice, but once you get the hang of it, you'll love how beautifully simple—and customizable—they are. The ingredients here are suggestions; feel free to play with other seasonal fillings like cucumber, asparagus, scallions, etc. You could also add a protein such as edamame, tofu, or shrimp. Look for the rice paper wrappers and noodles at Vietnamese or Chinese markets or in the Asian food aisle of the supermarket. Three Ladies brand is particularly good.

Yield: 8 rolls

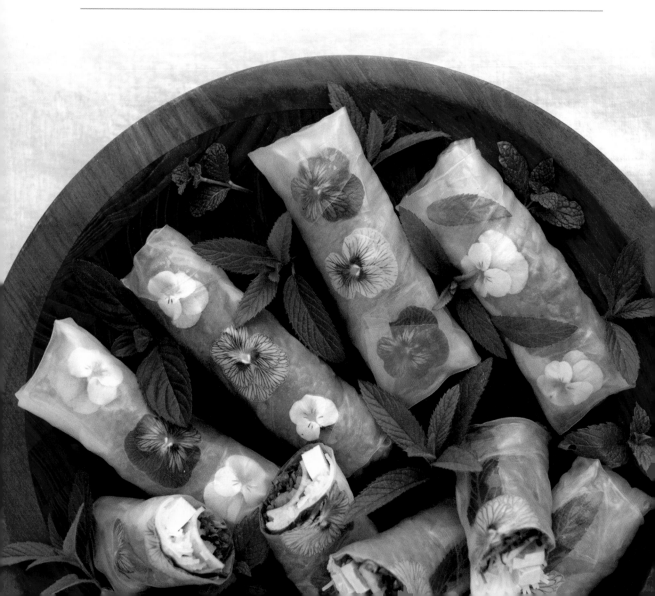

For the dipping sauce:

1. Combine the lime juice, soy sauce, brown sugar, and lukewarm water and stir to dissolve the sugar. Taste and adjust the balance of sour, salty, and sweet as desired. Stir in the chile and garlic, if using. Set aside until ready to serve.

For the summer rolls:

1. Put the noodles in a heatproof bowl and cover with boiling water. Soak the noodles until softened, 10 to 15 minutes. Drain and pat dry.

2. Set up your work area with a flat surface, such as a cutting board, for assembling the rolls and a serving platter nearby. Place the noodles, rice paper wrappers, and vegetables and herbs within reach.

3. Fill a pie pan or other wide, shallow dish with room-temperature water. Take one rice paper wrapper and dip it in the water until it becomes pliable but not gummy, about 10–30 seconds. Lay the wrapper on your work surface.

4. Place a piece of lettuce on the bottom third of the wrapper closest to you. Top the lettuce with the greens, mint leaves, radishes, carrots, snap peas, and noodles, taking care not to overstuff the roll. Gently lift the bottom edge of the wrapper away from you and up over the filling. Roll it once, using your fingers to keep the fillings tightly tucked in as you roll. Fold in the sides of the wrapper and roll it once more.

5. Right above the crease of the roll, arrange a row of 3 flowers or mint leaves with the tops facing down. Continue rolling to close the roll. Transfer the roll to a serving platter.

6. Repeat to make the rest of the rolls. Keep the rolls from touching each other on the platter, or they will stick to each other.

7. Serve the rolls whole or cut in half, with dipping sauce on the side.

Make ahead: The rolls can be made up to 2 hours ahead, covered, and stored at cool room temperature. (Refrigerated rolls might get hard and crack.)

Dipping sauce

3 tablespoons fresh lime juice (from about 2 limes)

3 tablespoons soy sauce

2 tablespoons brown sugar or honey

⅓ cup lukewarm water

1 Thai or serrano chile, thinly sliced (optional)

1 garlic clove, minced (optional)

Summer rolls

2 ounces dried rice stick noodles (maifun)

4 green or red lettuce leaves, ribs removed and leaves halved

1 cup tender greens such as chickweed, violet leaves, pea shoots, or microgreens

30 to 40 fresh mint leaves

½ cup thinly sliced red radishes (about 3 radishes)

½ cup carrots (about 2 carrots), cut into matchsticks

16 sugar snap peas

24 fresh edible flowers such as violets, violas, or pansies (or substitute mint leaves)

Eight 8-inch round rice paper wrappers, plus a few extra in case of tearing

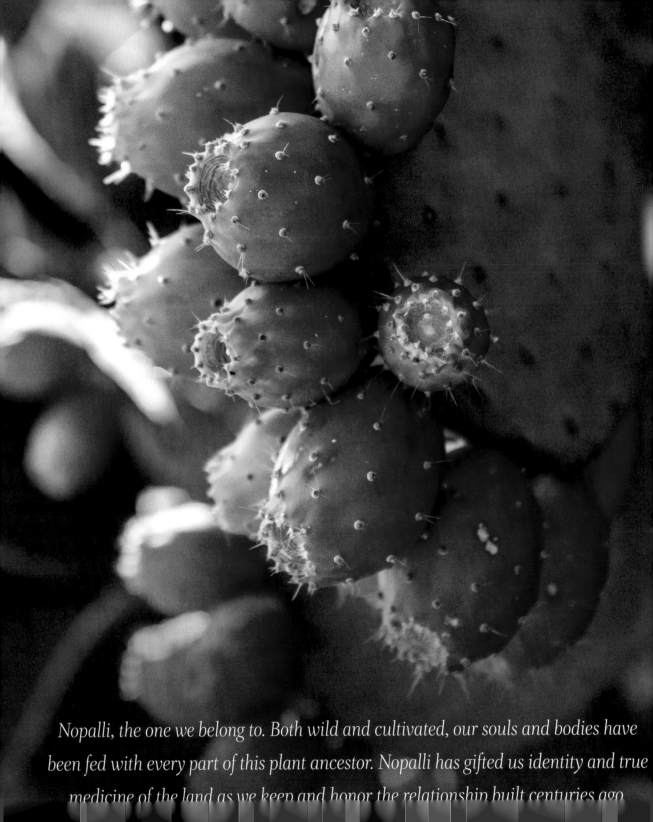

Nopalli, the one we belong to. Both wild and cultivated, our souls and bodies have been fed with every part of this plant ancestor. Nopalli has gifted us identity and true medicine of the land as we keep and honor the relationship built centuries ago.

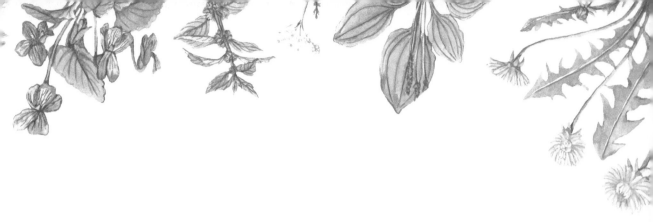

PRICKLY PEAR

On the outside, prickly pear is tougher than tough. It thrives in rugged, dry soils and marginal lands, and its spines will jab you if you aren't paying attention or rush in too fast. But this is just a layer of protection. Given patience and respect, this cactus can be one of the most soothing herbs you'll meet. From its green pads to its delicate flower petals and vibrant fruits, prickly pear offers bountiful food and medicine.

Other common names: nohpalli, nopal, nopalli, tuna, cactus fig, cactus pear

Botanical names: *Opuntia* spp. (including *O. engelmannii*, *O. ficus-indica*, *O. humifusa*, *O. stricta*, and many other species)

Family: Cactaceae (cactus)

Parts used: stem pads, flowers, fruits, seeds

Energetics: cooling, moistening

Taste: sour, sweet

Properties: antioxidant, astringent, diuretic, demulcent, febrifuge, inflammatory modulator

Uses: acid reflux/gastritis, bruises, burns, edema, food, inflammation, insect bites, sprains, type 2 diabetes, urinary tract infections, wounds

Preparations: food, succus (juice), poultice, tea

Native to Mexico, prickly pear has long offered food and medicine to the peoples of northern Mexico and the southwestern United States. In Texas, archaeologists have found evidence of *Opuntia* consumption dating from before 7000 B.C.E.[1] Prickly pear played a central role in the story of the Culhua-Mexica (Aztec) Empire, and the name of their capital city, Tenochtitlan, can be translated to "place of the prickly pear cactus." The pads (nopales) and fruits (tunas) continue to be staples in these parts of the world and farther afield. Prickly pear now grows in various habitats across North America as well as Africa, Australia, and the Mediterranean. It is also commercially grown and can be found in many grocery stores and farmers markets.

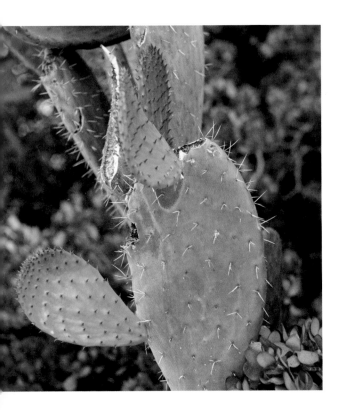

MEDICINAL PROPERTIES AND ENERGETICS

Prickly pear is a demulcent herb rich in mucilage, a juicy, slimy substance that cools and moistens inflamed and irritated tissues. The entire plant also offers high levels of nutrients. The pads contain calcium, potassium, carotenoids, and ascorbic acid (vitamin C). The fruits are rich in antioxidants (betacyanins) and flavonols and contain ascorbic acid, tocopherols (fat-soluble vitamin E), calcium, magnesium, potassium, and beta-carotene.[2]

PLANT GIFTS

Heals the Skin and Soft-Tissue Injuries

Like aloe vera gel, prickly pear's gooey pulp can be used topically to soothe irritated skin conditions, including sunburns, bug bites, and rashes. Prickly pear can also help modulate inflammation and swelling in sprains and bruises. In *Working the Roots*, Michele E. Lee writes that African American healing traditions have used prickly pear gel topically "to maintain healthy scalp, hair, and skin. It was also applied to burns, cuts and insect bites."[3] The pulp can be scraped out of the pads, or the pads can simply be sliced and applied directly, but take care to remove all spines and glochids first (see Using Prickly Pear in Your Life on page 186). Crushed flower petals can also be used topically.

Soothes the Digestive System

As a demulcent and mucilaginous herb, prickly pear can coat and soothe mucous membranes,

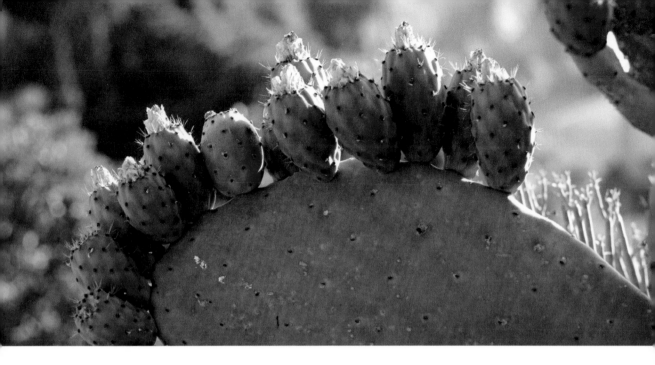

providing relief for gastrointestinal inflammation. Pulp from the pads as well as infusions of the flowers have been used internally for this purpose. Herbalist Charles Kane writes, "Several ounces of pulp mixed with a small amount of water has a cooling effect on esophageal and stomach irritations, be they from acid reflux or gastritis. . . . Not only does prickly pear mucilage serve as a protectant to damaged stomach lining, it also has the ability of augmenting the quality of gastric mucus, making it useful as a stomach ulcer healer."[4]

Supports the Urinary System

Thanks to that demulcent quality, prickly pear can also cool and soothe painful burning associated with urinary tract infections. Although prickly pear doesn't address the bacteria causing the infection, it can relieve the inflammation. The flowers can be used in an infusion, or the pads or fruits can be juiced to drink. Herbalist Michael Moore recommends taking a teaspoon of the pad juice "every two hours until the pain is gone."[5]

Treats Diabetes

Prickly pear has a long history of use in traditional Mexican medicine to treat type 2 diabetes, and preliminary clinical evidence supports this. In one study, researchers found that after patients with type 2 diabetes ate a high-carbohydrate breakfast, consumption of steamed *Opuntia ficus-indica* pads significantly reduced spikes in blood glucose and serum insulin levels.[6] Another study of prediabetics focused on an aqueous extract of *O. ficus-indica* pad and fruit skin. Researchers found that it decreased blood glucose spikes 60, 90, and 120 minutes after ingestion of a 75-gram glucose drink. The authors concluded that the study supported the traditional use of *Opuntia ficus-indica* for blood glucose management.[7] This ability to lower blood sugar is attributed to prickly pear's high fibrous polysaccharide and pectin content.[8]

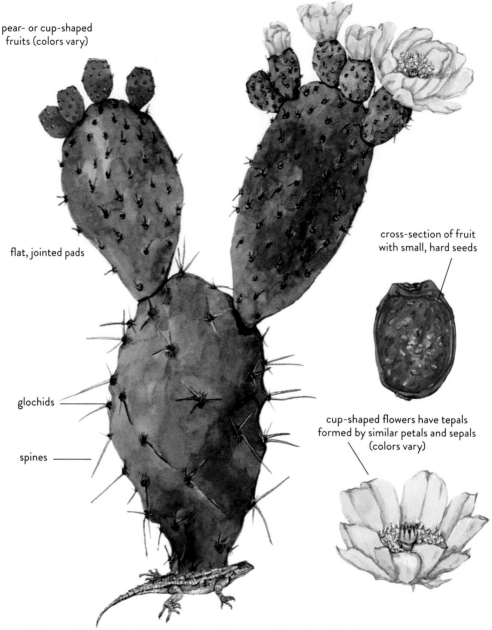

pear- or cup-shaped
fruits (colors vary)

flat, jointed pads

glochids

spines

cross-section of fruit
with small, hard seeds

cup-shaped flowers have tepals
formed by similar petals and sepals
(colors vary)

prickly pear (*Opuntia ficus-indica*), shown with western fence lizard (*Sceloporus occidentalis*)

Life cycle: evergreen herbaceous perennial
Reproduces by: vegetative cloning, seed
Growth habit: succulent shrub, up to 15 feet tall and wide
Habitat: canyon bottoms, coastal areas, deserts, fencerows, grasslands, hillsides,
   prairies, roadsides, rocky cliffs, woodlands, yards
Sun: full sun
Soil: dry, sandy or rocky
USDA Hardiness Zones: 6–11, depending on species

HOW TO IDENTIFY

There are more than 150 species of *Opuntia* worldwide. Each has its own identifying characteristics, so you should consult a field guide for specific information. Generally speaking, prickly pears are composed of flat, jointed cladodes, or pads. These oval pads are covered in groups of larger spines (these are actually modified leaves) and clusters of fine, hairlike spines called glochids. The flowers are yellow, orange, or pink. These produce spiny pear- or cup-shaped fruits along the edges of the pad. When the fruits are ripe, their exterior and their pulp can range in color from green to yellow, orange, red, and purple. Inside are many small, hard seeds.

ECOLOGICAL CONNECTIONS

Prickly pear mounds provide shelter for animals, including rodents, snakes, and lizards. The northern bobwhite, a species of quail, uses prickly pear for nesting cover. Animals ranging from bighorn sheep to stink bugs and moth larvae suck on the pads for moisture and food. Bees, ants, wasps, hoverflies, beetles, hawk moths, and other animals visit the flowers for nectar and pollen. Wild native bees are particularly important pollinators, and some genera, such as *Diadasia* and *Lithurgus*, may have coevolved with *Opuntia*. The fruits are eaten by birds, deer, peccaries, rodents, tortoises, and cycluras (rock iguanas), which help to disperse the seeds. Prickly pear is also a host plant for cochineal insects (*Dactylopius* spp.), which form a cottonlike web on the pads.

HOW TO HARVEST

We recommend wearing heavy gloves to protect yourself when harvesting. Prickly pear pads may be gathered at any time of year, but the new, bright green pads of spring and early summer are more palatable. Pads harvested early in the morning tend to be more sour, as the malic acid content is higher. Harvest each pad by holding it with tongs and using a knife to cut it across the base.

Flower petals may be gathered when fresh and then dried at home, or collected once they have dried on the plant. The fruits typically ripen from midsummer to autumn. Depending on the species, they may taste sweet, sour, or bland, so you'll want to test them first. Harvest each fruit by grabbing it with tongs and gently twisting it off the pad. If it doesn't twist off easily, it is not yet ripe.

Avoid taking too many pads from any one plant, and leave enough flowers and fruits for wildlife and for the plant to seed. Prickly pear can be propagated by breaking off a pad and planting it (see Gardening Tips on page 186).

Harvesting Cautions

Certain species of *Opuntia* are vulnerable or endangered. Learn about the species in your area, be able to identify them, and avoid harvesting those that are of concern.

Large spines are relatively easy to pick out of the skin, but the fine glochids are more difficult to remove and can be very irritating. Always wear heavy gloves when handling prickly pear. If you do get poked, first remove as many spines as you can with tweezers. Evergreen conifer resin or duct tape can help draw out the glochids. Then use the prickly pear pad or fruit pulp to soothe your irritated skin!

GARDENING TIPS

This perennial succulent is drought tolerant, cold tolerant, and low maintenance, making it the ideal garden guest for a variety of climates. It can also be container-grown indoors (with strong light). Propagation is done by cutting a pad: With heavy work gloves, a sharp knife, and temperatures above 60°F, cut a pad from the main cactus and then rest it in a warm room to allow the cut area to callus. Plant directly in the ground, or plant in a container for one year and then transplant outdoors.

USING PRICKLY PEAR IN YOUR LIFE

The pads have been compared in flavor and texture to okra, asparagus, green beans, and cucumber. They can be used whole, sliced, or diced. We especially like them grilled or pickled, and they can also be fried, boiled, dehydrated, or pureed. Abe Sanchez, a promoter of indigenous arts, mixes the pureed pads with masa harina to make beautiful green tortillas.[9]

The fruits vary from bland to sweet and can be reminiscent of watermelon, strawberries, and even bubble gum. After you peel the fruit and strain out the seeds, the pulp can be used raw or cooked in drinks, syrups, sauces, infused vinegars and shrubs, desserts, and fruit leather. The seeds can be dried and ground into flour.

The fresh pads and fruits can be mashed, pureed, juiced, or simply cut open and used as poultices. Fresh flower petals can be used as poultices and dried flower petals can be used in teas and infusions.

To clean the pads: Hold the base of the pad with tongs or a wad of newspaper or cloth to protect your hand. Using a sharp knife, scrape the spines and glochids off both sides of the pad. (You can also burn off the glochids over an open flame.) Cut along the perimeter of the pad to trim off the sides and base. Then rinse the pad with water and use as desired.

To clean the fruit: Hold the fruit with tongs and scrub the glochids off with a scrub brush (or burn them off over an open flame). Using a knife, cut off the top and bottom ends and make a shallow incision (about ¼ inch deep) down the length of the fruit. Use your fingers to peel back the skin and remove the flesh.

Recommended Amounts

Recommended therapeutic amounts are as follows:

- *Pad (cooked or pulp slurry):* 1 to 2 ounces before meals[10]

- *Flower infusion:* 4 to 8 ounces, 2 to 3 times daily[11]

Special Considerations

Prickly pear is very cooling. Eating large amounts of the raw pads, fruits, or juice has been known to cause chills and fever. If you are new to prickly pear or have a cold constitution, we recommend starting with a small amount.

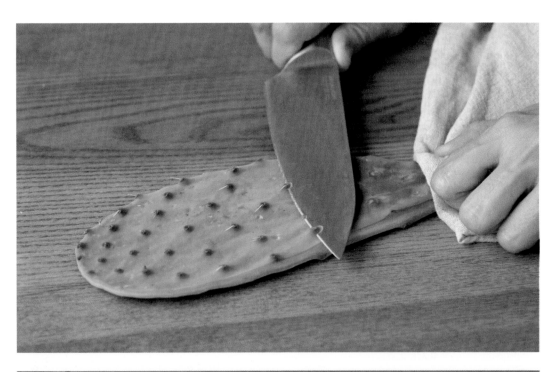

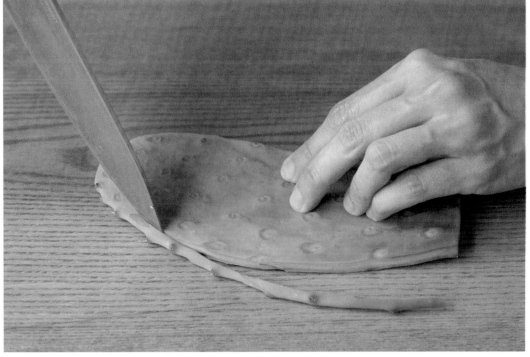

GRILLED NOPALES TACOS

This recipe was inspired by the bright and refreshing nopalitos (cactus pad salads) and tacos con nopales (cactus pad tacos) from Mexico. Like a cross between okra and green beans, nopales have a tart flavor and a texture that's both crisp and slippery. Grilling them gives a nice smoky flavor and balances out the slime. You can boil the pads to remove mucilage, but the flavor won't be as good as grilled. We say embrace the goo! It's wonderfully nourishing on a hot summer day.

Yield: 8 tacos

1 pound (about 8 medium) fresh prickly pear pads, cleaned and spines removed (see page 186)

Olive oil

Salt

Freshly ground black pepper

1 medium tomato, seeded and chopped

½ cup chopped cilantro

¼ cup chopped onion

1 serrano chile, seeds and ribs removed and finely chopped

2 teaspoons dried Mexican oregano (optional)

Juice of ½ lime (about 1 tablespoon)

Eight 6-inch corn tortillas

1 avocado, sliced

Salsa verde, store-bought or homemade (see note below)

Crumbled queso fresco (optional)

Lime wedges for serving (optional)

1. Cut each prickly pear pad into ¼-inch-wide strips, leaving the base intact. It should resemble a fan or hand. Brush each pad with olive oil and season with salt and pepper.

2. Prepare a charcoal or gas grill for medium-heat grilling. (Alternatively, use a grill pan.) Grill the pads until tender and slightly charred, about 4 minutes on each side. The color will change from bright green to a more faded olive green. Remove from the grill. When cool enough to handle, chop each pad into ¼-inch pieces.

3. Place the nopales in a large bowl and toss with the tomato, cilantro, onion, serrano, Mexican oregano (if using), lime juice, and a pinch of salt. Taste and adjust seasonings as desired. (This filling can be made a couple of days ahead and stored in the refrigerator. It can also be eaten on its own as a salad.)

4. Warm the tortillas, then fill with the nopales mixture, followed by avocado, salsa verde, and queso fresco if desired. Serve immediately, with lime wedges on the side if you like.

> *Note:* To make your own quick, fresh salsa verde, combine in a blender: ½ pound husked tomatillos, ¼ cup chopped cilantro, ¼ cup chopped onion, 1 garlic clove, 1 serrano chile (seeds and ribs removed, or leave them in for extra heat), and ¾ teaspoon salt. Blend until smooth. Makes about 1¼ cups.

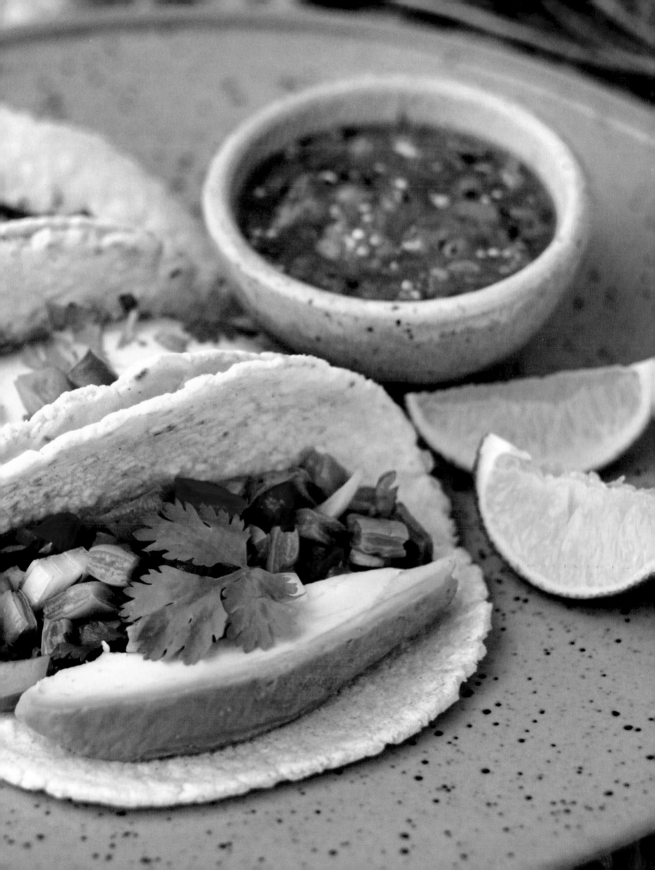

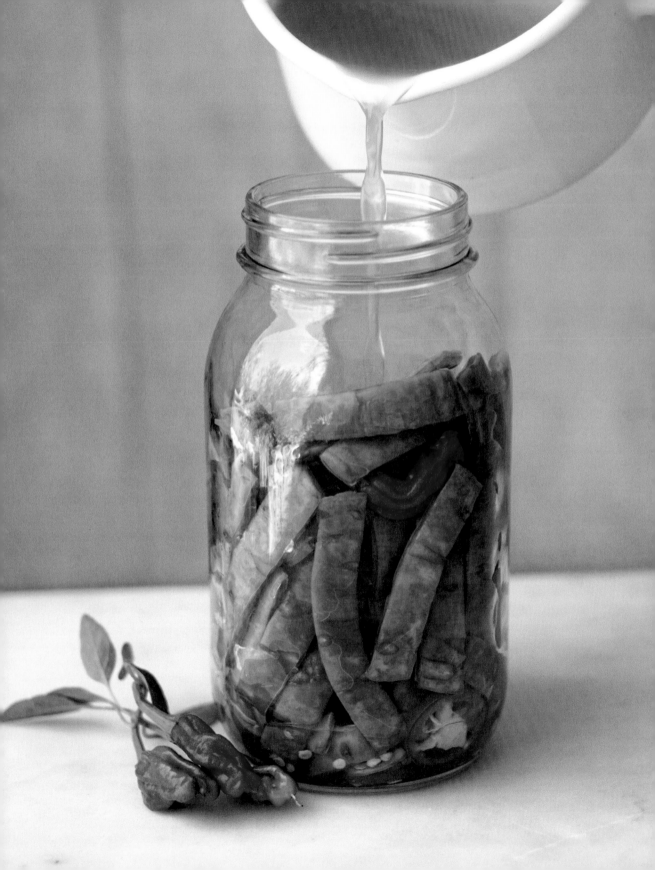

PICKLED NOPALES

Tangy and spicy with a nice bite, these nopales pickles are reminiscent of pickled green beans. Tossing the cactus in salt helps to draw out the slime, giving the pickles a more crisp texture than using fresh or boiled cactus. Enjoy these like any other pickle—with a sandwich, chopped up in a salad, as a relish, or simply as a snack.

Yield: 2 cups

---

1 pound (about 8 medium) fresh prickly pear pads, cleaned and spines removed (see page 186)

Kosher salt

1 cup apple cider vinegar (at least 5% acidity)

1 cup water

2 garlic cloves, peeled

1 jalapeño, sliced

1. Slice the prickly pear pads crosswise into ½-inch-wide strips. Place the strips in a nonreactive bowl and toss with a generous amount of salt. Let stand for 1 hour. Rinse the nopales, rubbing away the salt and slime. Drain and pat dry.

2. Place 1 garlic clove and half of the jalapeño slices in each jar. Tightly pack the nopales in the jars, leaving at least ¾ inch of space at the top. If necessary, trim the strips to fit.

3. Combine the apple cider vinegar, water, and 2 tablespoons of salt in a nonreactive saucepan and bring to a boil.

4. Pour the hot brine over the vegetables in the jars, leaving ½ inch of space at the top. Wipe the jar rims with a clean towel. Cover the jars without screwing the lids on too tightly (to allow gases to escape during the pickling process). Let cool to room temperature, then refrigerate.

5. The pickles will be ready to eat after 3 days but are more tender and flavorful after a couple of weeks. Store in the refrigerator for up to 3 months.

Variations: Depending on your taste and what you have on hand, you can experiment with other fresh or dried chile peppers, or leave out the chile if you prefer a milder pickle. To make dill pickles, add 1 teaspoon of dill seeds to each jar and, if desired, omit the jalapeño.

PRICKLY PEAR FRUIT JUICE

Sweet prickly pear juice enlivens fizzy water, lemonade, margaritas, and more. Although bright pink fruits (also known as tunas) make the most colorful juice, you can use fruits of any color to make this refreshing treat. You can also turn the juice into a syrup, which is delightful in drinks and desserts.

Yield: About 1 cup

2 pounds (about 12 large) prickly pear fruits, cleaned and spines removed (see page 186)

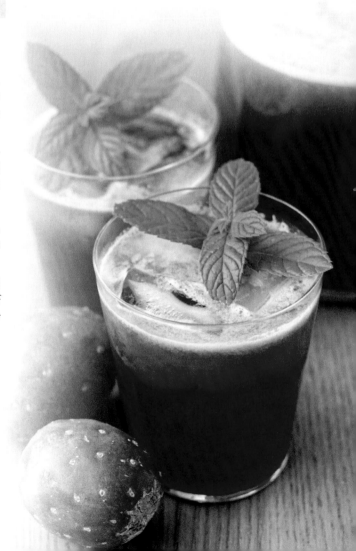

1. Slice the ends off the prickly pear fruits. Cut a ¼-inch-deep slit down the length of each fruit. Slide your fingers into the incision and peel off the skin.

2. Place the peeled fruits in a blender or food processor and process until pureed. (The seeds are very hard and will stay whole.)

3. Strain through a fine-mesh strainer, pressing with a flexible spatula or the back of a spoon to extract the juice.

4. Store the juice in the refrigerator and use within 1 to 2 days. For a longer shelf life, freeze the juice in ice cube trays for up to 6 months.

PRICKLY PEAR LEMONADE

Yield: About 6 cups

1 cup Prickly Pear Fruit Juice
(see page 192)

1 cup freshly squeezed lemon
juice (from about 8 lemons)

½ cup honey

4 cups cold water

1. Combine the prickly pear juice, lemon juice, and honey in a large pitcher, stirring to dissolve the honey. Add water and stir to combine. Taste and add more lemon juice or honey, if desired.

2. Serve over ice. This lemonade also makes delicious, colorful ice pops.

> *To make a cocktail:* Add 2 cups of silver tequila to the pitcher of prickly pear lemonade just before serving. This can also be blended with ice to make a frozen cocktail. Or, for a single serving, fill a glass with ice and add 6 ounces of prickly pear lemonade and 2 ounces of silver tequila.

PRICKLY PEAR SYRUP

Yield: About 1½ cups

1 cup Prickly Pear Fruit Juice
(see page 192)

1 tablespoon freshly squeezed
lemon juice (from about ½ lemon)

1 cup honey

1. Combine the prickly pear juice and lemon juice in a saucepan and bring to a boil over medium heat. Reduce the heat to low and simmer for 5 minutes.

2. Remove from the heat. Stir in the honey and let cool.

3. Transfer the syrup to a clean jar or bottle. Store in the refrigerator for up to 2 weeks.

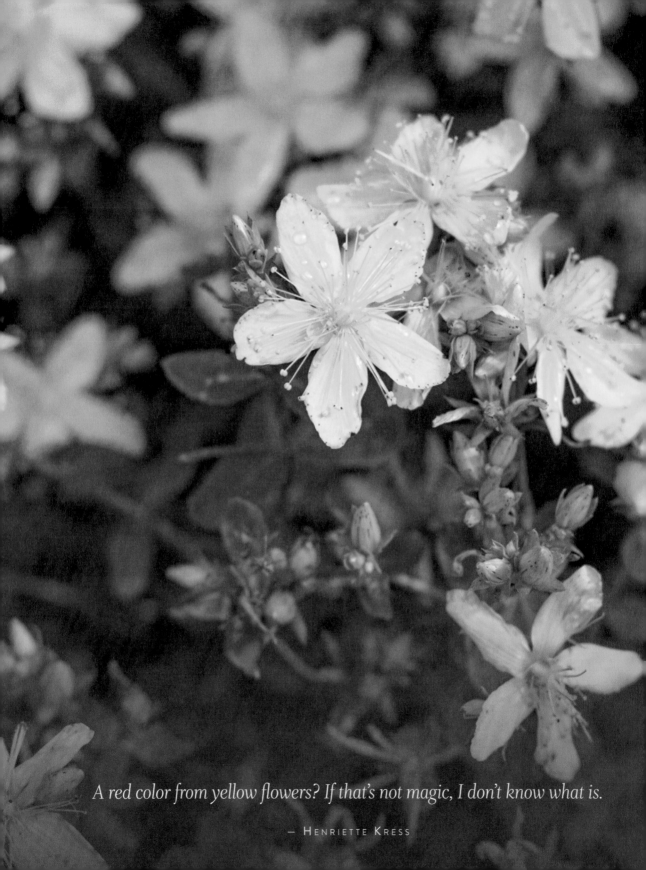

A red color from yellow flowers? If that's not magic, I don't know what is.

— HENRIETTE KRESS

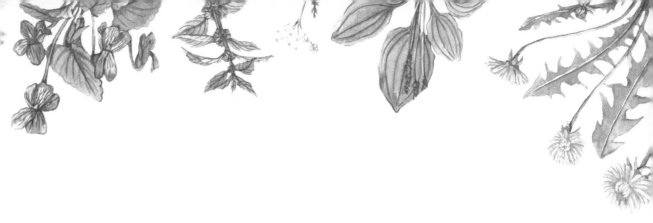

CHAPTER 18

ST. JOHN'S WORT

As high summer approaches, St. John's wort flowers begin to pay homage to the sun. Often blooming around the solstice, these bright yellow flowers shine back their luminescence to the skies above. Grab your basket and head to the meadows, fields, and stream banks to search for this sun-filled plant. Once you find St. John's wort flowers, the magic really begins. This wayside weed has a special trick: Pick a flower bud and crush it between your fingers. That surprising reddish-purple stain tells you this is powerful herbal medicine.

Botanical name: *Hypericum perforatum*
Family: Hypericaceae (St. John's wort)
Parts used: flowering tips including buds (preferred), flowers, and leaves
Energetics: cooling, drying
Taste: slightly bitter, pungent, sweet
Properties: alterative, antiviral, astringent, hepatic, inflammatory modulator, nervous system trophorestorative, relaxing nervine, vulnerary
Uses: cold sores, liver stagnation, nerve pain, stagnant depression, viruses
Preparations: oil, tea, tincture

Hypericum perforatum is native to Europe, northern Africa, and western Asia. It has been used since ancient times in Europe and often appears in folklore with fairies, witches, and saints. First Nations people use several native species of Hypericum for wounds, diarrhea, aching feet, sore eyes, and weak lungs.[1]

Modern scientists have taken an interest as well. In the 1990s, researchers announced they had found the bioactive chemical constituent in St. John's wort: hypericin. Herbal companies rushed to make products featuring that isolated extract. Fast-forward a few years, and researchers said they had found another bioactive constituent of St. John's wort: hyperforin. Again isolated chemical constituents were made into nutraceutical products. But herbalists know that plant medicine can rarely be reduced to a single constituent (or two). Instead, it's the herbs' complexity that makes them so powerful.

MEDICINAL PROPERTIES AND ENERGETICS

St. John's wort is slightly cooling and moderately drying. It has a poetic relationship with the sun: it blooms on the solstice, can protect your skin from excessive sun exposure, and is commonly used to lift the spirits of someone who is missing the sun. It also relieves hot nerve pain, heals wounds, stimulates the liver, and works against a virus that can be triggered by the sun.

PLANT GIFTS

Relieves Nerve Pain

Have you ever had nerve pain? It's a hot, shooting kind of pain that can be absolutely debilitating. Common nerve pain complaints include sciatica, foot neuropathy, and thoracic outlet syndrome. St. John's wort can calm nerve irritation and relieve that intense pain. It was recommended for spinal injuries by the Eclectic physicians of the late 1800s and continues to be used that way today. Oil-based topical preparations work especially well to relieve nerve pain.

Treats Depression Caused by Light Deprivation

St. John's wort is a popular herbal remedy for depression. A meta review of St. John's wort for depression looked at 27 clinical trials with a total of 3,308 people enrolled. The researchers

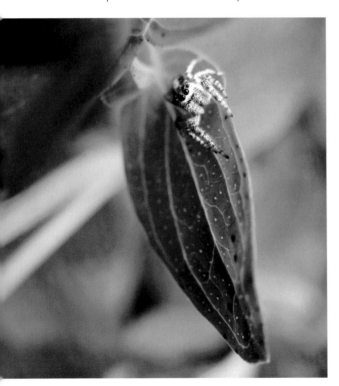

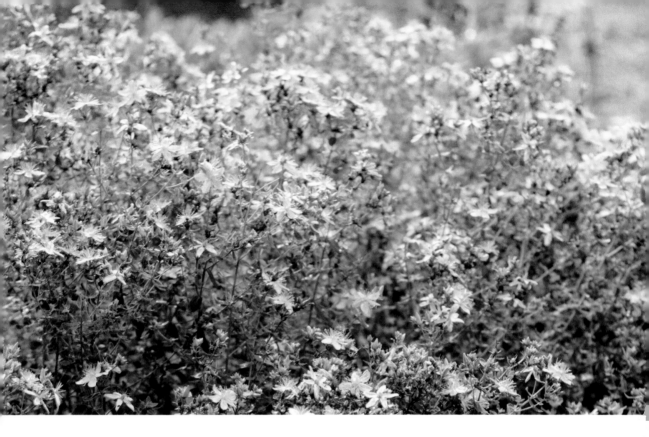

concluded that St. John's wort was as effective as prescription medication for depression for those with mild to moderate symptoms.[2] As promising as those results are, the studies don't reflect how herbalists tend to work with people who have depression. Herbalists recognize that depression is a complicated disease and regularly approach it with a holistic mind-set that includes therapies beyond herbs.

Herbalists often advise the use of St. John's wort for particular types of depression, which have their own specific indications. For example, herbalist David Winston recommends St. John's wort for gastrointestinal-based or hepatic depression, when a person may have a sour stomach and a sour attitude.[3] French herbalist Christophe Bernard specifically uses it for the elderly who have lost interest in life and have a dark view of the world. Many herbalists use St. John's wort for seasonal affective disorder and anyone who generally struggles to find joy in the dark winter months.

Acts as an Antiviral

As soon as you feel that first tingle of a cold sore, St. John's wort can be applied topically and taken liberally internally to either stop the cold sore from appearing or shorten its duration. St. John's wort can even be taken preventively to avoid future outbreaks. It's effective against many herpes viruses, including herpes 1, herpes 2, and shingles. In one clinical trial, volunteers with active herpes skin lesions were given a topical formula containing St. John's wort and copper sulfate, while others were given acyclovir (the pharmaceutical antiviral drug often used for herpes). The herb and copper formula was found to be more effective with fewer side effects than the topical acyclovir.[4]

Promotes Liver Health

St. John's wort is a powerful herb for supporting the liver—so powerful, in fact, that it can clear pharmaceuticals from the system before they've had a chance to work. It does this by speeding up one of the major CYP450 enzymes, CYP3A4, which is responsible for metabolizing a number of drugs. It's so effective that St. John's wort is contraindicated for use with many pharmaceuticals. See the Special Considerations section for more information.

Herbalists often consider a sluggish liver the root cause of many illnesses, ranging from depression to imbalanced hormones, digestive problems, and even cholesterol imbalances. St. John's wort can be used to support your liver's natural function, and this can have a wide range of beneficial effects.

Restores Hormonal Balance

Hormonal imbalance is frequently seen as a symptom of a sluggish liver, and herbs for the liver are often used as part of a larger protocol to restore healthy hormone levels. St. John's wort has been shown to be beneficial for people with polycystic ovary syndrome and for people with mild premenstrual syndrome.[5]

In a randomized, double-blind, placebo-controlled clinical trial, volunteers who had been diagnosed with mild PMS were split into two groups. One group was given St. John's wort while the other was given a placebo. The results showed that daily use of the St. John's wort was more effective than placebo for the most common physical and behavioral symptoms associated with PMS.[6] This may be due to St. John's wort's ability to restore liver function,

its known effect on the nervous system, its ability to mildly reduce cramping, or, more likely, a combination of all three actions plus several others we aren't even aware of. This synergy of actions illustrates the beauty of our complex herbs and is a great example of why a plant can't be reduced to isolated constituents like hypericin or hyperforin.

Heals Wounds, Bumps, and Bruises

St. John's wort can speed up the healing of bumps and bruises. It's often compared to arnica (a popular herb used for injuries) in both its use and effectiveness. According to the 1898 *King's American Dispensatory*, "St. John's wort is valued by many practitioners as a vulnerary, much as Arnica is employed. Therefore it has been used extensively as a local application to bruises, contusions, sprains, lacerations, swellings, ecchymoses, and in acute mammitis."[7] The infused oil can be made into a salve for easy application.

St. John's wort can heal wounds as well as reduce scarring. One study found that a combination of St. John's wort and yarrow reduced the pain, redness, edema, and ecchymosis (discoloration) of an episiotomy incision.[8] Another study concluded that St. John's wort was a safe treatment to facilitate the healing of a cesarean section to minimize scarring as well as reduce pain.[9]

Offers Protection from the Sun

For many people, whole St. John's wort preparations can help protect them from the harmful effects of the sun. A St. John's wort–infused oil can be used as a light sunscreen. This seems to work best when applied daily for mild sun exposure (in other words, don't assume it will work as all-day protection on a tropical beach). It can also be used to heal skin that has been exposed to excessive sun.

Modern clinical trials have verified that a cream made from St. John's wort can protect the skin from sunburn. In this study, the UV-protective effect of the St. John's wort cream was tested on 20 volunteers in a randomized, double-blind, vehicle-controlled study. The herbal cream was found to significantly reduce UVB-induced erythema (redness) as opposed to a placebo.[10]

However, St. John's wort—especially products that contain isolated chemical constituents (as opposed to the whole plant)—have the potential to increase photosensitivity. This risk is increased when those products are taken in large amounts. If you are taking a lot of St. John's wort daily, use caution in exposing your skin to sunlight.

HOW TO IDENTIFY

St. John's wort is a branching plant that often has dozens of woody stems rising from the base. Its leaves may be lanceolate, ovate, elliptic, or oblong, and they measure 0.5 to 1 inch long. They are oppositely arranged at nodes along the stem. When held up to the light, the leaves appear perforated with translucent dots, hence the species name *perforatum*.

Numerous star-shaped yellow flowers grow on terminal clusters called cymes. Each flower is 0.75 to 1 inch across and has five petals, five sepals, and many stamens. Tiny black dots pepper the margins of the petals. The seed capsule has three sections containing round, resinous seeds that can stick to fur and clothing, helping their dispersal.

ECOLOGICAL CONNECTIONS

Insects such as honeybees, bumblebees, sweat bees, hoverflies, and beetles collect the pollen. Moth and butterfly caterpillars, such as the gray hairstreak (*Strymon melinus*), eat the foliage and seed capsules.

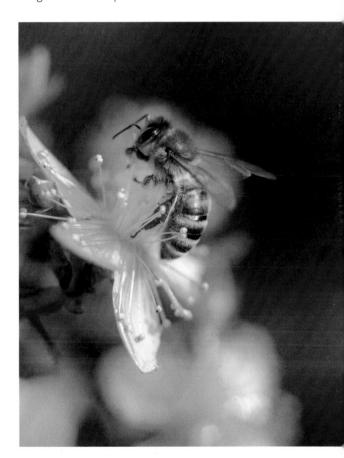

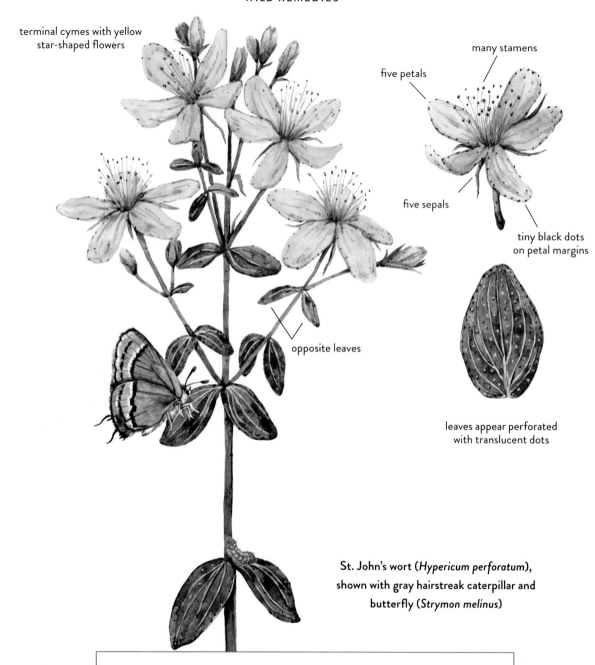

terminal cymes with yellow
star-shaped flowers

many stamens

five petals

five sepals

tiny black dots
on petal margins

opposite leaves

leaves appear perforated
with translucent dots

St. John's wort (*Hypericum perforatum*),
shown with gray hairstreak caterpillar and
butterfly (*Strymon melinus*)

Life cycle: partially woody perennial
Reproduces by: seed, rhizome, stolon
Growth habit: upright, branching, 1–3 feet tall
Habitat: abandoned fields, disturbed areas, forest clearings, grasslands, lakeshores,
    meadows, pastures, railways, riverbanks
Sun: full sun to partial shade
Soil: sandy or gravelly, well drained, moist; can tolerate some drought
USDA Hardiness Zones: 3–8

HOW TO HARVEST

Gather individual flowers by hand or use pruning shears to clip the upper aerial parts of the plant. All of the aerial portions of St. John's wort are medicinally active; however, we often prefer the unopened flower buds. If you have access to large amounts of fresh St. John's wort, then we recommend harvesting a lot of flower buds. If your supply is lower, then use both buds and flowers. If your supply is really low, use buds, flowers, and upper leaves.

St. John's wort reproduces by seed and also spreads aggressively from aboveground runners and underground rhizomes. Leave enough flowers for it to go to seed, or propagate it through stem cuttings. Note, however, that in some locations St. John's wort is considered "invasive" and people are advised not to grow it.

Harvesting Cautions

A look-alike plant is *Hypericum punctatum*, or spotted St. John's wort. This plant can be differentiated by the black dots that cover the flower's entire petal, not just the edges.

GARDENING TIPS

Start with seeds that have been stratified for four weeks. Sow indoors and transplant, or sow directly in early spring. St. John's wort is considered a "noxious" weed in some states, so seeds cannot be purchased in those states. It can be propagated by root divisions of existing plants in the spring or fall. For future harvests, allow some flowers to go to seed.

USING ST. JOHN'S WORT IN YOUR LIFE

Due to concerns that isolated extracts of St. John's wort could have negative effects (one study found a 36 percent risk of adulteration in commercial St. John's wort products), we strongly recommend harvesting St. John's wort and making your own remedies with it.[11]

Whether to select fresh or dried St. John's wort depends on how you are planning to use the plant. Dried St. John's wort works well as a tea or powder (e.g., in capsules). Dried does not work well as an oil infusion and isn't great for an alcohol extraction or tincture (though it *could* work as a tincture if you have access only to dried). Fresh is the only choice for an oil infusion, which can be used for a variety of topical applications ranging from lip balms to face creams to salves.

Recommended Amounts

- *Tea or powder (recently dried herb):* 3 to 6 grams daily

- *Tincture (fresh flowers and leaves):* 1:2, 75%+ alcohol; 3 to 5 ml daily

- *Oil:* apply as often as desired or deemed necessary

Special Considerations

St. John's wort is contraindicated with many pharmaceutical drugs. According to the *Botanical Safety Handbook*, pharmaceutical drugs that are affected by internal use of St. John's wort include the following:

- Immunosuppressants
- Anticoagulants
- Antiarrhythmics
- Calcium channel blockers
- Anti-anginals
- Hormonal contraceptives*
- Anxiolytics
- Antidepressants
- Antivirals
- Statins
- Anticancer drugs, such as chemotherapies
- Beta-adrenergic blockers
- Hypoglycemics
- Antiulcer agents
- Antifungals
- Anticonvulsants
- Skeletal muscle relaxants
- Antihistamines[12]

*While there have been some concerns that St. John's wort may reduce the effectiveness of female hormonal birth control, more recent studies have shown that this is unlikely.[13]

St. John's wort has also been shown to greatly reduce the plasma concentrations of oral oxycodone.[14]

Due to the complex nature of how St. John's wort interacts with liver function, we are constantly learning more about contraindications. If you take pharmaceutical medications, we recommend that you consult with an experienced practitioner as well as do your own research regarding the herb's safety and your unique situation.

Some people find that taking St. John's wort (especially standardized extracts) causes photosensitivity. Do not use artificial light, such as a tanning bed, while taking St. John's wort internally or applying it externally. Do not concurrently use St. John's wort with other photosensitizing drugs.

ST. JOHN'S WORT OIL

Infusing fresh St. John's wort buds and flowers into oil gives you a brilliantly red oil with deeply heal-ing benefits. If you have access to a lot of St. John's wort, then use only the flower buds for an especially vibrant oil. However, using buds, flowers, and the top leaves will still result in a lovely and healing oil. If using it in salves, olive oil is an ideal carrier oil because it is shelf stable and affordable. If using it as a facial treat-ment, then a lighter carrier oil such as apricot kernel or jojoba is a better choice.

Yield: About 2 cups

---

2 cups tightly packed fresh St. John's wort

Up to 2 cups carrier oil

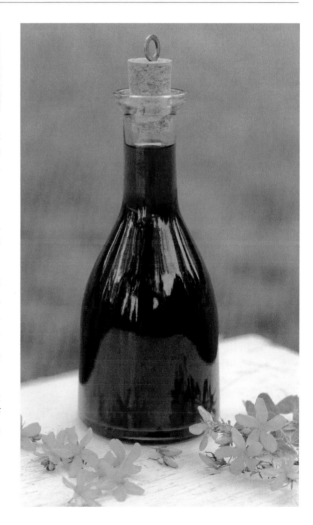

1. Chop the St. John's wort well and place it in a pint jar. Pour in enough oil to fill the jar and submerge the herbs completely. (You might not use the entire 2 cups.)

2. Using a clean instrument, stir well, mak-ing sure to push the herb under the oil. Tightly cover the jar and label it. Place the jar in a sunny window.

3. Every day open the jar and make sure the herbal material is still below the oil line. Stir or add more oil, as needed to cover. Herbs above the oil can easily grow mold.

4. Infuse the oil for about 1 month, until the oil has turned a dark red.

5. Strain the oil through cheesecloth. Let the oil sit for 24 hours. Then pour most of the oil into a clean container, leaving the bottom residue behind.

6. Store in a cool, dark place.

ALL-PURPOSE HEALING SALVE

This is a wonderful salve to have on hand for many purposes, including bumps, bruises, clean cuts, rashes, bug bites, and more. It is truly all purpose as it can relieve pain, modulate inflammation, and prevent infection. To make the yarrow- and plantain-infused oils, follow the process described in steps 1 through 7 of the Chickweed Salve on page 88.

Yield: 8 ounces

1 ounce (28 grams) beeswax

⅓ cup St. John's Wort Oil (page 203)

⅓ cup yarrow-infused oil

⅓ cup plantain-infused oil

30 to 50 drops (¼ to ½ teaspoon) lavender (*Lavandula angustifolia*) essential oil (optional)

1. Melt the beeswax in the top of a double boiler or a pan on very low heat. (*Tip:* The smaller your beeswax pieces, the more easily they will melt.)

2. Once the beeswax has melted, add the infused oils. Stir well to combine, using as little heat as possible to keep the mixture liquid. (*Note:* It's normal for the beeswax to harden slightly when you add the oil. Allow it to melt again.)

3. Add the lavender essential oil, if using. Stir, then immediately pour into tins or glass jars.

4. Let the salve sit until it hardens. Label and store in a cool place. This salve will last for a year, if not longer.

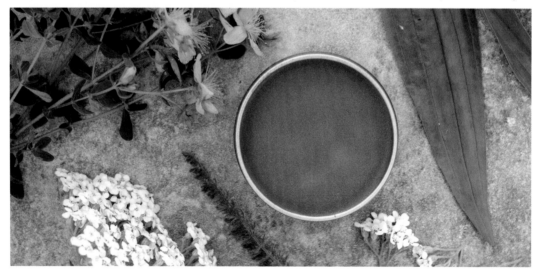

Cleanup tip: Use a paper towel to wipe out any container that held oil or salve. Remove as much as possible, then wash with hot, soapy water.

ST. JOHN'S WORT AND LEMON BALM TEA

The sunny and aromatic combination of St. John's wort and lemon balm is a simple way to soothe your nerves and uplift your mood. (However, remember that St. John's wort is not appropriate for people taking antidepressants.) This combination can also be taken daily to help prevent herpes outbreaks or to address symptoms of a cold or flu such as a sore throat.

Yield: 1½ cups

1½ cups water

1 teaspoon dried St. John's wort leaves and flowers

2 teaspoons dried lemon balm leaves

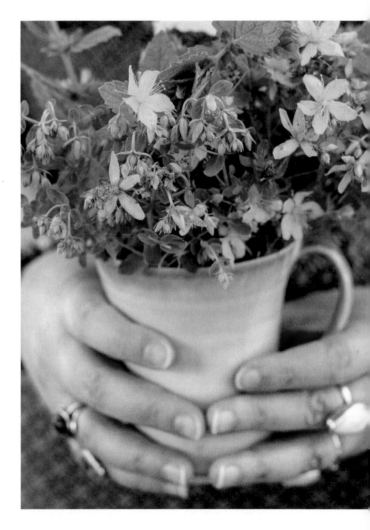

1. Heat 1½ cups of water in a small saucepan until boiling. Turn off the heat. Add the herbs and stir well. Cover and let infuse for 5 to 7 minutes.

2. Strain. Drink warm or lukewarm within 24 hours.

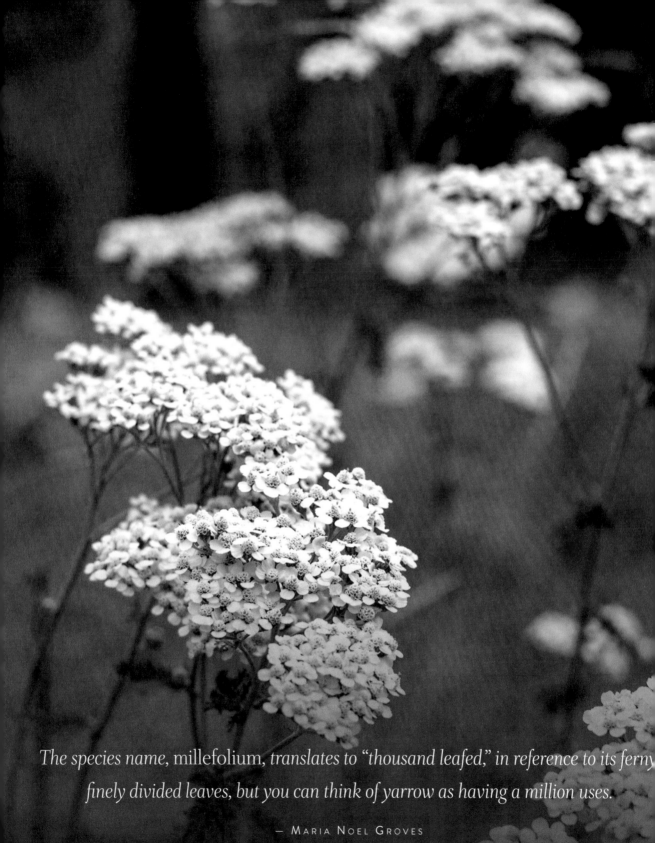

The species name, millefolium, translates to "thousand leafed," in reference to its ferny, finely divided leaves, but you can think of yarrow as having a million uses.

— MARIA NOEL GROVES

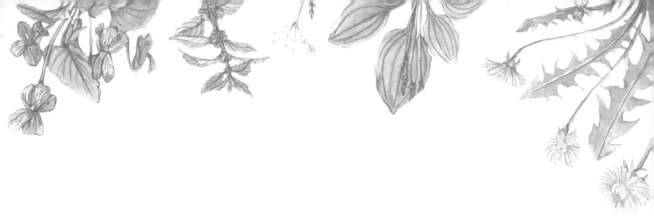

CHAPTER 19

YARROW

Commonly found all over the Northern Hemisphere, yarrow offers us a myriad of healing remedies for both acute and chronic conditions. This plant is especially worth knowing if you spend any time outdoors, as it can be used fresh in a variety of first-aid situations, from stopping bleeding to preventing the infection of wounds.

Botanical name: *Achillea millefolium*
Family: Asteraceae (aster)
Parts used: leaves, flowers, roots
Energetics: drying, cooling
Taste: bitter, pungent
Properties: antiseptic, anodyne, antimicrobial, aromatic, astringent, carminative, diuretic, inflammatory modulator, relaxing diaphoretic, styptic, vulnerary
Uses: dysmenorrhea, fevers, urinary tract and other infections, varicose veins, wounds
Preparations: oil, poultice, salve, smoke, steam, suppository, tea, tincture

As herbalist Guido Masé has pointed out, yarrow has been helping us since long before we were even human.[1] Archaeologists in Spain analyzed the dental tartar of a Neanderthal who lived 50,000 years ago and found that they had eaten yarrow![2] Because of yarrow's bitter taste, it's unlikely it would have been eaten as food; its presence is thought to have been an early sign of hominids using medicine.

Yarrow is seen frequently throughout human history as both a spiritual and a medicinal herb. Historical accounts say 50 yarrow stalks were used to configure hexagrams in the *I Ching*, or the Chinese *Book of Changes*. In the Western world, yarrow was revered as a battlefield herb and called many descriptive names such as staunchweed, woundwort, and herba militaris.

MEDICINAL PROPERTIES AND ENERGETICS

Energetically yarrow is a harmonizer that shows us how nuanced and complex herbal medicine can be. It doesn't simply do one thing or act in one way. Instead it can promote flow, or it can bring fluids to a stop. Although mostly cooling, it has some warming qualities. And while it is drying through its diuretic and diaphoretic qualities, it can also be moistening. Yarrow sidesteps any attempts to easily categorize its many gifts.

PLANT GIFTS

Harmonizes the Blood and Heals Wounds

Yarrow is perhaps most famous for its ability to stop external bleeding and heal wounds.

In Greek mythology, the centaur Chiron, who is credited with the creation of botany and herbal medicine, taught Achilles to use yarrow on warriors' wounds. This is the origin of the plant's genus name, *Achillea*. Yarrow has many virtues that make it the perfect wound herb. Used as a poultice, either fresh or dried, it promotes blood clotting and can stop bleeding. It's mildly astringent, helping to pull tissues together. And it is broadly antimicrobial, helping either to keep wounds clear of infection or to address signs of infection such as redness, heat, and pus. Herbalist 7Song has used yarrow extensively for first aid, including as a hot tea soak for wounds as well as animal bites and scratches that are prone to infection.[3]

Recent studies have confirmed yarrow's gifts for healing wounds. One study showed that oil infused with yarrow was effective in reducing skin inflammation.[4] Another demonstrated that yarrow in combination with St. John's wort increased the healing of episiotomy incisions.[5]

Yarrow is also used to heal wounds and infections in the mouth. In *Medicinal Plants of the Mountain West*, Michael Moore shares how he used yarrow root to relieve a toothache.[6] A distillate of yarrow has been found to heal the symptoms of oral mucositis in chemotherapy patients faster than simply using the routine solution.[7]

While yarrow is best known for stopping blood flow, herbalists also use it to move stagnant blood and promote blood flow. It is commonly used on varicose veins and hemorrhoids, both signs of stagnant blood. Physician Aviva Romm recommends yarrow as a topical treatment for varicosities related to pregnancy.[8] It is also used as a pelvic decongestant for uterine fibroids and delayed menses. One

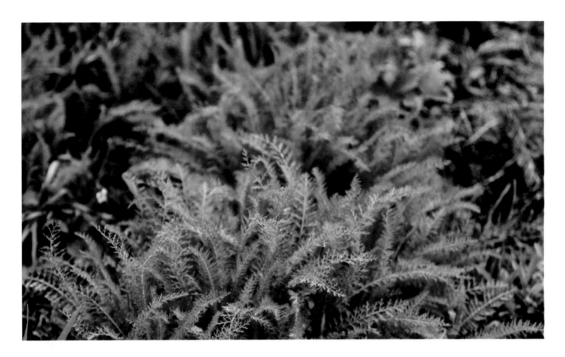

double-blind clinical trial found that yarrow was effective at relieving pain associated with menstrual cramps.[9]

Soothes Cold and Flu Symptoms

Taken as a hot tea, yarrow can make you sweat. It promotes circulation to the periphery, dilating capillaries and letting heat escape through the skin. Used in this way, it can be a powerful treatment supporting the fever process when someone is feeling hot and restless but isn't sweating. This is similar to how elderflowers are used (see Supports the Fever Process on page 152).

Yarrow tea, yarrow throat spray, or yarrow-infused honey can soothe a sore throat. The herb can also be used to dispel a cough. Eclectic herbalists used it specifically for coughs accompanied by a bloody sputum (although we recommend you consult a doctor for this).

Supports the Urinary System

Taken as a cool or lukewarm tea, yarrow acts as a diuretic and promotes the flow of urine. It's also antimicrobial and is frequently used to address urinary tract infections, often in combination with other herbs for best effects. It is commonly formulated with herbs like bearberry (*Arctostaphylos uva-ursi*), juniper (*Juniperus communis*), and echinacea (*Echinacea* spp.). Eclectic herbalists used yarrow for a variety of urinary complaints, including irritation of the kidneys and urethra, suppression of urine, and "chronic diseases of the urinary apparatus."[10]

Supports Digestion

Yarrow is aromatic and bitter, making it a wonderful ally to support digestion. It can be used in bitters blends or taken as a tea. Eclectic herbalists used yarrow for people with dysentery.

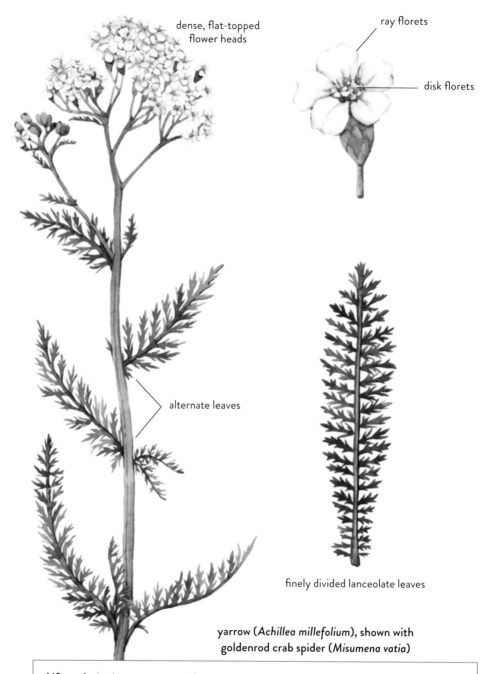

dense, flat-topped flower heads

ray florets

disk florets

alternate leaves

finely divided lanceolate leaves

yarrow (*Achillea millefolium*), shown with goldenrod crab spider (*Misumena vatia*)

Life cycle: herbaceous perennial
Reproduces by: seed, rhizome
Growth habit: clumping, with upright stems 1–3 feet tall
Habitat: coastal areas, disturbed areas, fields, forests, meadows, roadsides, rocky slopes
Sun: full sun to partial shade
Soil: variable; prefers dry or moist but well drained
USDA Hardiness Zones: 3–9

Repels Insects

The spicy aromatics of yarrow can be employed to deter insects such as mosquitoes. In a pinch we've seen this work simply by taking fresh yarrow leaves and flowers and rubbing them against our skin and clothes. You can also brew up your own bug spray using yarrow (see recipe on page 215).

HOW TO IDENTIFY

Yarrow may be found in various locations and elevations, from open fields to mountaintops to seashores. Spreading by rhizomes to form clumps, it has aromatic, dark-green or gray-green leaves. The leaves start from a basal rosette and grow alternately up an erect stem, becoming smaller toward the top. The lanceolate leaves are finely divided, giving them a feathery or fernlike appearance.

The flat-topped inflorescence consists of many small "flowers," each of which is actually a composite of small disk florets surrounded by petal-like ray florets. Although wild yarrow flowers are generally white, they can also be pink tinged. Cultivars of yarrow come in many colors and may also offer some medicinal benefits; however, since the taste and scent vary widely, it's best to stick with the wilder white variety.

ECOLOGICAL CONNECTIONS

Yarrow is a host plant for butterflies, including the painted lady (*Vanessa cardui*). Its flowers provide nectar and pollen to moths, butterflies, skippers, bees, wasps, hoverflies, and beetles. Yarrow can also attract predatory wasps, ladybugs, and spiders. Sheep and deer have been known to graze on the flower heads, and the foliage is an important food source for sage grouse (*Centrocercus urophasianus*) chicks.

The plant's extensive rhizomes can stabilize soil and prevent erosion. It can draw up nutrients from the soil, including potassium, phosphorus, and copper, and some gardeners use yarrow as a nutrient-rich mulch.

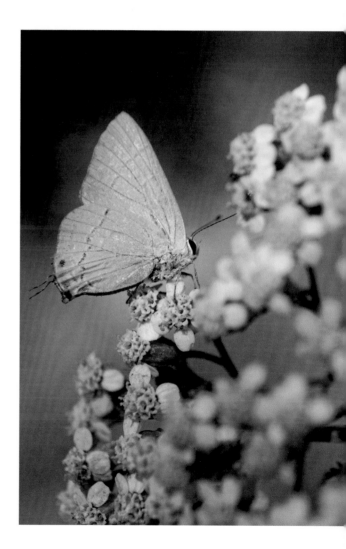

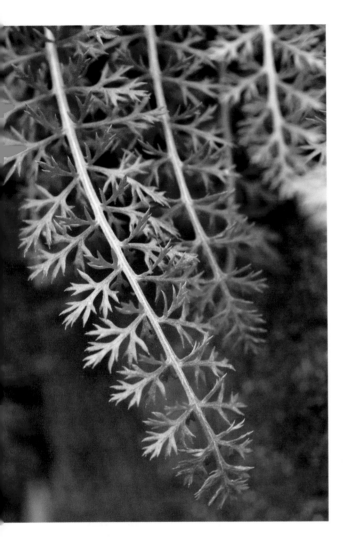

Yarrow reproduces by rhizomes and seeds. Encourage future generations by keeping the roots intact and leaving enough flowers so the plant can produce seeds, which are dispersed primarily by the wind.

Harvesting Cautions

Yarrow is superficially similar to Apiaceae family flowers like wild carrot (*Daucus carota*) and poison hemlock (*Conium maculatum*) (see Common Poisonous Plants on pages 36 to 37). Carefully examine the flowers to distinguish them. Unlike Apiaceae flowers, each small yarrow flower is composed of disk and ray florets.

GARDENING TIPS

Drought-tolerant yarrow can be propagated by root divisions of nearby plants in spring or fall. Direct seed in the garden from early spring through autumn. Yarrow likes to slowly spread via underground rhizomes, so give it the space it desires but be prepared to restrain it now and then. Avoid colorful cultivars if using medicinally.

HOW TO HARVEST

The leaves can be gathered throughout the growing season as needed. Harvest the flowers just after they bloom or as long as they remain aromatic. To gather leaves, use your fingers to pluck just a few leaves from each plant. To harvest both flowers and leaves, use scissors or pruning shears to snip stalks near the base, leaving the roots so the plant can regrow.

USING YARROW IN YOUR LIFE

Yarrow can be made into herbal medicine in many ways. It is soluble in water, oil, alcohol, and witch hazel distillate. It can simply be used as an external poultice for addressing injuries and wounds. Or it can be made into a tea or infused into an oil or alcohol to use on wounds. Prepared as a hot tea, yarrow promotes sweating. As a cool tea, it promotes diuresis. As an herbal steam, it can decrease congestion in the lungs and sinuses as well as promote healthy skin; see Mullein and Yarrow Facial Steam on page 263.

Recommended Amounts

- *Tea (dried):* 3 to 9 grams daily

- *Tincture (fresh leaves and flowers):* 1:2, 95% alcohol; 2 to 4 ml, 3 times daily

- *Tincture (dried leaves and flowers):* 1:5, 40% alcohol

Special Considerations

- Yarrow may not be safe during pregnancy.

- Rarely, some people find they are allergic to yarrow; those with severe allergies to the Asteraceae family should approach yarrow with caution.

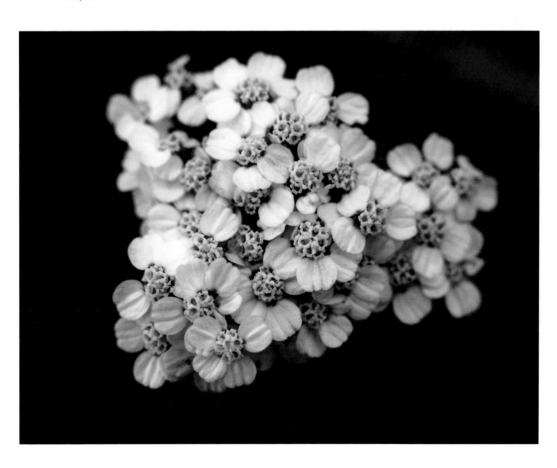

YARROW AND ELDERFLOWER TEA

This is our version of a very old Western herbal formula for colds and flu. It's effective for relieving general discomfort, but gentle enough for most people and even children. Both elderflowers and yarrow are relaxing diaphoretics, making this blend especially well suited for people with fevers who feel hot and restless. For best results, sip this frequently over the course of an hour or so, rather than all at once. Putting it in a small thermos will keep it warm.

Peppermint, spearmint, lemon balm, or even bee balm (*Monarda fistulosa*) are wonderful mints to use in this blend. This is a strong-tasting tea. If you have a sensitive palate, you might want to start with less yarrow or steep it for less time.

Yield: 2 cups

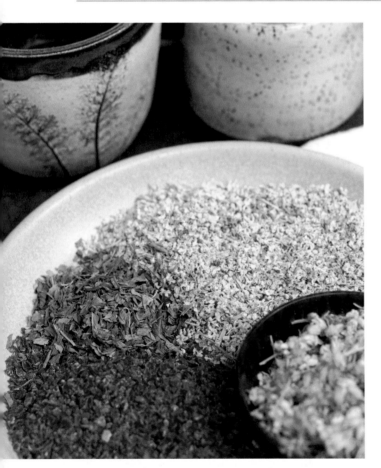

¼ cup dried yarrow leaves and flowers

¼ cup dried elderflowers

2 tablespoons dried rose hips, cut and sifted, or ¼ cup dried whole rose hips

Big pinch of dried mint, any type

2 cups water

Honey, to taste (optional)

1. Place all of the herbs in a pint jar.

2. Bring 2 cups of water to a boil. Pour the water over the herbs, cover, and let steep for 30 minutes.

3. Strain. Add honey to taste, if desired. Sip while warm.

YARROW BUG SPRAY

The strong aromatics of yarrow leaves and flowers are an excellent bug deterrent. We recommend that you crush and smell the yarrow you're using to make sure it has a strong scent. If not, find fresher yarrow. This spray is a convenient, safe, and effective way to keep mosquitoes at bay. The oil and vegetable glycerin keep yarrow's scent on your skin longer than witch hazel alone will. This is best applied directly to the skin; it could leave oil stains if sprayed on clothing. For best results, reapply every couple of hours.

Yield: 1½ cups

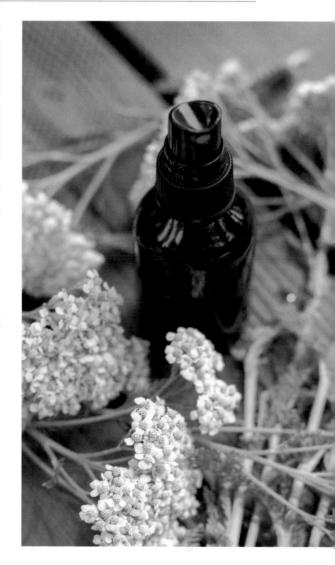

1½ cups (approximately 22 grams) freshly dried yarrow leaves and flowers

2 cups witch hazel distillate

1 tablespoon carrier oil (e.g., olive oil, apricot kernel oil)

1 tablespoon vegetable glycerin

45 to 60 drops (0.4 to 0.6 teaspoons) lavender (*Lavandula angustifolia*) essential oil (optional)

1. Place the yarrow in a pint jar.

2. Mix the witch hazel distillate, carrier oil, and vegetable glycerin in a small bowl. Pour enough of this mixture into the jar to fill the jar and submerge the herbs completely. Stir well, then tightly cover and label it.

3. Store the jar in a cool, dark place for at least 2 weeks. Shake the jar daily for the first week. In the first few days, the dried yarrow will soak up some of the liquid. Add more witch hazel as necessary to keep the jar full.

4. Strain the tincture through cheesecloth, squeezing it well to extract all the liquid. If desired, add the lavender essential oil and stir well.

5. Use a funnel to pour the bug spray into clean spray bottles. Label and store in a cool, dark place.

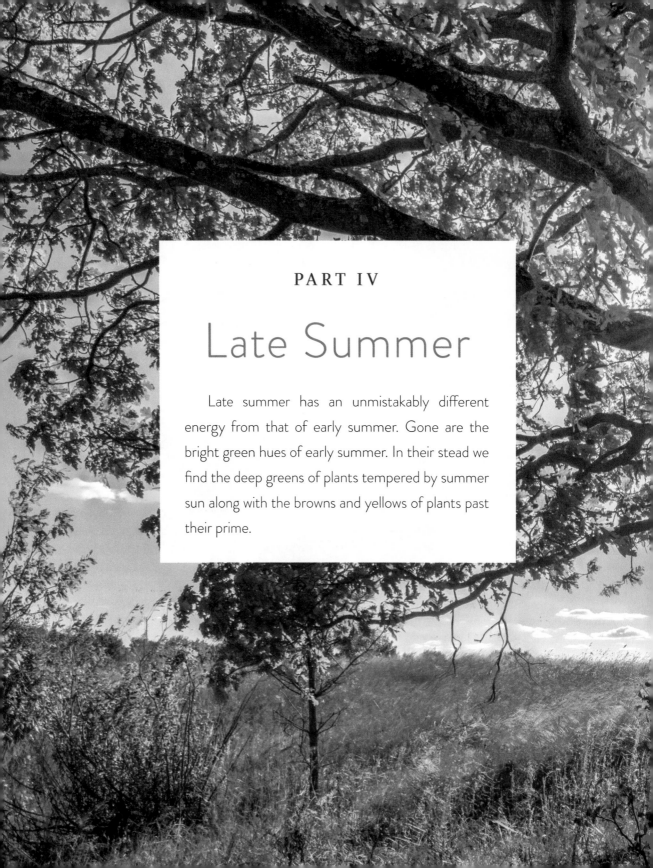

PART IV

Late Summer

Late summer has an unmistakably different energy from that of early summer. Gone are the bright green hues of early summer. In their stead we find the deep greens of plants tempered by summer sun along with the browns and yellows of plants past their prime.

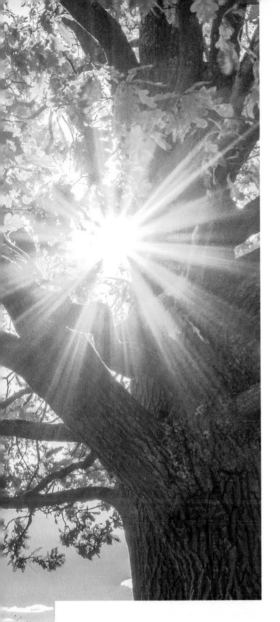

While spring and early-summer wildflowers have withered, late-blooming flowers persevere, bringing a last hurrah of color to fields and roadsides. Yellow hues permeate the landscape, from sprays of goldenrod to the lengthening rays of the sun.

In some places late summer is a time of harvest, a time to reap and celebrate the energy we've sown. Farmers markets explode with produce like peppers, melons, and okra. Like diligent squirrels preparing for winter, we preserve, can, dehydrate, and freeze the plants we have gathered. Harvest dinners bring together communities as we offer gratitude for the growing season.

In other places late summer is a time of slowness as both people and plants languish in the heat. Here we feel the pause between the bounty of early summer and the harvest of fall crops. This is a season to nourish ourselves with foods and remedies that offer cooling refreshment. With our wildcrafting tools set aside, we can fill our evenings with gatherings of family and friends.

Are you already longing for cooler temperatures, cozy sweaters, and pumpkin flavors? Or are you savoring the last days of summer warmth? In nature the only certainty is change; autumn will come soon enough. Resist the urge to look ahead, and instead immerse yourself in this golden time.

Late-Summer Activities

- Hike or swim
- Pick a plant bouquet
- Listen to cicadas or crickets
- Watch the clouds
- Sleep under the stars

- Make jams, pickles, or canned tomatoes
- Draw pictures of seeds
- Throw a cocktail party
- Keep a journal (see Chapter 7)

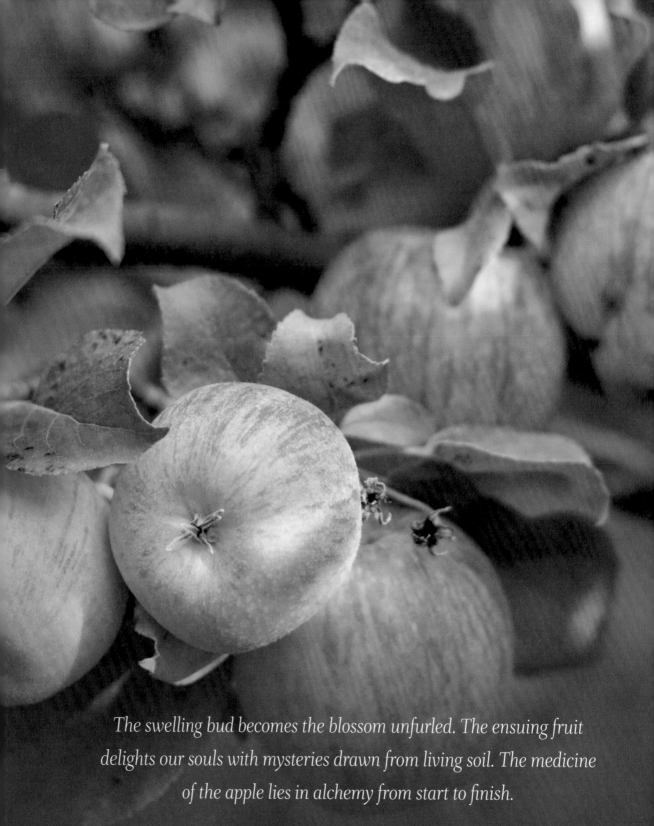

The swelling bud becomes the blossom unfurled. The ensuing fruit delights our souls with mysteries drawn from living soil. The medicine of the apple lies in alchemy from start to finish.

— MICHAEL PHILLIPS

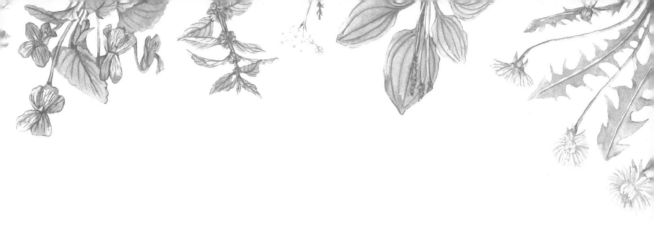

CHAPTER 20

APPLE

Those large, sweet fruits of the cultivated apple tree get all the love and attention. Millions of tons are grown and shipped around the world every single year. But what these mass-produced fruits offer in convenience, they often lack in style. Apples from feral apple trees or artisanal orchards most likely have more flavor and nutrients. Access to an abundant supply of local apples can be a blessing of many treats, from apple desserts to apple cider vinegar to homemade fermented hard ciders.

Botanical name: *Malus* spp.
Family: Rosaceae (rose)
Parts used: fruit, twigs, bark, leaves
Energetics: fruit: cooling, moistening; twigs/bark/leaves: cooling, drying
Taste: sour, sweet
Properties: astringent, digestive, nutritive
Uses: constipation (fruit), diarrhea (twigs, bark), food, "keep the doctor away," tighten and tone tissues
Preparations: apple cider vinegar, fermented alcohol, food, tincture, wash

Apple trees originated in central Asia, in the mountains of Kazakhstan. Spread through the spice trade and then by colonialists, the apple is now found in every temperate climate in the world. It has been carefully cultivated for hard cider and sweet fruit for as many as 9,000 years.[1] Crab apples, the small, bitter, and more astringent cousins to domesticated apples, are often more nutrient dense but aren't as likely to be palatable.

MEDICINAL PROPERTIES AND ENERGETICS

Apples are delicious, nutritive, and cooling. The twigs and leaves are astringent and drying in nature, while the fruits are juicy and flavorful. Apple-based preparations have been used for hundreds of years to address digestive complaints and fevers and to satisfy a sweet tooth.

PLANT GIFTS

Leaves and Bark Act as Astringents

Like other members of the rose family, apples are astringent plants that can be used to tighten and tone lax tissues. The leaves are less astringent than the bark (but easier to harvest). A tea made from the leaves and bark can be swished to address mouth sores. It can also be ingested to tone the tissues of the digestive tract, part of a formula for addressing ulcers or excessive diarrhea.

The astringent qualities of apple can also tighten and tone the esophageal sphincter.

When this sphincter doesn't close tightly, acid from the stomach can leak into the esophagus, causing heartburn. Herbalist jim mcdonald, who has written and taught extensively about using apples as medicine, suggests a formula of apple leaves and bark, plantain, and mallow as a multipronged approach to addressing heartburn.[2]

A tea made from the leaves and bark can be used as a wash to address skin wounds and inflammation, including cuts, scratches, insect bites, and rashes.

Fruits Keep the Doctor Away

Apples have long been valued for their nutrients. They are notably high in vitamins C and E, fiber, and minerals like potassium and magnesium. They also contain a wide range of phytonutrients, especially in their peels.[3] However, not all apples are created equal. Different types vary widely in how many nutrients they contain. Wild apples or crab apples can contain hundreds more phytonutrients than their domesticated cousins. Unfortunately, those varieties can be super sour, astringent, or bitter and a challenge to eat. Tastier crab apples do exist, however. The only way to know is by taking a small bite out of the crab apples you find.

Author Jo Robinson, in her book *Eating on the Wild Side*, reports that Braeburn, Fuji, Gala, Granny Smith, Honeycrisp, and McIntosh apple cultivars are high in phytonutrients.[4] Among those with the least phytonutrients are Golden Delicious and Pink Lady. Commercial growers often heavily spray apples with chemicals. When possible, buy organic apples (or apples that you know haven't been sprayed) so you can eat the peels, which are full of phytonutrients.

Fruits Can Be Medicine for Children

Apple's sweet taste and healing gifts make it a good match for children, especially when dealing with a variety of digestive complaints. Applesauce is a delicious and easy-to-digest food that can be especially helpful after stomach upset. Taken by itself, it can gently support bowel movements to address constipation. If loose stools or diarrhea is the issue, then stir some ground cinnamon into the sauce. One study showed that children with mild dehydration caused by gastritis were better hydrated with diluted apple juice followed by preferred fluids than children given an electrolyte blend.[5]

HOW TO IDENTIFY

Apple trees have grayish-brown bark that may be scaly or smooth. The leaves grow alternately and are elliptic or ovate with serrate or crenate margins. They may have fuzzy or downy undersides. The flowers grow in clusters, are white to pink in color, and each have five petals. Fruits range in color from greenish yellow to red. When cut in half along the equator, a fruit will have five seeds arranged in a star shape. Fruit size varies: crab apples grow to less than 2 inches in diameter, while other species are generally 3 to 4 inches in diameter.

THE COSTS OF SPRAYING CHEMICALS

Many years ago apple blossoms helped me (Rosalee) make the switch to buying only organic foods. I was driving through eastern Washington in May, giddy with all the beautiful orchards full of apple blossoms. What a sight!

I pulled into a park to eat lunch, and just as I got out of the car, I noticed a sign that warned pregnant people and other sensitive populations to avoid this park while the surrounding orchards were being sprayed, as the chemicals would be carried by the wind.

I got back in my car. Shortly after that I saw people in hazmat suits warning passersby that chemicals were being sprayed. Through the trees I could see other people, also in hazmat suits, driving large tank trucks with huge, billowing blasts of chemicals surrounding them. I became a lot less giddy about all those beautiful blossoms.

I was fairly young at that point, and I didn't have a lot of money. But from that moment on, I only shopped organic. I realized that not only did I not want my own food sprayed with harmful chemicals, but I didn't want to support those chemicals being blown into the air, seeping into our soils, poisoning farmworkers, or even being produced in a factory.

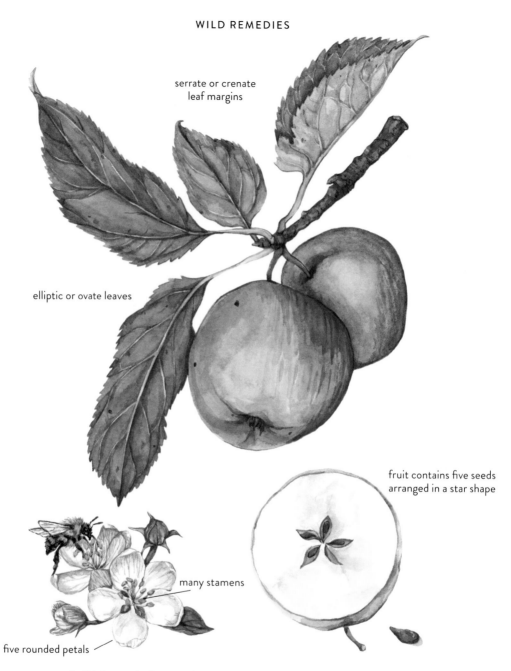

serrate or crenate
leaf margins

elliptic or ovate leaves

fruit contains five seeds
arranged in a star shape

many stamens

five rounded petals

apple (*Malus* spp.), shown with common eastern bumble bee (*Bombus impatiens*)

Life cycle: deciduous woody perennial
Reproduces by: seed, sucker
Growth habit: tree up to 40 feet tall but often smaller
Habitat: fields, hedgerows, orchards, parks, forests
Sun: full sun
Soil: well drained, moist, slightly acidic
USDA Hardiness Zones: 4–8

What's in a Name? Juice versus Cider

In the United States, the word *cider* typically describes fresh, raw, and unfiltered apple juice. In all other parts of the world, cider is more commonly used to describe a fermented and alcoholic beverage (aka *hard cider* in the United States). Commercial apple juice in the United States is often made from a concentrate or is highly filtered. Unfortunately, that filtering process removes a lot of the phytonutrients in the juice. Jo Robinson says that unfiltered apple juice contains up to four times more nutrients than filtered.[6] If you can see through the juice, it has been filtered. Look for a cloudy variety instead.

ECOLOGICAL CONNECTIONS

Some apple trees are self-pollinating, but most need to be cross-pollinated with an apple tree of a different variety growing nearby. The fragrant flowers attract pollinators such as hoverflies, honeybees, bumblebees, and solitary bees that may nest in the ground near the tree. Certain moths lay eggs on the leaves and fruit, which serve as food for the larvae. Wasps may then hunt these larvae as well as other insects on the tree. Birds and mammals like to eat the fruits and help to disperse the seeds through their droppings.

HOW TO HARVEST

If apples grow near you, go beyond the grocery store to find feral trees or buy direct from orchardists. Feral trees may be found in old orchards and along trails and in parks where people toss apple cores.

Twigs and leaves may be gathered at any time, but the best medicine will come from new growth in the spring. To gather twigs, use pruning shears to clip the tips of new growth. Leaves may be gathered by hand. Apples are ripe when they have reached their mature color

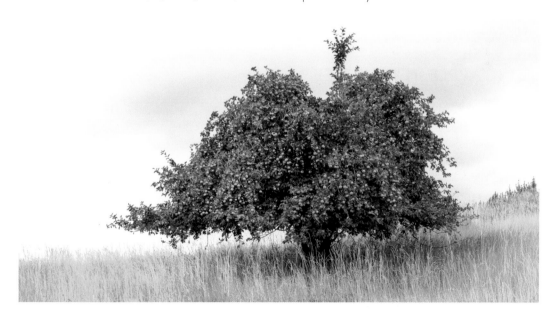

(this varies by cultivar); you can also taste an apple or two to find out whether they are ripe. To pick an apple, use your hands or a fruit picker to gently twist—not yank or pull—the fruit. You can also take apples from the ground as long as they aren't too bruised or insect damaged.

Be sure to leave some fruit on the tree (or windfall apples on the ground) so it can reproduce—and for the benefit of wildlife.

GARDENING TIPS

Apple is the most widely adapted deciduous fruit, grown in almost every climate, but most standard varieties do require 900 to 1,200 hours of temperatures below 45°F for most standard varieties. Pollination benefits from two or more varieties. To remain productive, apple trees require annual winter pruning and control for codling moth and apple maggot. Dwarf apples are ideal for small urban settings but do need support of a fence or trellis. If you live in the United States, select the state Cooperative Extension's recommended cultivars for your region.

USING APPLE IN YOUR LIFE

Fresh from the tree or baked into dessert, apples are a delicious treat, like candy straight from nature. See above for tips on how to get the most nutrient-dense apples. Apples that ripen later in the season will keep in your refrigerator for many months, while those that ripen in the summer tend to have a much shorter storage life. If you have a bountiful harvest, consider making applesauce or apple butter. To retain the most nutrients, don't peel the apples. Instead, use an immersion blender to puree the skins. Apples can also be cut into thin slices and dehydrated.

Crab apples vary widely in flavor. They are high in pectin and can be boiled down to make a homemade pectin for jams and jellies. They can also be used to make verjus, hard cider, and vinegar.

Apple bark and leaves can be used as a decoction, both internally and externally. They can also be made into an alcohol extract.

Recommended Amounts

- *Decoction (bark):* 1 to 4 fluid ounces, 3 times daily[7]

- *Tincture (bark):* 1:2, 40% alcohol; 5 to 15 drops, 3 to 5 times daily[8]

Special Considerations

- Avoid eating apple seeds as they have concentrated amounts of toxins called cyanogenic glycosides.

- Smaller amounts of hydrocyanic acid are found in the leaves and bark but should not be a problem when used in reasonable amounts.

WILD ROASTED APPLES

Here's a sweet taste of harvest season with some wild sidekicks! The mallow fruits add a chewy texture to the soft roasted apples, while the roasted dandelion roots offer a slightly bitter taste that balances all that sweetness. Wrap it all up in cinnamon, and you've got your new favorite treat!

Yield: 2 to 4 servings

1 tablespoon honey

1 tablespoon butter

2 teaspoons ground cinnamon

1 tablespoon fresh mallow fruits, papery coverings removed if desired

1 tablespoon minced fresh dandelion root

2 medium apples

1. Preheat the oven to 350°F.

2. Gently heat the honey and butter in a small saucepan. Once melted, add the cinnamon and stir well.

3. Mix the mallow fruits and dandelion root into the honey–butter mixture. Stir until everything is well coated.

4. Core and cut the apples into ¼-inch slices. Place the apple slices in an oven-safe baking pan. Pour the honey–butter mixture over the apples and stir well.

5. Bake for 30 minutes, stirring halfway through, or until the apples are tender.

6. Serve warm.

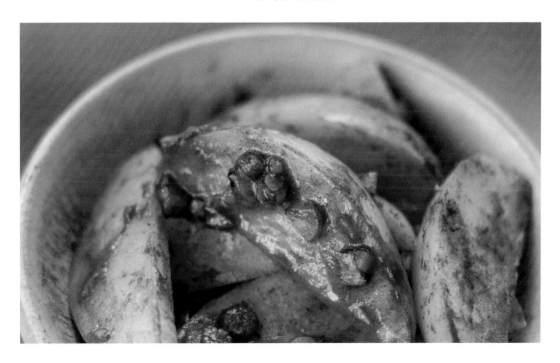

APPLE AND BERRY CONCENTRATE

This mixture concentrates both the delicious flavor and the medicinal qualities of apples, blueberries, and hawthorn (*Crataegus* spp.). Think of it as an antioxidant-rich spoonful of yumminess that you can take as is or drizzle on yogurt, bread, or ice cream. Hawthorn berries can be foraged or purchased dried from apothecaries.

This recipe came to us from jim mcdonald, who says, "You can absolutely add spices like cinnamon, allspice, clove, or whatever suits your tastes, though I do suggest trying it with just the apple juice and berries to start. When the apple juice is reduced, the mildly spicy flavors naturally found in apples are concentrated, and it's nice to taste those on their own." See more from jim at herbcraft.org.

Yield: 1 quart

1 gallon apple juice, filtered or unfiltered

1 pound blueberries, frozen or fresh

1 pound dried hawthorn berries

1. Combine the apple juice, blueberries, and hawthorn berries in a pot. Bring to a very low simmer and reduce the juice to about half a gallon. This may take 90 to 120 minutes.

2. Strain out the berries.

3. Return the juice to the pot and, again over low heat, reduce the juice down to 4 cups. This may take 45 to 90 minutes.

4. Transfer to a container for storage. This syrup will last in the refrigerator for 2 weeks. Consider reserving some for immediate use and freezing the rest for later. Take 1 to 2 spoonfuls a day, or as desired.

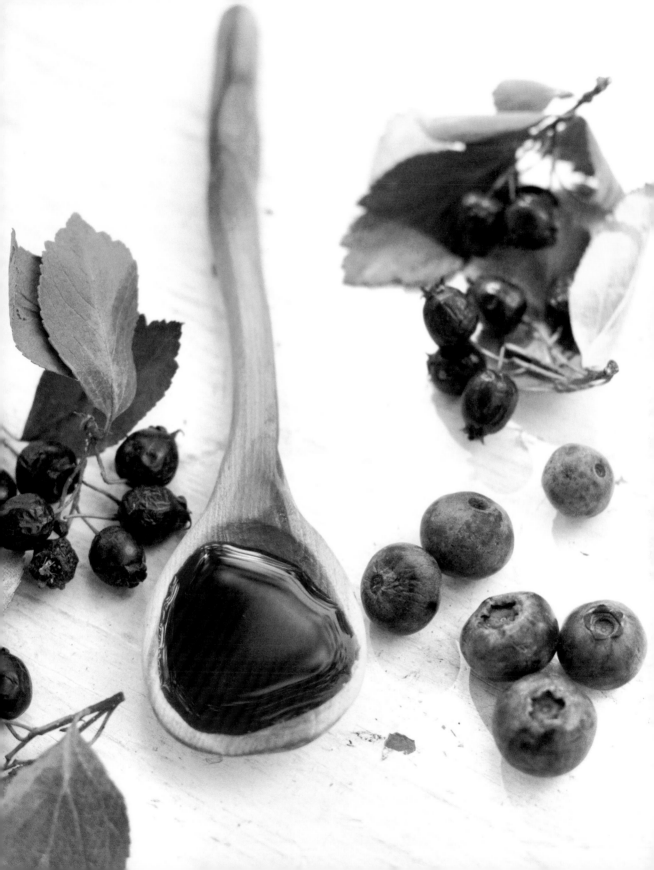

APPLE SCRAP VINEGAR

Making your own fruit scrap vinegar can be a deeply sensory process as you see, smell, and taste the different stages of your ferment. First there's the funky phase, when wild yeasts consume the fruit and sugar, spawning curious smells and bubbles. In the next phase, *Acetobacter* bacteria get to work, and your brew turns increasingly sour until, voilà, you have vinegar!

You can make this vinegar using apple cores, peels, or bruised fruit as long as it is not rotten or moldy. Sugar aids fermentation, and we've had success using plain white sugar, coconut sugar, molasses, and even honey (though it may take longer).

Yield: Variable

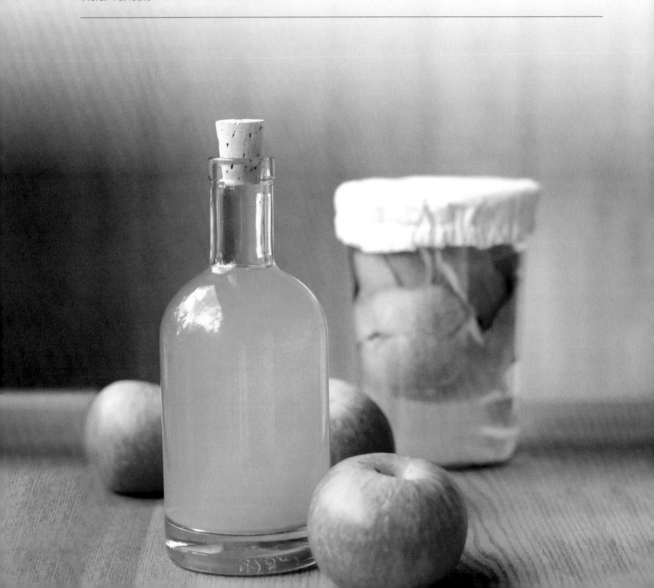

1. Put the apple scraps in a glass jar, ceramic crock, or other nonreactive container. They should more or less fill the container halfway. (*Tip:* If you don't have enough apple scraps ready at once, collect them in the freezer.)

2. Dissolve sugar in chlorine-free water, using a ratio of 1 tablespoon of sugar per 1 cup of water. Pour the sugar water over the apples, leaving a few inches of space at the top of the container. Cover the container so that it is exposed to oxygen yet protected from flies; we recommend cheesecloth, a dish towel, or a coffee filter secured with a rubber band.

3. Let the jar sit at room temperature, out of direct sunlight, for 1 week. At least once a day, vigorously stir the mixture with a nonmetal utensil; this helps to prevent mold from growing. Eventually bubbles will form, the liquid will turn darker and cloudy, and it will smell a bit alcoholic—this is fermentation in action!

4. After 1 week, strain out the fruit. Pour the liquid into a nonreactive container and loosely cover it as before. Let it sit at room temperature, out of direct sunlight, for another 2 to 4 weeks (we usually keep it in a cupboard). Check it from time to time, using your senses. As the *Acetobacter* bacteria convert the alcohol into acetic acid, the smell and taste will become more sour. You may also see a gelatinous, gray-brown substance on the surface; this is a vinegar "mother" and a good sign.

5. When the liquid smells and tastes like vinegar, it's ready. Strain it if you wish, and transfer it to a clean, airtight bottle. (If you strained out a vinegar mother, you can use it to jump-start a new batch of vinegar.) Store the vinegar in a cool, dark place.

Apple scraps to half-fill a container of your choosing

Sugar

Chlorine-free water (see note on water, page 67)

Note: Homemade vinegar is best used for cooking, salad dressings, and other recipes that will be eaten promptly. We do not recommend using it for canning and other types of food preservation, unless you have an acid test kit and are able to determine that your vinegar has at least 5 percent acetic acid.

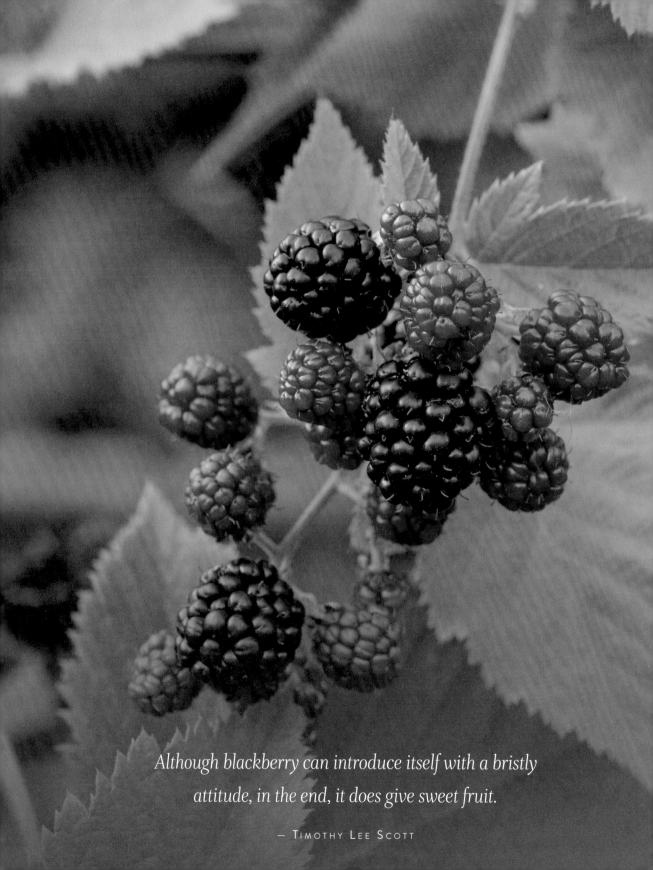

Although blackberry can introduce itself with a bristly attitude, in the end, it does give sweet fruit.

— TIMOTHY LEE SCOTT

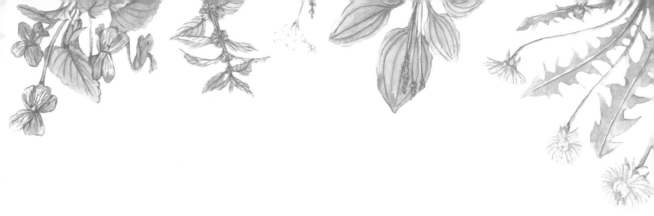

CHAPTER 21

BLACKBERRY AND RASPBERRY

When plump, juicy berries are dripping from the prickly vines of wild brambles, you know the harvest season is here. If you are lucky enough to spend some time at a large berry patch, you'll find it offers food and refuge to many, from the birds gorging on the sweet fruits to the pollinators visiting the abundant flowers to the rabbits who've created a maze through the thorny thicket. With some caution and awareness of the thorns, those ripe fruits can be easily plucked off the bush and, more than likely, into your mouth. If you're able to bring a basket of berries to your kitchen, you can create countless sweet treats.

Botanical names: *Rubus* spp. (including *R. allegheniensis*, *R. armeniacus*, *R. idaeus*, *R. occidentalis*, *R. ursinus*, and many other species)

Family: Rosaceae (rose)

Parts used: leaves, berries, roots

Energetics: cooling, drying

Taste: sour

Properties: astringent, nutritive, tissue toner

Uses: diarrhea, dysmenorrhea, food, leukorrhea, mouth sores, preparation for labor, type 2 diabetes

Preparations: food, tea, tincture

Hundreds of different kinds of *Rubus* berries may be found throughout the temperate Northern Hemisphere, and people have assuredly been using them as food and medicine for as long as we've existed. Through the help of humans, other mammals, and birds, the seeds have been eaten and then deposited, creating many berry briars across the world.

MEDICINAL PROPERTIES AND ENERGETICS

The many species of blackberries and raspberries each have their own gifts, but their similar chemical makeup gives them many common uses. High in tannins, these plants are often used as medicine for their astringent nature. Astringent herbs tighten and tone tissues. You've probably experienced this sensation if you've ever eaten an unripe banana or had a strong cup of black tea. That dry feeling that comes with astringency is your tissues tightening and not allowing fluids to pass through. This effect happens not only in your mouth, but also in the mucous membranes throughout your body. Astringent herbs can be used to reduce excess discharges and hold moisture within the body.

PLANT GIFTS

Leaves and Roots Act as Astringents

Astringency is an important action in herbal medicine. Many plants that are high in tannins have some degree of astringency. Oaks are heavy hitters on the astringency scale, but strong doesn't necessarily mean better, as their bark can cause adverse effects when taken over time or in high doses. Herbalists prize blackberries and raspberries for being just right on that astringency scale. The leaves and roots noticeably tighten and tone tissues without overdoing it. They can often be taken long term.

A tea from the leaves can be used as a mouthwash and gargle to reduce inflammation (swollen gums, sore throat) and to tighten tissues like spongy gums and mouth ulcers (canker sores). If seasonal allergies have you feeling like a leaky faucet, blackberries and raspberries can tone sinus tissues to arrest that copious clear mucus. They can be taken as a tea to encourage sphincters to pull together, which can be an important protocol for heartburn (to prevent stomach acids from escaping the stomach through the esophageal sphincter). They can be combined with wound-healing herbs (like plantain) to address ulcers within the digestive system. And they can tighten and tone the lower digestive tract to resolve noninfectious diarrhea and shrink hemorrhoids. Like the Eclectic herbalists of the late 1800s, modern-day herbalists use it for leukorrhea (excessive noninfectious vaginal discharge) and spermatorrhea (excessive involuntary ejaculation). Phew! That's a lot of benefits from astringency!

Berries and Leaves Provide Nutrition

Both the leaves and the berries of various species are nutrient dense. The most detailed nutritional information is known about red raspberry (*Rubus idaeus*). The leaves are high in magnesium and manganese.[1] They also contain phytonutrients like flavonoids and tannins. Red raspberries, black raspberries, and blackberries are exceptionally high in fiber for a fruit, containing about five to six grams of fiber per half cup.[2] They are also rich in flavonoids and vitamin C. In *Eating on the Wild Side*, Jo Robinson writes, "As a rough estimate, berries have four times more antioxidant activity than the majority of other fruits, ten times more than most vegetables, and forty times more than some cereals. We need to eat more of them."[3]

Berries and Leaves Benefit Heart Health and Type 2 Diabetes

Eating berries can be a delicious way to support a healthy heart as well as address inflammation and high blood sugar in people with insulin resistance and type 2 diabetes. Numerous studies have shown that regularly eating red and black raspberries can improve heart health by reducing high blood pressure and improving cholesterol levels.[4] Black raspberries have been shown to have health benefits for people with prediabetes and type 2 diabetes. One study showed that they controlled blood sugar and reduced vascular inflammation in patients with prediabetes.[5] Another trial showed numerous improvements, including reduced arterial stiffness, for people with metabolic syndrome, a cluster of conditions that increase the risk for cardiovascular disease and diabetes.[6]

And it's not just the berries that have benefits. One study cautions that red raspberry leaf is so effective at addressing blood sugar levels that it may lead to a reduced dependency on insulin. This study was aimed at people with gestational diabetes and recommends they keep their insulin levels closely monitored.[7]

Red Raspberry Leaves Tone the Uterus

References to using red raspberry leaves in Western herbalism date back hundreds of years. However, only recently have the leaves been used to support uterine health. Herbalists recommend regularly drinking red raspberry leaf tea to alleviate painful cramps during menstruation. The leaves are often combined with nettle and spearmint and taken long term for the best benefit.

Red raspberry is often used to support the uterus in the last trimester of pregnancy and to help prepare for birth. It is also valued for its ability to restore uterine integrity during postpartum recovery. Eclectic herbalists recommended red raspberry for uterine prolapse (however, we recommend seeing a doctor for this).[8]

HOW TO IDENTIFY

Each *Rubus* species has its own identifying characteristics, and you should consult a local guide for specific information. Fortunately, all are edible. Generally speaking, blackberries and raspberries have thorny stems or canes that can trail on the ground or grow into dense thickets. Depending on the species, the leaves may be trifoliate or palmate with each leaf having three, five, or seven ovate leaflets. The leaflets have serrate or doubly serrate margins. Flowers are white or pink with five petals, five sepals, and many stamens. The fruits are composed of drupelets, each containing a seed. Blackberries have a fleshy white or green core, while raspberries are hollow in the center.

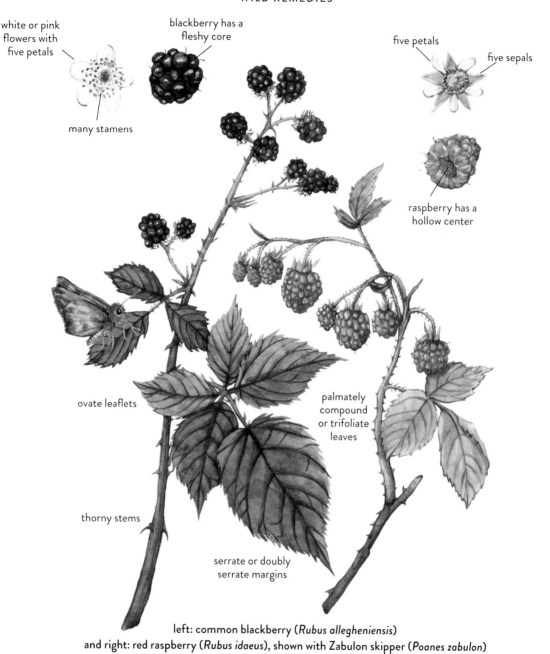

white or pink flowers with five petals

blackberry has a fleshy core

many stamens

five petals

five sepals

raspberry has a hollow center

ovate leaflets

palmately compound or trifoliate leaves

thorny stems

serrate or doubly serrate margins

left: common blackberry (*Rubus allegheniensis*)
and right: red raspberry (*Rubus idaeus*), shown with Zabulon skipper (*Poanes zabulon*)

Life cycle: woody perennial with biennial canes
Reproduces by: seed, stolon
Growth habit: thorny, sprawling bushes up to 20 feet
Habitat: disturbed areas, fields, forests, hedgerows, moist slopes and canyons, old homesteads, riparian areas, riverbanks, roadsides, thickets, vacant lots, woodlands
Sun: full sun to partial shade
Soil: fertile, well drained, moist
USDA Hardiness Zones: 3–9, depending on variety

ECOLOGICAL CONNECTIONS

Blackberry and raspberry plants provide shelter for birds as well as rabbits, squirrels, and other small mammals. The flowers attract pollinators like honeybees, native bees, butterflies, and skippers. Moth caterpillars eat the foliage and stems. Many animals eat the fruits and disperse the seeds, including birds, chipmunks, squirrels, raccoons, skunks, foxes, and coyotes. Passing through a bird's gut can even improve the germination rate of blackberry seeds.

In the United States, the nonnative Himalayan blackberry (*R. armeniacus*) has spread vigorously, disrupting ecosystems and crowding out native plants. At the same time, we may consider its ecological benefits. In *Invasive Plant Medicine*, Timothy Lee Scott writes that blackberry "protects those places that have been ravaged by improper logging, clearing, or other human actions. Its presence in these areas helps minimize soil erosion and creates a barrier to allow the land to rest and rejuvenate."[9]

HOW TO HARVEST

Blackberry and raspberry leaves are best picked before the plant flowers. Use your fingers or pruning shears to clip the leaves, taking care not to take too many from any one plant. The berries may be harvested whenever they taste ripe and come off the bush easily. They may not all ripen at the same time, so you can return to the bush several times throughout the season. Place the berries in a shallow layer in a sturdy container so they don't get crushed. Harvest the roots in autumn, after the plant has fruited and starts to die back. Use pruning shears to clear out the aboveground parts and a shovel to dig the root.

If the *Rubus* species is native to your area, harvest judiciously and leave enough flowers for pollinators and fruits for wildlife to eat and disperse the seeds. In addition to reproducing by seed, some blackberries and raspberries send out runners, which you can transplant. If the *Rubus* species is considered invasive, you may be doing local native plants a favor by harvesting leaves, berries, and roots more zealously—and avoiding propagation.

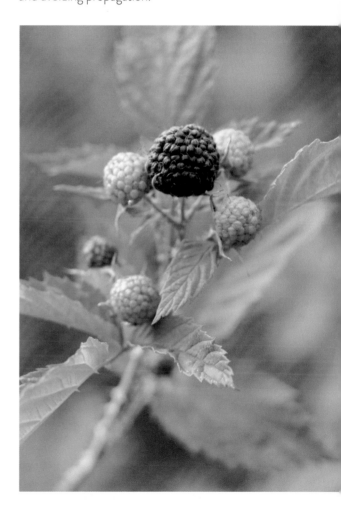

Harvesting Cautions

Gather carefully to avoid the thorns. Long sleeves, long pants, and gloves come in handy here.

GARDENING TIPS

For blackberries, selecting regionally adapted varieties is the key to growing success, but choose thornless blackberries whenever possible! Many varieties produce canes with trailing tendencies and are best grown on a trellis. Canes are biennial, and the berries appear on the second-year canes. To maintain steady production, early-autumn pruning of second-year canes is needed. First-year canes are trained (secured) to the trellis for the following year's production. Regular watering is necessary.

For raspberries, there are two types: summer bearing, which fruits once in early summer, and ever bearing (aka fall bearing), which fruits in early autumn and the following summer. Both types require annual pruning to remove older, dead canes, but the ever-bearing type has the easier option of cutting all canes after harvest. A trellis makes harvesting and pruning easier. Raspberries are self-fertile and do not require additional varieties for pollination. Well-drained soil is critical; regular watering and mulch help maintain moisture. If you live in the United States, select the state Cooperative Extension's recommended cultivars for your region.

USING BLACKBERRY AND RASPBERRY IN YOUR LIFE

The berries are undoubtedly food as medicine! Both blackberries and raspberries have delicate fruits that crush easily and spoil just days after harvest. This makes them costly for farmers to produce. Often the best way to get berries is to pick them yourself. Berries may be eaten fresh or made into jams, juices, wines, desserts, and more. We recommend harvesting an abundance and freezing them for use in the winter months. Frozen berries are almost as nutritious as fresh.

The roots and leaves are also used as medicine and can be made into a tea.

Recommended Amounts

- *Red raspberry leaf tea:* 7 to 10 grams daily

- *Red raspberry leaf tincture (dried):* 1:5, 30% alcohol; 3 to 5 ml, 3 times daily

- *Blackberry root tea:* 15 grams daily

Special Considerations

Excessive use of astringent herbs can cause constipation, which is normally resolved when amounts are lessened.

RASPBERRY LEAF INFUSION

This potent brew blends the nourishing qualities of raspberry leaves with the loving embrace of roses. Herbalists have long relied on raspberry leaves to strengthen and tone the uterus to relieve menstrual cramps and to assist in healing after giving birth. Drink warm or cold and, for best results, frequently.

Yield: 3 cups

⅓ cup (10 grams) finely crumbled dried raspberry leaves

⅓ cup (5 grams) dried rose petals

1 teaspoon (1 gram) dried hibiscus

1 teaspoon (1 gram) dried mint

3 cups water

1. Place all of the herbs in a quart jar (or quart-sized tea press).

2. Bring 3 cups of water to a boil. Pour the water over the herbs, stir well, and then cover. Infuse for 30 minutes.

3. Strain well and drink within 24 hours.

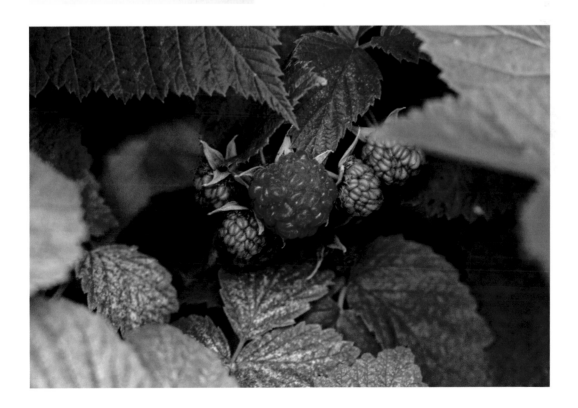

BRAMBLEBERRY SHRUB

A splash of this shrub, or drinking vinegar, can turn a glass of sparkling water into a refreshing home-made soda. This is a fairly straightforward recipe using blackberries and raspberries (or other *Rubus* species), but feel free to jazz it up with a handful of rose petals, a cinnamon stick, or a piece of vanilla bean. For best results, use raw vinegar and raw honey.

Yield: About 1¼ cups

1 cup blackberries or raspberries, or a combination

1 cup apple cider vinegar (at least 5% acidity)

½ cup mild honey, or to taste

1. Put the berries in a pint jar and lightly crush them with a fork. Pour the vinegar over the berries.

2. Wipe the rim of the jar with a clean cloth. Cover the jar, preferably with a glass or plastic lid. If using a metal lid, place parchment paper between the lid and the jar (vinegar will corrode metal). Label the jar.

3. Store the jar in a cool, dark place for 1 to 2 weeks, shaking it daily.

4. Strain the vinegar. (You can discard the berries or eat them in other dishes.) Add honey to taste and stir to combine. Transfer the shrub to a clean jar or bottle with a nonreactive lid and label it.

5. Store in the refrigerator and use within 1 year. To serve, mix 1 part shrub with 4 parts sparkling water, or adjust proportions to taste.

BRAMBLEBERRY SHRUB COCKTAIL

Yield: 1 cocktail

2 ounces white or gold rum

1 ounce Brambleberry Shrub (see recipe, above)

4 ounces club soda

Mint sprig for garnish (optional)

1. Fill a tall glass with ice. Add the rum and shrub. (You may want to adjust the amount of shrub, depending on how much you sweetened it.)

2. Top with club soda and stir gently to combine. Garnish with mint, if desired.

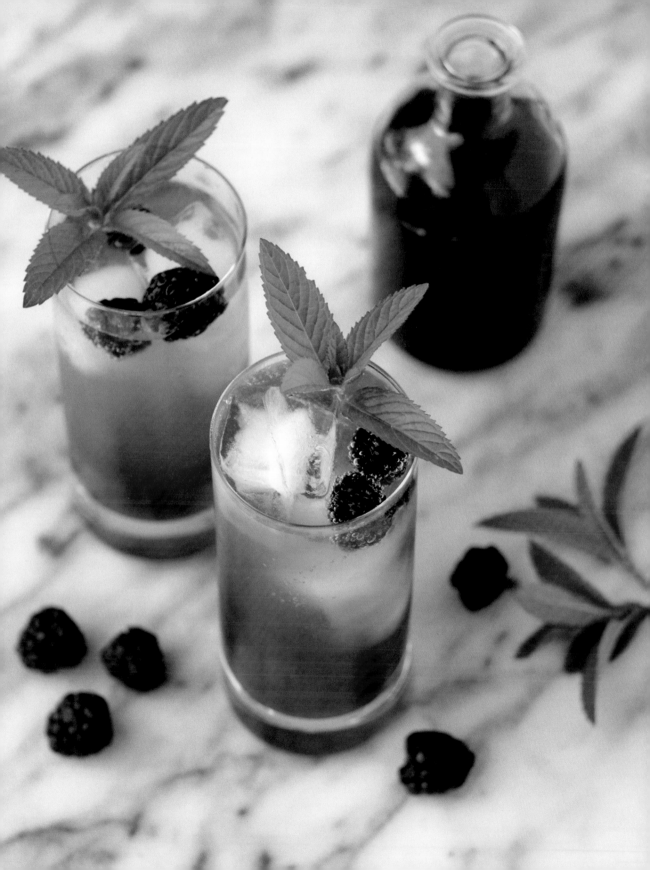

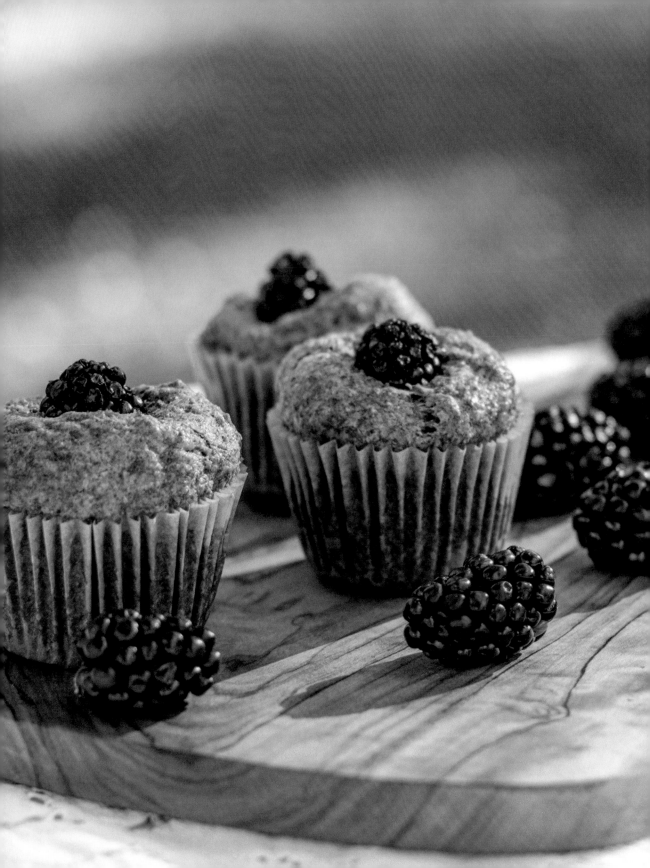

HIGH-FIBER BLACKBERRY MUFFINS

These dense muffins are a moist and fiber-rich treat that we love for breakfast, as a midmorning or afternoon tea snack, or as a dessert. Any berries can be used here, but we especially enjoy big, plump blackberries freshly picked from the vine.

Yield: 12 muffins

¼ cup chia seeds

¼ cup flaxseeds

1 cup oat bran

1 teaspoon baking powder

½ teaspoon baking soda

2 teaspoons ground cinnamon

½ teaspoon ground nutmeg

¼ teaspoon salt

¼ cup butter, melted

¼ cup honey

4 large eggs

¾ cup coconut milk

1 teaspoon vanilla extract

1 cup large blackberries

1. Preheat the oven to 350°F. Line a 12-cup muffin pan with baking cups.

2. Using a spice grinder, grind the chia seeds and the flaxseeds into a fine powder.

3. Whisk the powdered seeds, oat bran, baking powder, baking soda, cinnamon, nutmeg, and salt in a medium bowl.

4. In a separate large bowl, whisk the melted butter, honey, eggs, coconut milk, and vanilla extract.

5. Add the dry ingredients to the wet ingredients and stir thoroughly with a large wooden spoon. The mixture should be moist and sticky. Gently fold in the blackberries.

6. Divide the batter equally among the baking cups.

7. Bake for 30 minutes, or until a tester inserted in the center of one comes out clean. Let cool slightly before eating.

8. Cool the muffins completely before storing them in an airtight container in the fridge. We like these best when they've been reheated. Eat within 3 days.

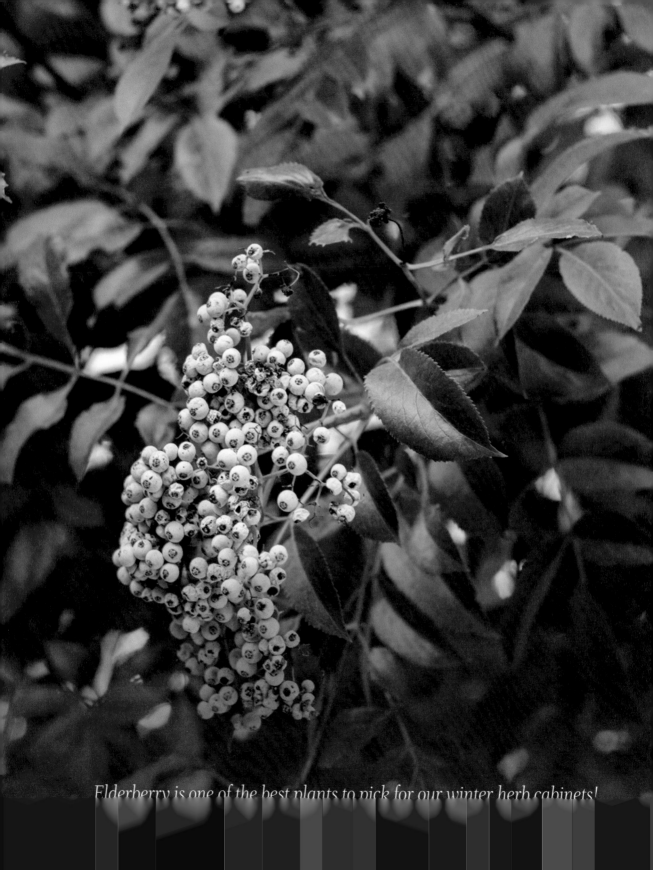

Elderberry is one of the best plants to pick for our winter herb cabinets!

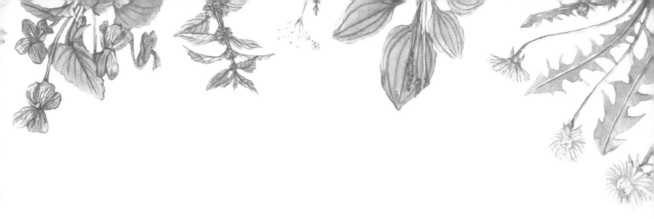

CHAPTER 22

ELDERBERRY

As warm weather continues, the once-creamy white blossoms of elder slowly transform into large, drooping clusters of dark fruits or berries. This bounty feeds birds and bears and shows us that some of our best medicines grow on trees.

Botanical names: *Sambucus nigra, S. nigra* ssp. *canadensis, S. nigra* ssp. *caerulea, S. ebulus*
Family: Adoxaceae (moschatel)
Parts used: berries, flowers (see Chapter 14)
Energetics: cooling, drying
Taste: sour
Berry properties: antioxidant rich, antiviral, immunomodulator, inflammatory modulator
Berry uses: colds and flu, food, herpes, weak eyes
Berry preparations: dye, elixir, food, glycerite, oxymel, syrup, tea, tincture

The elder shrub has a long history of use for food, medicine, and tools. The berries have been a traditional remedy for symptoms of a cold or flu. In the 1990s this popular folk remedy caught the attention of Israeli virologist Madeleine Mumcuoglu. Clinical trials confirmed elderberry's powerful abilities. Today you can commonly find elderberry preparations in health food stores, grocery stores, and pharmacies.

MEDICINAL PROPERTIES AND ENERGETICS

Elderberries are filled with phytonutrients that modulate inflammation and ward off infection. And while they can be prepared as medicine, they are also a delicious food that can be used in baked goods or made into syrup and drizzled on pancakes.

PLANT GIFTS

Stops or Shortens the Duration of Cold and Flu

Imagine if there were a potent medicine that you could take to prevent an upper respiratory infection, stop it at the first sign of illness, or shorten the duration of an illness. To answer all our dreams, let's say it was an abundant plant that grew all over the Northern Hemisphere and that it was safe to use, easy to find, and simple to harvest. And just to be totally crazy, let's say it tasted good. Meet elderberry. For many, it's a winter medicine chest all rolled into one

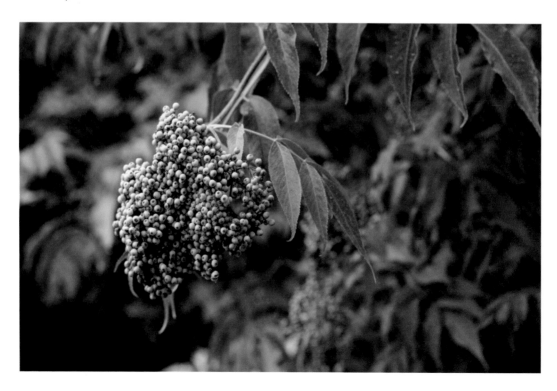

plant. French herbalist Bernard Bertrand says elder has so many properties, it's often simply called the house pharmacy.[1]

Elderberries and elderflowers have long been used to treat symptoms of a cold or flu. Today many herbalists rely on these phytonutrient berries. Elderberries especially shine when taken just at the onset of a cold or flu. When you feel that first tingle in your throat or a telltale sign of fatigue or chills, frequent doses of elderberry can often stop the illness from progressing. It's also taken preventively to ward off illness and can help shorten the duration of an illness.

Several studies have confirmed elderberry's powerful abilities and given us some insight into how it works. One of the first studies was a human clinical trial that showed that 93.3 percent of people with flu symptoms who took elderberries saw a significant improvement within two days, while those taking a placebo did not see improvement until six days later.[2] Another study, in Norway, confirmed these findings in a randomized, double-blind, placebo-controlled study: Researchers gave 60 people who had had influenza-like symptoms for less than 48 hours either 15 ml (roughly 1 tablespoon) of elderberry syrup or a placebo syrup four times a day. On average, those receiving the elderberry reported that their symptoms were relieved four days earlier than those taking the placebo. Moreover, those taking the elderberry reported using significantly less over-the-counter medication to relieve their symptoms.[3]

While it's rarely convenient to get sick, catching a cold or flu when traveling can be especially bothersome. Elderberry to the rescue! One study followed 312 airline passengers flying overseas from Australia. Half were given an elderberry preparation and the other half got a placebo. Those taking the placebo had slightly more occurrences of a cold or flu during their trip than did those taking the elderberry. More significantly, those taking the elderberry who did get a cold reported a marked reduction of cold duration and severity compared with those taking the placebo.[4] We always travel with a tincture of elderberry and echinacea and take it preventively as we go.

We could simply call elderberry an antiviral and leave it at that, but glimpses into how it works are fascinating. One mechanism is a protein within the berries that has been shown to inhibit a virus from penetrating a cell wall, which then stops its ability to replicate. This hints at why elderberries may be so effective at the very beginning of a cold or flu. As the virus is revving up, it's suddenly stopped in its tracks.

Eases Pain and Inflammation

These phytonutrient-rich berries can modulate inflammation and decrease associated pain. In her 1931 book, *A Modern Herbal*, Maude Grieve relates the story of a sailor who claimed that dark red port was an effective remedy for rheumatic pains. This led to an investigation that found that while actual port wine didn't seem to have those benefits, the sailor had been drinking cheap port made with elderberries.[5] Another way this can be applied is to support the eyes. Eyes are sensitive to inflammation, and elder's strong inflammation-modulating ability can protect and strengthen them (similar to bilberry and blueberry).

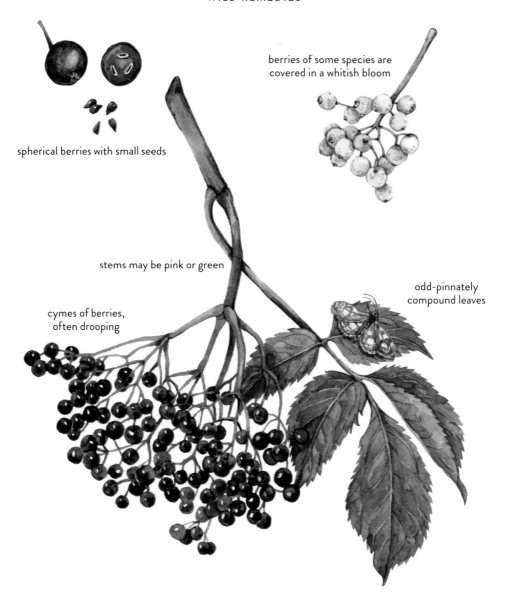

spherical berries with small seeds

berries of some species are covered in a whitish bloom

stems may be pink or green

cymes of berries, often drooping

odd-pinnately compound leaves

elder (*Sambucus nigra*), shown with elderberry pearl moth (*Anania coronata*)

Life cycle: deciduous woody perennial
Reproduces by: seed, root
Growth habit: shrub or small tree, 5–30 feet tall
Habitat: ditches, fencerows, fields, forest edges, hedgerows, hillsides, low-lying areas, meadows, riparian areas, roadsides, stream banks, thickets, wetland margins
Sun: full sun to partial shade
Soil: moist, well drained; can tolerate some drought or wet sites
USDA Hardiness Zones: 3–9

HOW TO IDENTIFY

Each *Sambucus* species or subspecies has its own identifying characteristics, and you should consult a local guide for specific information. (It's also not uncommon for them to hybridize.) For a general description of the elder shrub, including leaves and flowers, see page 153. After the flowers have been pollinated, they develop into clusters or cymes of spherical fruits or berries. The berries may be blue, purple, or black, and in some species they are covered in a whitish glaucous bloom. Each berry is typically about 1 centimeter in diameter and contains several tiny seeds. The weight of all the juicy berries can make the clusters droop dramatically from the branches.

ECOLOGICAL CONNECTIONS

Elderberries are eaten by many birds, including waxwings, mockingbirds, warblers, thrashers, and vireos. Mammals like squirrels and mice also eat the berries. This is mutually beneficial, as the tree gets to have its seeds dispersed through the animals' droppings.

HOW TO HARVEST

Gather the berries when they are completely ripe and juicy, using your fingers or pruning shears to cut entire clusters at the base. Place them in a sturdy container to prevent them from getting crushed. Also be mindful of spiders that may be hanging out in the berries; gently shake them off at your gathering spot, and check again when you get home.

Elders reproduce by seed and spread by root suckers. Leave enough berries on the plant

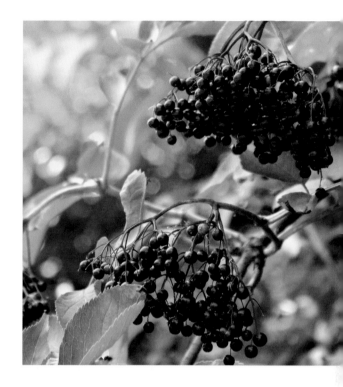

so it can reseed, and also for the benefit of birds and other wildlife.

Before using the berries in food or medicine, completely separate them from the stems and leaves, which contain cyanogenic glycosides and can make you sick. You can stick the clusters in the freezer for a few hours to make the berries easier to remove. Some people like using a fork to shuck off the berries.

Harvesting Cautions

The berries of red elder (*Sambucus racemosa*) are quite different from blue or black varieties; they have a mealy consistency and don't taste very good. Even so, some people do make jams out of the red berries. Keep in mind that the red berries contain more cyanogenic glycosides and need to be thoroughly cooked before eating. Someone who is sensitive may

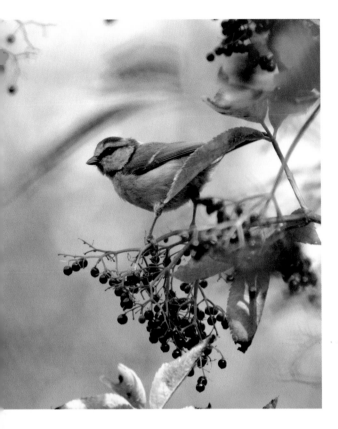

USING ELDERBERRY IN YOUR LIFE

Elderberries can be used fresh or dried. The small berries have relatively large seeds, so they are often made into preparations that extract the juice and strain the seeds. Elderberry syrup can be drizzled on sweet breakfasts and desserts. The berries can be cooked into foods or made into jams, sauces, baked goods, and even a delicious wine. Eating lots of raw berries can make you sick, but cooking or fermenting them renders them safe.

Elderberry medicines include syrups, tinctures, and elixirs. When taking elderberries to address a cold or flu, use it at the very beginning stages in order to get the best results. It is also best to take it frequently throughout the day rather than consuming a large amount only once or twice a day. Elderberries can be eaten as food, so the dosage can be fairly high.

Recommended Amounts

- *Decoction/Syrup:* 30 to 60 grams prepared as a decoction/syrup daily

- *Tincture (dried berries):* 1:5, 40% alcohol; 30 to 90 drops (¼ to 1 teaspoon) per hour during acute situations

Special Considerations

Elderberries are generally safe for everyone. The raw seeds contain toxic substances that can cause nausea and vomiting; cooking them diminishes this effect.

experience more discomfort, nausea, or even vomiting when using the red berries. *S. racemosa* can be distinguished from other species by the color of its berries and its cone-shaped (instead of flat) flower clusters.

It may be possible to confuse the toxic devil's walking stick (*Aralia spinosa*) and poke (*Phytolacca americana*) for elderberry. However, with careful observation of the berry cluster shapes along with other characteristics, they are not hard to differentiate.

GARDENING TIPS

See Elderflower, Chapter 14.

ELDERBERRY SYRUP

This classic herbal remedy can help shorten the duration of a cold or flu or ward it off altogether. We usually take a teaspoon of elderberry syrup every 30 to 60 minutes until the sickness subsides. It can also be taken as a daily preventative during cold and flu season—or simply enjoyed on pancakes or stirred into sparkling water! You can make the syrup with water or juice; apple, pomegranate, or tart cherry juice are good choices. Other add-ins might include spices like black pepper and ginger, aromatics like rosemary and thyme, and orange or lemon peel.

Yield: Varies; about 2 to 4 cups

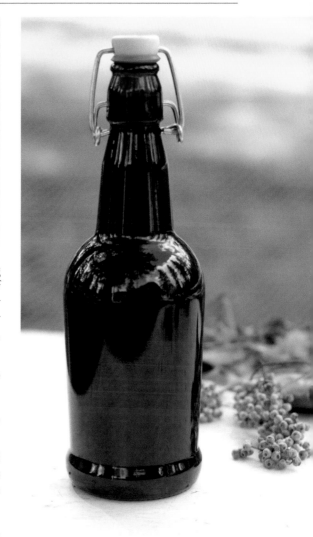

1 cup fresh elderberries (150 grams), or 1 cup frozen elderberries (130 grams), or ½ cup dried elderberries (55 grams)

¼ cup dried rose hips, cut and sifted (35 grams) (optional)

2 teaspoons cinnamon chips (3 grams) (optional)

2 whole cloves (optional)

2 or 3 cups water or juice (see instructions)

Honey, to taste

1. Place the elderberries in a medium saucepan along with the rose hips, cinnamon, and cloves, if using. If using fresh or frozen elderberries, add 2 cups of water or juice. If using dried elderberries, add 3 cups of water or juice. Bring to a boil over high heat. Cover the pan, reduce the heat to low, and simmer for 20 minutes.

2. Turn off the heat, remove the lid, and let the mixture cool until you can comfortably process it further.

3. Strain the mixture through a jelly bag or cheesecloth, squeezing it well to extract all the liquid.

4. Measure the resulting liquid, then add honey to taste and mix well. If you add an equal volume of honey, the syrup will last for up to a year in the refrigerator. If you add less honey, you will need to use the syrup more quickly.

5. Transfer the syrup to a clean jar or bottle and label it. Store in the refrigerator.

ELDERBERRY GUMMIES

Made with elderberry juice and little to no added sweeteners, these gummies are a tasty snack for all ages. You can shape them using silicone molds, or simply cut them into bite-size cubes. We recommend eating 1 to 3 small gummies a day.

If you choose to make these with gelatin, we suggest using a good-quality gelatin from grass-fed, pasture-raised animals. You can also use vegan-friendly agar-agar, which is made from red algae; look for it at health food stores and Asian grocers. Gelatin gummies will be softer and less chewy than store-bought gummy candies, while agar gummies will be firmer and less springy.

Yield: Variable; fills about 184 2.5-ml gummy molds

---

1 batch elderberry juice (refer to step 1 below)

3 tablespoons gelatin powder or 2 tablespoons agar-agar powder

Honey or maple syrup, to taste (optional)

1. To make elderberry juice, follow the Elderberry Syrup recipe (page 249), steps 1 through 3.

2. Measure out 2 cups of juice. If you don't have 2 full cups, top it off with water or juice.

3. Proceed as directed for gelatin or agar-agar:

   To use gelatin: Pour ½ cup of the elderberry juice into a large bowl. If the juice is still warm, let it come to room temperature. Sprinkle the gelatin on top of the juice and let it sit for 1 minute. Meanwhile, pour the remaining elderberry juice into a saucepan and bring it to a simmer. Add the hot juice to the bowl, stirring constantly with a whisk. Continue to whisk until the gelatin has dissolved, about 2 minutes. Stir in honey or maple syrup, if desired (we usually add about 2 tablespoons). Skim off any foam.

   To use agar-agar: Start with room-temperature elderberry juice. Pour the juice into a saucepan, sprinkle the agar-agar on top, and let it sit for 5 minutes. Simmer the mixture over medium heat, whisking frequently, until it has thickened to the consistency of syrup, about 5 minutes. Remove from the heat and stir in honey or maple syrup, if desired (we usually add about 2 tablespoons).

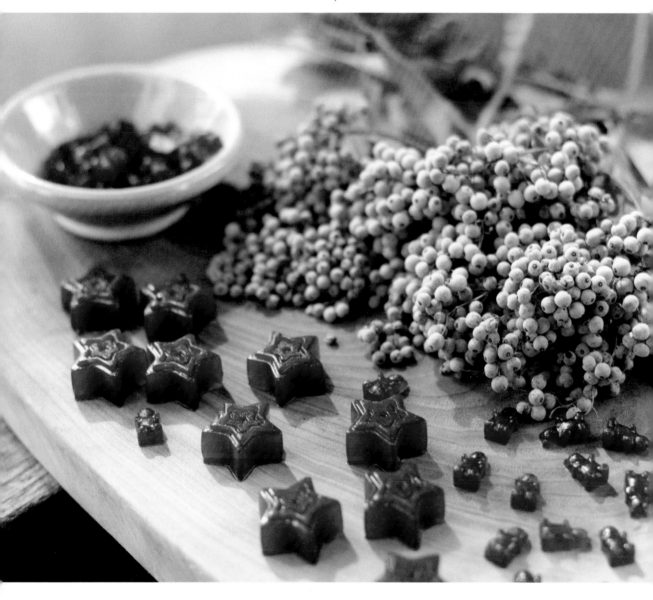

4. Pour the mixture into molds (a dropper is handy for filling small molds), or an 8 x 8-inch baking dish lined with parchment paper. Pop any air bubbles with your finger or a toothpick. Refrigerate until set, about 1 hour.

5. If you used molds, pop out the gummies. If you used a pan, slice the gummies into small cubes. Store the gummies in an airtight container in the refrigerator for up to 2 weeks.

ELDER ELIXIR

As with Elderberry Syrup (page 249), you can take this frequently by the teaspoonful at the onset of a cold or flu and continue until you feel better. It's also a delicious preventive medicine; enjoy it as is, or add it to a hot toddy. Or use it to put an herbalist's spin on the classic sidecar cocktail (see Elder Sidecar, below).

Yield: About 2 cups

1½ cups dried elderberries or 3 cups fresh elderberries

½ cup dried elderflowers or 1 cup fresh elderflowers

⅔ cup honey

About 2 cups brandy (XO or VSOP)

1. Place the elderberries, elderflowers, and honey in a 1-quart jar.

2. Pour brandy into the jar, leaving an inch of space at the top. Using a chopstick or butter knife, stir to combine the ingredients and release any air bubbles. Tightly cover the jar and label it.

3. Store the jar in a cool, dark place for 6 weeks. Shake the jar daily for the first week. If you used fresh berries or flowers, make sure the plant material stays submerged in the alcohol for the entire macerating time.

4. Strain through a fine-mesh strainer, and discard the solids.

5. Transfer the liquid to a clean jar or bottle and label it. Store in a cool, dark place and use within 1 year.

ELDER SIDECAR

Yield: 1 cocktail

2 ounces Elder Elixir (see recipe above)

1 ounce Cointreau

½ ounce fresh lemon juice

Lemon twist for garnish (optional)

1. Combine all ingredients in a cocktail shaker. Fill the shaker with ice and shake until chilled. Strain into a chilled cocktail glass. Garnish with a lemon twist, if desired.

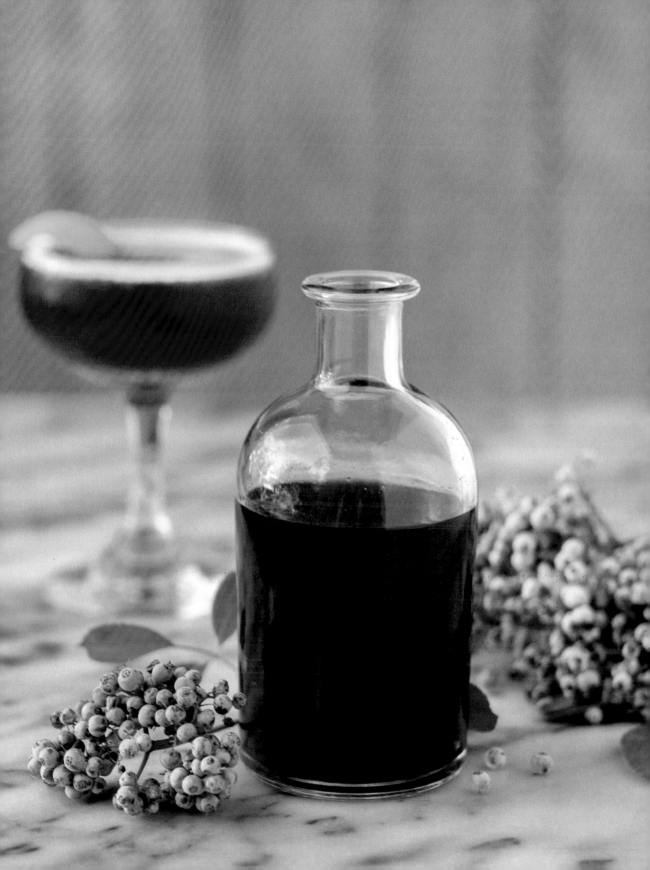

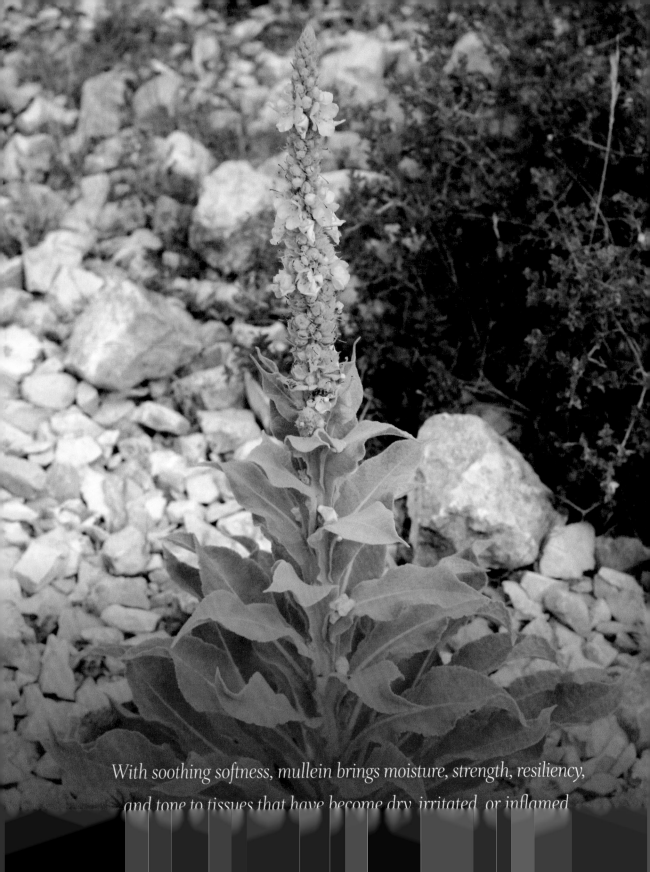

With soothing softness, mullein brings moisture, strength, resiliency, and tone to tissues that have become dry, irritated, or inflamed.

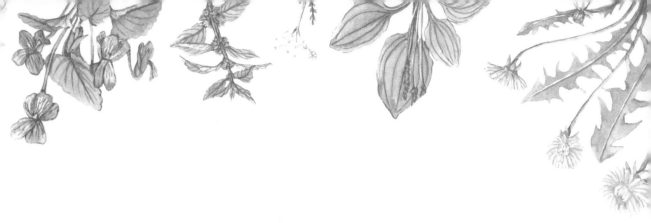

CHAPTER 23

MULLEIN

As a generous restorer of disturbed soils, mullein offers refuge, food, and medicine to many creatures. The thick, large leaves provide a cool, protected habitat for small beings like mice or voles. Ants and other insects commonly patrol the flowers. In the fall, woodpeckers are frequently spotted moving up and down the mullein stalks, foraging the many insects found there. In some ways mullein becomes its own microcosm of a habitat.

Botanical names: *Verbascum thapsus, V. densiflorum, V. olympicum, V. virgatum*
Family: Scrophulariaceae (figwort)
Parts used: roots, leaves, flowers
Energetics: leaves and flowers: cooling, moistening; roots: warming, drying
Taste: sweet, salty
Properties: antiviral, demulcent, inflammatory modulator, lymphatic
Uses: asthma, back pain, dry coughs, earaches, relaxes lungs, sore lungs, weak bladder muscles
Preparations: decoction (roots), fomentation (leaves), nourishing herbal infusion (leaves), oil (flowers), smoke (leaves), tea (flowers), tincture (all parts)

Originally native to Europe and Asia, mullein has spread across the globe and is frequently found in disturbed soils. It has been used as medicine for thousands of years. Greek physician Dioscorides was recommending it for coughs more than 2,000 years ago!

MEDICINAL PROPERTIES AND ENERGETICS

Every part of mullein has medicinal virtues. The leaves and flowers are used to soften and soothe, while the roots have a more warming and drying energy. The word *mullein* is related to the French *molle*, meaning "soft." Gently touching the large, fuzzy leaves, you can understand the inspiration. However, when you strongly rub those leaves, the soft hairs become an irritant or rubefacient and can be used to bring circulation to an area.

PLANT GIFTS

Leaves Support the Lungs

Mullein leaves are nourishing and nutritive. They can be taken as a tea to support long-term lung health or used in the short term for more acute situations. Mullein leaf acts as a mild relaxant as well as a demulcent, making an excellent remedy for dry, irritated lungs accompanied by a cough. Herbalists use mullein leaves to support people with asthma or bronchitis or for those inhaling irritants like pollution or wildfire smoke. We especially like it combined with other demulcent herbs such as mallow (see the Healthy Lungs Tea recipe on page 262).

Mullein's large, hairy leaves can feel like thick, dense wool. The complex web of plant fibers covering the leaves protects the plant from the strong rays of the sun. These same fibers are a bit irritating to human skin, which can be annoying, beneficial, or both. The action of irritating the skin is called rubefacient. This irritation dilates the capillaries, increasing circulation to the area, and has a wide variety of therapeutic applications. Used as a poultice on the chest, mullein leaves can help move stagnancy in the lungs, increasing a healthy, thin mucus that can be readily expelled.

Scientists may be finding new ways that mullein can support the lungs. A preliminary study isolated a constituent of mullein that was shown to be active against a type of lung cancer.[1] We look forward to future studies involving human clinical trials.

Roots Strengthen the Bladder

Mullein root can strengthen the bladder and is used for incontinence caused by stress, pregnancy, or menopause as well as childhood incontinence. Herbalist Christa Sinadinos also recommends mullein root for those with interstitial cystitis and benign prostatic hyperplasia (BPH, enlarged prostate).[2]

Roots Address Back and Joint Pain

Recently mullein root has become popularized for back pain. Herbalist Jim mcdonald says, "Prepared either as an infusion or taken in small doses as a tincture, [mullein root has] been a lifesaver for me when working a bit too gung-ho has me wake up the next morning with my back kinked and not quite able to straighten up. I usually take about seven drops of tincture, stretch out a bit, and the kink disappears and I feel perfectly aligned."[3]

Flowers Relieve Earaches and Infections

Mullein's biggest claim to fame is as an earache remedy. This historic use is backed up by the experiences of countless present-day parents and children. Mullein flower–infused oil acts as an anodyne to take away the pain of the earache while also exerting lymphatic action on the area around the ear to help resolve the infection. Mullein flower–infused oil is commonly found in health food stores and apothecaries.

Herbalist Michael Moore writes that mullein flower tea has a negative effect on the herpes simplex virus (HSV-1) and seems especially helpful for adults and children who have frequent outbreaks around the mouth triggered by sun, food allergies, or estrogen surges before ovulation.[4] Preliminary in vitro research shows some antiviral qualities against HSV-1 as well as influenza.[5]

HOW TO IDENTIFY

Mullein often grows in poor soils and neglected places, popping up early before successive vegetation moves in. In its first year, the plant forms a basal rosette of grayish green, feltlike leaves. Covered in fuzzy hairs, these leaves are oblong or lanceolate, 4 to 12 inches long, and 1 to 5 inches wide. The root is a taproot with fibrous secondary roots.

In the second year, the plant produces a tall, wandlike stalk up to 10 feet tall. This stalk has smaller, alternately arranged leaves that decrease in size toward the top. Sometimes a plant will develop one or two side stems. Toward the top of the stalk, five-petaled yellow flowers are arranged on a terminal spike. Only a few flowers bloom at a time, and each is open for one day, closing by midafternoon. The fruit is an oval capsule containing many seeds.

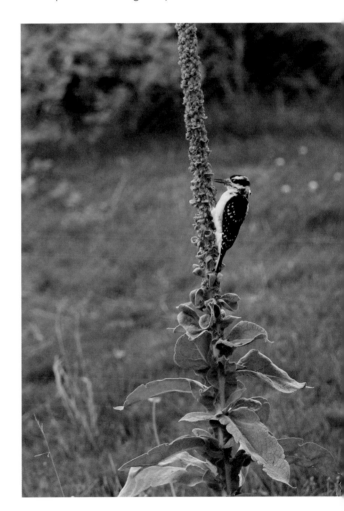

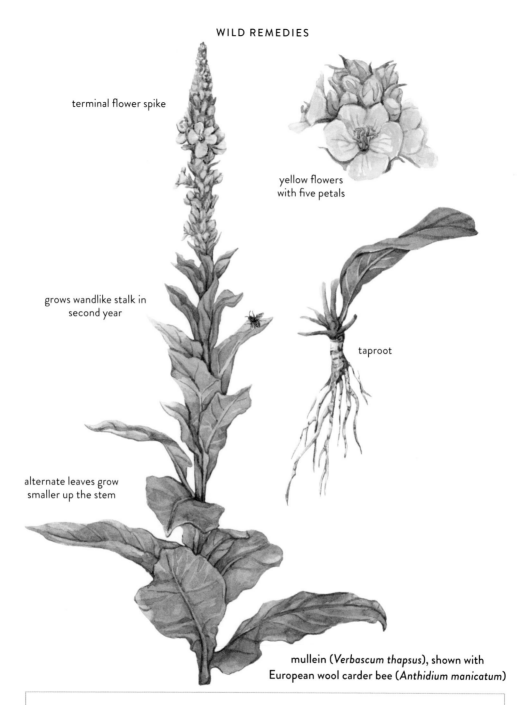

terminal flower spike

yellow flowers
with five petals

grows wandlike stalk in
second year

taproot

alternate leaves grow
smaller up the stem

mullein (*Verbascum thapsus*), shown with
European wool carder bee (*Anthidium manicatum*)

Life cycle: herbaceous biennial
Reproduces by: seed
Growth habit: low-growing rosette in first year; erect flower stalk in second year, 1–10 feet tall
Habitat: disturbed areas, dry hillsides, fields, forest clearings, meadows, old pastures, railways,
    roadsides, vacant lots, woodland edges
Sun: full sun
Soil: prefers dry and gravelly, well drained
USDA Hardiness Zones: 4–9

ECOLOGICAL CONNECTIONS

Mullein flowers are visited by various insects, including bees, flies, and butterflies. If a flower has not been cross-pollinated by the end of the day, it will self-pollinate. Carder bees (*Anthidium* spp.) gather the hairs from mullein leaves to line their nests. Birds such as downy woodpeckers and goldfinches visit mullein to feast on the seeds as well as insect larvae.

Mullein is a hyperaccumulator of heavy metals. This means it can uptake heavy metals from the earth and store them. This ability has led to some interesting research on using mullein for soil remediation. Researchers in Serbia tested five different plants for their ability to clean up a heavily contaminated site. Their research concluded, "Because mullein efficiently transported metal pollutants into the aboveground parts and because it fits well the desired characteristics for its use as a biomass, it is our plant of choice for further bioremediation use at the polluted industrial site."[6]

HOW TO HARVEST

Harvest the basal leaves using scissors or a knife, preferably in the autumn of the plant's first year or spring of the second year. Because the dense, woolly hairs on mullein leaves can be a bit irritating, you may want to wear gloves when processing a lot of leaves. Dig the taproot in the autumn of the first year to early spring of the second year, before the stalk

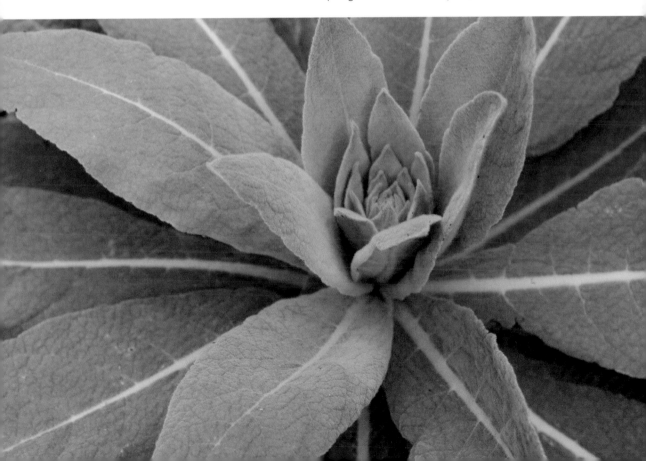

forms. Handpick the flowers individually as they bloom, early in the day before the flowers close.

Mullein reproduces by seeds, which can survive for decades in the soil. Make sure not to harvest all the flowers so the plant can form seeds, which it will drop nearby.

Harvesting Cautions

Lookalikes for the leaves include foxglove (*Digitalis purpurea*), which is poisonous, and lamb's ear (*Stachys byzantine*). Mullein is a hyperaccumulator of heavy metals. Be certain that the mullein you are harvesting and using comes from healthy soils that aren't contaminated with metals.

GARDENING TIPS

This tall biennial adapts to all kinds of soil and conditions, including rich garden soil. Classified as a "noxious" and "invasive" weed in several U.S. states, mullein forms small colonies on bare, disturbed soil if left unchecked. Propagation is by seeds that are light-dependent for germination and take two weeks to sprout. If allowed, mullein will vigorously self-sow, popping up throughout the garden the following year. The long taproot is not conducive to container growing except in very deep pots. There are many ornamental cultivars that are not used for medicinal purposes.

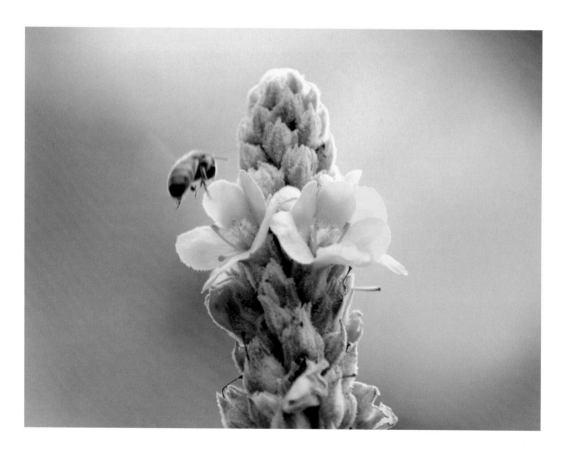

USING MULLEIN IN YOUR LIFE

Mullein leaves can be dried for use in teas and steams. Because the tiny hairs on mullein leaves can be irritating, strain teas through a coffee filter to avoid ingesting them. Fresh leaves can be used to make a poultice, and whole leaves can be frozen to preserve them for a future poultice. Fresh or dried leaves can be used to make an alcohol extract. Flowers can be dried for use in teas. Fresh flowers or freshly dried flowers can be infused into oil or made into an alcohol extract. Mullein roots can be used fresh or dried as an alcohol extract. They can also be chopped and dried for use in decoctions or powdered for use in capsules.

Recommended Amounts

Leaves:

- *Tea:* 10 to 30 grams daily (more if desired)

- *Tincture (dried):* 1:5, 40% alcohol; 90 to 120 drops (1 to 1¼ teaspoons), 3 times daily

Flowers:

- *Tea:* 5 to 10 flowers per cup, 3 cups a day

- *Tincture (fresh):* 1:2, 40% alcohol; 30 to 90 drops (¼ to 1 teaspoon), 3 times daily

Roots:

- *Decoction or powder:* 15 grams

- *Tincture (fresh):* 1:2, 50% alcohol; 30 to 60 drops (¼ to ½ teaspoon), 1 to 3 times daily

Special Considerations

- The *Botanical Safety Handbook* gives mullein its highest safety rating.

- Mullein oil should not be used in ear canals if the eardrum has been perforated.

HEALTHY LUNGS TEA

This blend offers soothing relief for the respiratory system and is perfect for when you have dry, irritated lungs that may be accompanied with spasmodic coughing. We like this blend when we are recovering from a cold or flu or when we've been exposed to air pathogens like wildfire smoke. For best results, drink throughout the day.

Yield: 3 cups

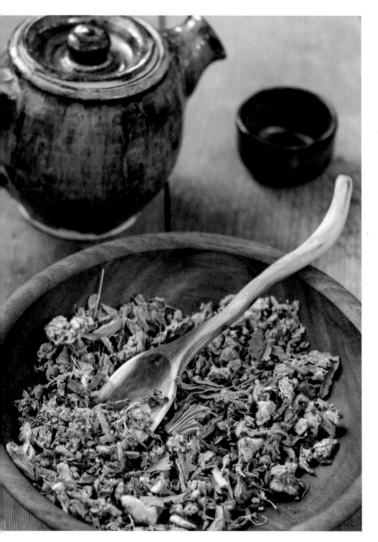

½ cup (10 grams) finely crumbled dried mullein leaves

2 tablespoons (4 grams) finely crumbled dried plantain leaves

2 tablespoons (4 grams) finely crumbled dried mallow leaves

2 tablespoons cut and sifted dried rose hips, or ¼ cup whole dried rose hips

2 teaspoons dried mint or tulsi leaves

3 cups water

1. Place all of the herbs in a quart jar (or quart-sized tea press).

2. Bring 3 cups of water to a boil. Pour the water over the herbs, stir well, and cover. Infuse for 30 minutes or as long as overnight.

3. Strain well, using a coffee filter or a couple of layers of cheesecloth to avoid the small, irritating hairs of the mullein leaf. Drink within 24 hours.

MULLEIN AND YARROW FACIAL STEAM

We like to do this facial steam when we have congested sinuses and/or lungs. In this case, keep a box of tissues nearby as it's quite effective. This facial steam can also be used to support healthy skin. For a complete facial experience, follow it up with St. John's Wort Oil (page 203) or Forest Facial Cream (page 358).

Yield: 1 treatment

---

1 large handful dried mullein leaves, crumbled

1 small handful dried yarrow leaves and flowers, crumbled

Water

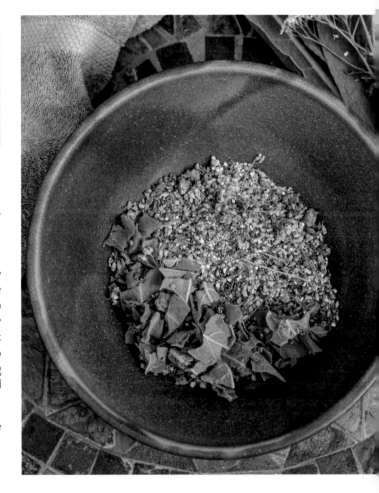

1. Place the herbs in a medium bowl.

2. Bring to a boil enough water to fill your bowl. Pour the water over the herbs, creating an herbal "soup."

3. Place your face over the bowl, then drape a towel over your head to capture the steam. Inhale deeply. Experiment with moving your head closer or farther away to find where it is most comfortable. If it gets too hot, allow a bit of the steam to escape. Enjoy the experience for as long as desired. We often do it for around 10 minutes.

4. If desired, add more hot water as time goes by to create more steam.

HERBAL BURNING BUNDLES

Herbalists, healers, Indigenous communities, the spiritually devoted, religious leaders, and others all over the world burn herbs and resins as part of their cultural, spiritual, and healing traditions. While it is common to find smoke bundles in shops, these are often unscrupulously harvested and marketed. Making your own from plants you have grown or sustainably gathered can be more ethically sound and is an opportunity to create intention and meaning specific to your life.

The herbs you choose can be aromatic, leaving wisps of sweet, spicy, or floral scent, or they can be medicinal in nature, like mullein burned for lung health. Mullein leaves make a wonderful base for smoke bundles, as they provide a solid and wide surface for other herbs to settle into. If your mullein leaves are large, you may want to cut them in half lengthwise, along the midrib of the leaf. Never burn poisonous plants, plants you are allergic to, or plants you can't identify.

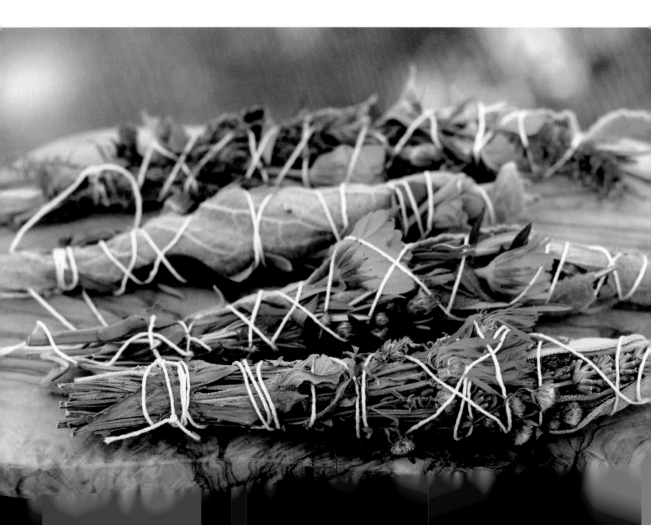

Making a Smoke Bundle

1. After harvesting your herbs, we find it's best to wilt them for 12 to 24 hours so they can lose some of their water content and be made into tighter bundles. If using plants in the Asteraceae family, harvest them as buds rather than blossoms to avoid the puffing out of the seed heads.

2. Gather a couple of handfuls of wilted herbs into a small bundle. Using 100 percent cotton string, tie a tight knot at the base of the bundle, leaving one end of the string about 3 inches long.

3. Take the other (long) end of the string and wrap it around the bundle, working your way up and securing everything together. Wrap this as tightly as possible, as the herbs will shrink as they dry. When you reach the top of the bundle, wrap the string around and continue back down again. If desired, you can do this one more time to really secure the bundle.

4. At the base, tie off the string. Then cut the end of the string you've been working with to match the length of the other (shorter) string. Tie the ends together to form a loop that you can use to hang the bundle as it dries. You can also place the bundle on a drying screen or in a dehydrator. In either case, you want good air circulation to aid the drying process (see Drying Plants on page 60).

Using Smoke Bundles

1. To light the smoke bundle, use a match, lighter, or fire to light one end. Let it catch fire and then lightly wave or blow out the flames, leaving the bundle to smolder.

2. Once you are done with the smoke bundle, place it in a fireproof container like a ceramic bowl or plate. You may also want to stamp the fire out to discourage it from burning further. Avoid leaving a burning bundle unattended. Also do not use water to extinguish the burning, as this will make it harder to burn again.

Here are some suggestions for plants to use:

Mullein leaves
(*Verbascum thapsus*)

Yarrow leaves, flowers, or stems (*Achillea millefolium*)

Calendula flowers
(*Calendula officinalis*)

New England aster leaves or flower buds (*Symphyotrichum novae-angliae*)

Common sage leaves or flowers (*Salvia officinalis*)

Thyme leaf sprigs
(*Thymus vulgaris*)

Rosemary leaf sprigs
(*Rosmarinus officinale*)

Lavender leaves, flowers, or stems (*Lavandula angustifolia*)

Anise hyssop leaves, flowers, or stems (*Agastache foeniculum*)

Big sagebrush leaves
(*Artemisia tridentata*)

Mugwort leaf sprigs
(*Artemisia* spp.)

Hyssop leaves, flowers, or stems (*Hyssopus officinalis*)

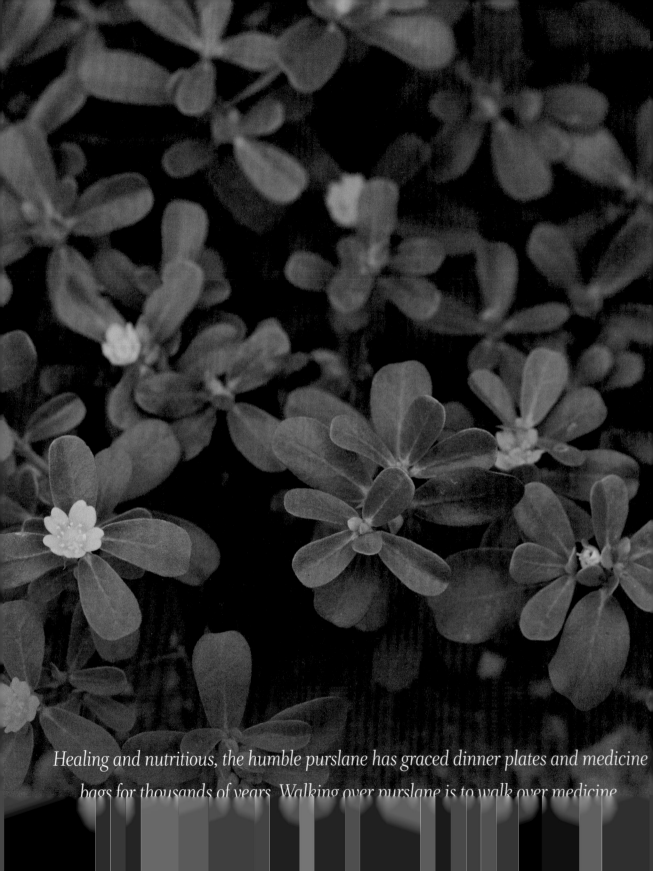

Healing and nutritious, the humble purslane has graced dinner plates and medicine bags for thousands of years. Walking over purslane is to walk over medicine.

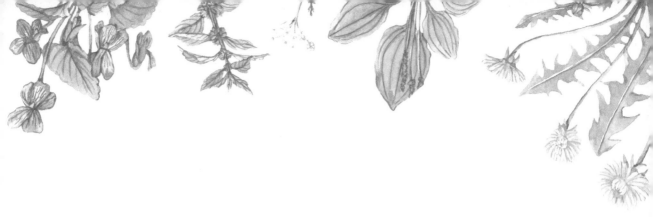

CHAPTER 24

PURSLANE

Springing up from cracks in the sidewalk, purslane softens concrete jungles.
Creeping over garden beds in summer, it offers relief from hot weather. This
succulent plant is an enthusiastic volunteer—some may consider it overenthusiastic—
determined to offer its gifts. We would do well to accept them, as the lives of
people and purslane have been interwoven for as long as we can remember.

Other common names: pigweed, portulaca, pursley, pussley, verdolaga

Botanical names: *Portulaca oleracea*; also *P. grandiflora*, *P. pilosa*, *P. sativa*, and
other species

Family: Portulacaceae

Parts used: leaves, stems, flower buds, seed capsules

Taste: sour

Energetics: cooling, moistening

Properties: analgesic, antimicrobial, antioxidant, antispasmodic, demulcent, diuretic, febrifuge, inflammatory modulator, laxative, vermifuge

Uses: burns, constipation, cough, dermatitis, diarrhea, dysentery, fever, food, headache,
inflammation, insect bites and stings, itchy skin, stomachache, ulcer, worms, wounds

Preparations: food, juice, poultice, tea, wash

Dozens of purslane varieties grow around the world, on every continent except Antarctica. *Portulaca oleracea* is the most commonly found species. The exact origin of purslane is unknown, and scientists have variously traced it to North Africa, India, western Asia, Europe, the Americas, and Australia! Early peoples most likely had a hand in spreading it far and wide. In North America, archaeologists have excavated purslane seeds dating from between 1000 B.C.E. and 750 C.E. It was used as a medicinal plant in ancient Egypt and has been cultivated on the Arabian Peninsula and in the Mediterranean region since the Middle Ages. All over the planet, purslane continues to be an accessible source of food and medicine.

MEDICINAL PROPERTIES AND ENERGETICS

Purslane is known for its ability to grow in hot, dry conditions, and it can be called on for heat and dryness in the body, too. When crushed, the leaves and stems are juicy, slippery, and mucilaginous or demulcent. Purslane is cooling and moistening, and it can be used to soothe hot, irritated tissues, as in the case of sunburn or a dry cough, or simply to cool down on a summer day. The taste of purslane is reflected in its Dhofari Arabic name, *humdeh*, which means "sour" or "acid."

PLANT GIFTS

Provides Nutrient-Dense Food

Every part of this exceptionally nutritious plant is edible. Researchers have identified purslane as the richest vegetable source of alpha-linolenic acid (ALA), an essential omega-3 fatty acid that has been shown to help prevent heart disease and stroke and may protect against cancer. Purslane has five times more omega-3 content than spinach and is considered a particularly good source of omega-3s for people who don't consume fish oils. In addition, purslane contains high amounts of vitamin A (from beta-carotene), vitamin C (from ascorbic acid), and vitamin E (from alpha-tocopherol), as well as potassium, magnesium, calcium, phosphorus, and iron.[1]

Fortunately, this nutrient-rich food is also tasty. As a result of its wide spread around the world, you can find ways to prepare this lemony herb in numerous culinary traditions. Although the leaves and stems are the parts most commonly eaten, aboriginal peoples in Australia have used the seeds for food. Clinical studies have shown purslane seeds to have promise for cardiovascular health and treatment of type 2 diabetes.[2]

Soothes the Skin

Purslane's demulcent qualities make it useful for hot, irritated skin conditions. Similar to aloe vera gel, purslane can soothe superficial burns, sunburns, insect bites and stings, heat rashes, and other inflamed or itchy skin. The leaves and stems can be mashed to make a poultice, or a wash can be made from the juice or a decoction. A mash can be applied to the face for a soothing and antioxidant-rich face mask. Purslane has also been used as a compress to alleviate headaches and fever discomfort.

Relaxes the Muscles

Purslane poultices, juices, and aqueous extracts have been used in traditional West African medicine for various conditions, including muscle aches. In a clinical study in Nigeria, researchers gave patients with muscle spasticity a topical extract prepared from fresh *Portulaca oleracea* leaves and stems. They found that it was an effective muscle relaxant, reducing spasms by 50 percent in some patients.[3] Researchers believe this antispasmodic property is due to purslane's high concentration of potassium.[4]

HOW TO IDENTIFY

Purslane thrives in a variety of conditions but particularly in disturbed soils. This low-growing plant has succulent leaves and thick stems that branch out from a central taproot and sprawl along the ground. Its fleshy leaves are ovate to oblong, flat, smooth, and arranged either oppositely or alternately along the stem. The stems, and sometimes the leaf edges, may be reddish. It has small yellow flowers with five petals. The fruit is a little capsule that splits to release numerous tiny black seeds.

ECOLOGICAL CONNECTIONS

As a living ground cover and companion plant, purslane can maintain moisture in soil, and its taproots can break up hard soil and bring up nutrients. Purslane flowers generally self-pollinate or pollinate by wind. Seeds are dispersed by wind as well as birds and small mammals that occasionally eat the seeds. Purslane is a host plant for the larvae of sawflies (*Schizocerella* spp.) and the portulaca leaf-mining weevil (*Hypurus bertrandiperris*), both of which can kill the plant if present in large numbers.

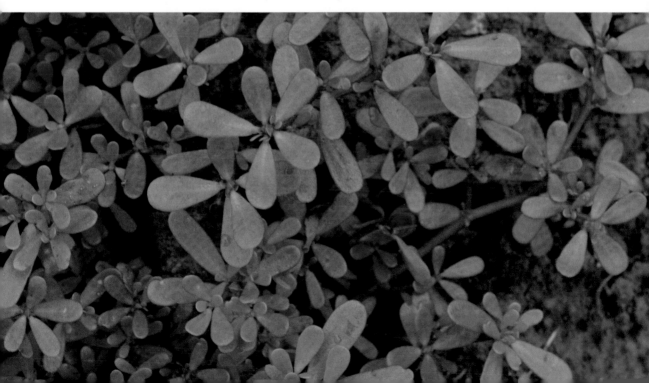

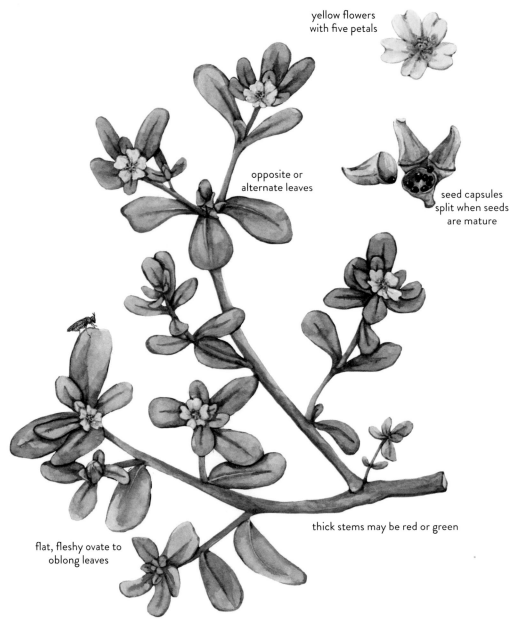

yellow flowers
with five petals

opposite or
alternate leaves

seed capsules
split when seeds
are mature

thick stems may be red or green

flat, fleshy ovate to
oblong leaves

purslane (*Portulaca oleracea*), shown with sawfly (*Schizocerella lineata*)

Life cycle: annual or tender perennial in frost-free zones
Reproduces by: seed, stem
Growth habit: crawling and spreading, 1–6 inches tall
Habitat: coastal areas, disturbed areas, driveways, fields, gardens, lawns, riverbanks,
    roadsides, sidewalk cracks
Sun: full sun to partial shade
Soil: variable; prefers well drained, sandy
USDA Hardiness Zones: 5–10

HOW TO HARVEST

Heat-loving purslane is typically a summer plant and may have several generations in one season. Gather it anytime, as long as the leaves and stems are tender and succulent; older purslane may be fibrous. Purslane picked early in the morning tastes more sour, as it has a higher malic acid content. Using your fingers or scissors, harvest individual leaves or tender sections of stem (or pull out the entire plant if weeding a garden). To encourage regrowth, pick only the tops, leaving at least a couple of inches behind. Flowers and seeds may also be eaten.

Purslane reproduces easily from seed. A single plant can produce 240,000 seeds, which can remain dormant for up to 40 years! To encourage future growth, allow it to self-seed. Conversely, do not let purslane go to seed if you're trying to prevent it from spreading. Broken stem fragments can also root naturally or with human help.

Harvesting Cautions

Be sure to avoid the poisonous spurge (*Euphorbia* spp.), which has a somewhat similar appearance and often grows near purslane. Spurge has thinner (and sometimes hairy) stems and flatter, nonsucculent leaves. A broken stem of spurge will exude milky white sap that can irritate the skin.

GARDENING TIPS

Purslane has adapted to all types of soils and can quickly cover an area with its trailing vines. Propagate by casting seed on the surface of soil, but do not cover; purslane seeds require light for germination. Stem cuttings can also be easily propagated: place cuttings on top of soil, press lightly, and keep moist until the plant begins to root. To produce large, juicy leaves, plant in rich soil, fertilize with composted manure in the spring, and water regularly. Purslane grows well in containers.

USING PURSLANE IN YOUR LIFE

Purslane may be eaten fresh or cooked and is a common ingredient in many global cuisines. The succulent, lemony leaves and stems make a great addition to green salads, potato salad, sandwiches, juices, smoothies, and cold soups like gazpacho. They can also be steamed, sautéed, boiled in soups, and pickled (a good use for leftover stems). Purslane turns slightly more mucilaginous when cooked.

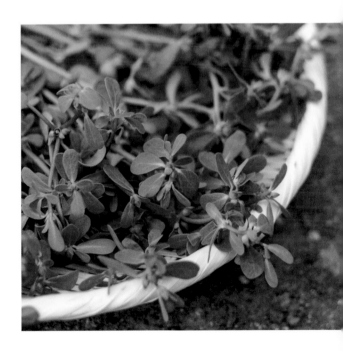

Fresh purslane leaves may be juiced to drink or for use as an external wash. The leaves can also be mashed to make a poultice. Other traditional uses include fresh or dried purslane infusions and decoctions taken internally or used as an external wash. Herbalist Briana Wiles recommends infusing purslane in vinegar to extract its mineral content, or infusing it in oil to make salves and serums.[5]

Recommended Amounts

Purslane is both medicine and food. As a result, the dosage can be quite high when eaten as a vegetable, with the caveats below.

Special Considerations

- Avoid eating large amounts of raw purslane, especially if you easily form calcium oxalate kidney stones. Cooking or blanching reduces the oxalates.

- Animal studies have shown that large amounts of purslane may induce uterine contractions. Medicinal use is not recommended during pregnancy except under the supervision of a qualified health-care practitioner.[6]

- Animal studies have shown that purslane may modify glucose regulation. People with diabetes are advised to consult a qualified health-care practitioner before use.[7]

PURSLANE INSPIRES CONNECTIONS

"We have verdolagas!" I (Emily) was eight years old, and my teacher, Felipe, had just pulled a handful of succulent plants from the edge of our school garden bed. It wasn't one of the vegetables we had intentionally planted; in fact, I no longer remember what those were (radishes? carrots?). But the memory of our weedy volunteer endures. Felipe, who had moved to Texas from Guadalajara, eagerly introduced us to this plant he knew from home. He ushered us into the kitchen and fried up the verdolagas, or purslane, with scrambled eggs—a traditional Mexican dish that delighted me with its ingenuity and that I still enjoy today.

As it turns out, I had tasted purslane before. When my *ba noi* (grandmother), a Vietnamese refugee, came to the United States, she, too, recognized this weed growing in front of our house in Massachusetts. Grateful to find the vegetable she had known in Southeast Asia as *rau sam*, she harvested and cooked it into soups for family dinners.

Over the years I have encountered similar stories about this humble plant making itself available to immigrants and refugees from places as diverse as Burma and Palestine. *Purslane. Verdolagas. Rau sam.* It goes by many names, including "noxious weed" to some people. But for many, this plant is a touchstone of familiarity, one that offers nourishment on many levels.

PURSLANE COOLER

Purslane is juicy, tart, and succulent, making it a welcome ingredient for summertime beverages. This refreshing drink combines purslane with chia seeds for hydration and omega-3s. The chia seeds also add visual and textural interest; however, if you don't like chia seeds in drinks, you can leave them out or substitute basil seeds.

Yield: 4 servings

1 cup fresh purslane (leaves and tender stems), coarsely chopped

Juice of 2 limes (about ¼ cup)

¼ cup honey, or to taste

4 cups cold water

1 tablespoon black or white chia seeds

Purslane, mint, or lemon balm sprig for garnish (optional)

1. Combine the purslane, lime juice, honey, and water in a blender. Blend until smooth. You can strain the mixture through a fine-mesh strainer if you don't want any pulp in your drink, but we usually leave it in.

2. Transfer the juice to a pitcher. Stir in the chia seeds. Let stand for about 15 minutes so the chia seeds can plump up.

3. Serve immediately or store in the refrigerator for up to 1 day. Just before serving, stir to evenly disperse the chia seeds. Pour the drink into ice-filled glasses and garnish as desired.

> *Variation:* For a fizzy drink, blend the purslane with just 2 cups of cold water. Before serving, stir in 2 cups of chilled sparkling water.

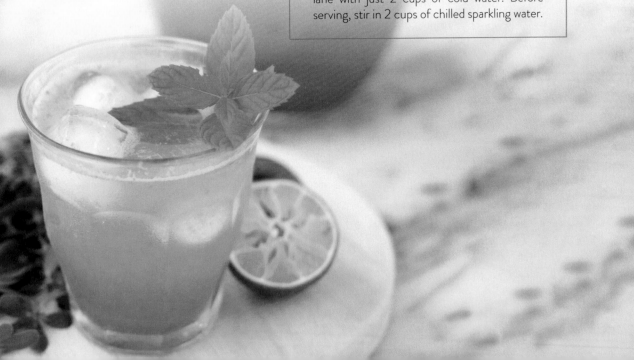

PURSLANE AND CUCUMBER SALAD

This crisp salad makes a refreshing addition to summer meals and barbecues and is excellent alongside grilled foods. The Vietnamese-inspired dressing is tangy and sweet with a hint of spice. If you like more kick, you can leave in the jalapeño seeds.

If you are using Persian or English cucumbers, the peel is not likely to be bitter and you do not need to remove it. However, if you are substituting another cucumber variety, you may wish to peel them.

Yield: 4 to 6 servings

Dressing

1 tablespoon fresh lime juice

1 tablespoon unseasoned rice vinegar

2 teaspoons brown sugar or coconut sugar

¼ teaspoon salt

1 teaspoon avocado oil (or other mild-tasting oil)

1 garlic clove, crushed

1 large jalapeño (seeds and ribs removed), thinly sliced

Salad

3 Persian cucumbers or 1 English cucumber

2 cups purslane sprigs and leaves (thick stems removed)

¼ cup packed chopped cilantro

2 tablespoons packed chopped mint

2 scallions, thinly sliced

¼ cup unsalted, roasted peanuts, coarsely chopped

1. Combine the lime juice, rice vinegar, sugar, and salt in a small bowl and stir to dissolve the sugar. Stir in the oil, garlic, and jalapeño. Set this dressing aside while preparing the vegetables; this will give the flavors time to marry.

2. Thinly slice the cucumbers, then toss them with the purslane, cilantro, mint, and scallions in a large bowl. Add the dressing and toss to coat.

3. Garnish with the peanuts and serve.

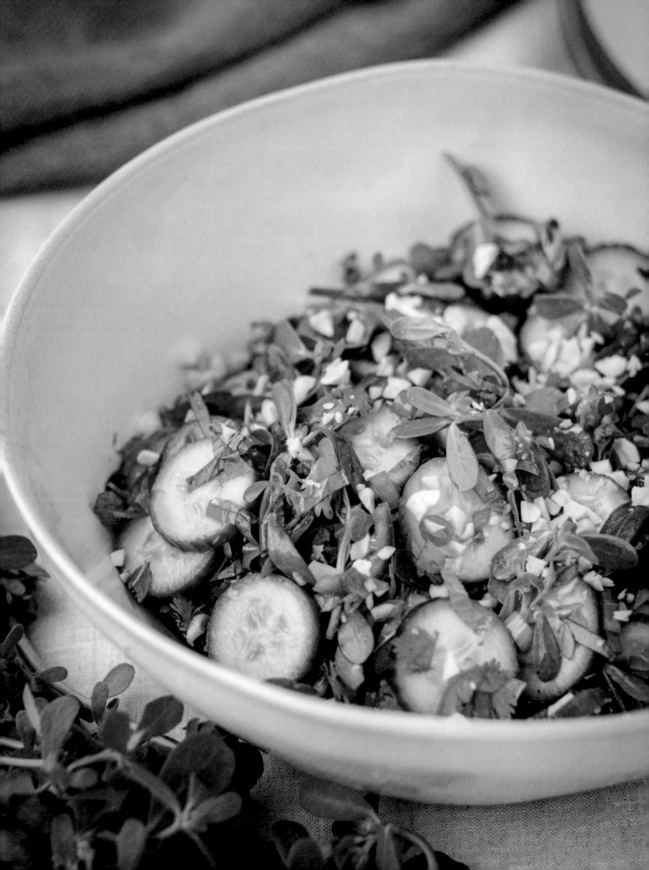

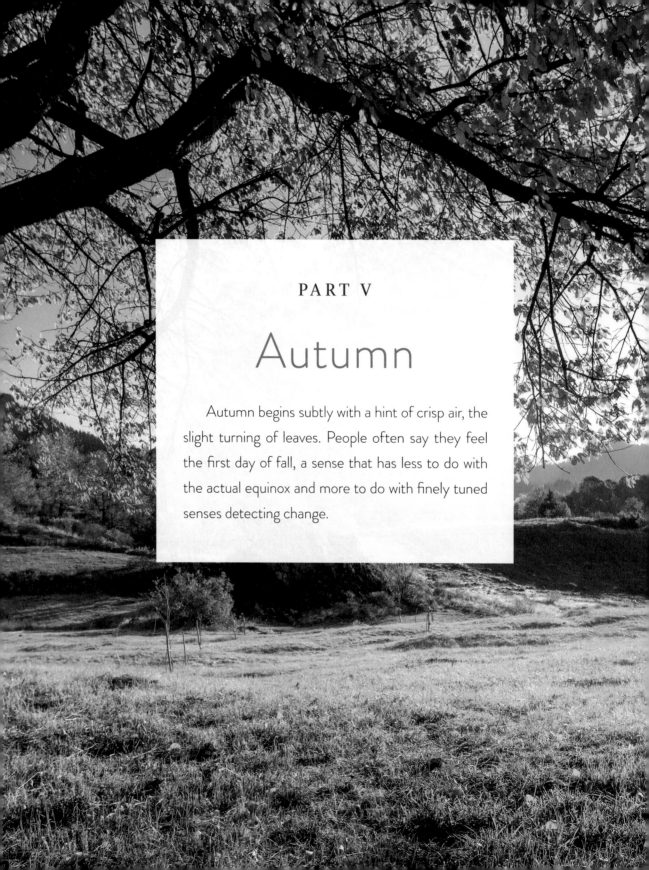

PART V

Autumn

Autumn begins subtly with a hint of crisp air, the slight turning of leaves. People often say they feel the first day of fall, a sense that has less to do with the actual equinox and more to do with finely tuned senses detecting change.

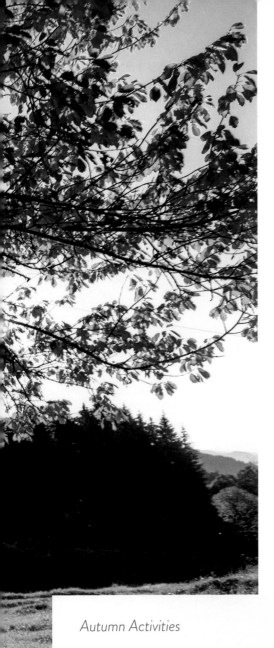

As the subdued colors of late summer fade, rains may return to soften soils, stimulating the fruiting of fungi. Awakened by the cool and moist earth, some plants like dandelion and chickweed return with tender leaves. With gratitude and a trowel, we dig to unearth roots that offer toning and building foods and medicines.

Like a finely tuned orchestra, the climax of fall begins to build. Birds, bats, and dragonflies leave their annual summer homes and travel to winter habitats. As more leaves turn, gold cottonwoods and orange and red oaks and maples stand out against a deep blue sky. Our foods blend into the flame-colored trees as we prepare feasts with squash, pumpkins, and sweet potatoes.

Just as your heart overflows with fall's colors, winds whip through the trees, pulling and tugging to release the fading currency of summer's hard work. Leaves littering the ground remind us that the wheel is constantly turning; nothing is permanent. In many cultures late autumn is a time to connect with those who came before in recognition that death is but one part of a continuing cycle. In what ways do you turn inward? How can you harness this time to connect to your ancestral roots?

Autumn Activities

- Take an outdoor stroll
- Breathe in the crisp air
- Make a nature arrangement
- Jump in a pile of leaves
- Sip warm beverages

- Carve a pumpkin and roast the seeds
- Draw roots or mushrooms
- Plant seeds and bulbs for next spring
- Have an autumn feast
- Keep a journal (see Chapter 7)

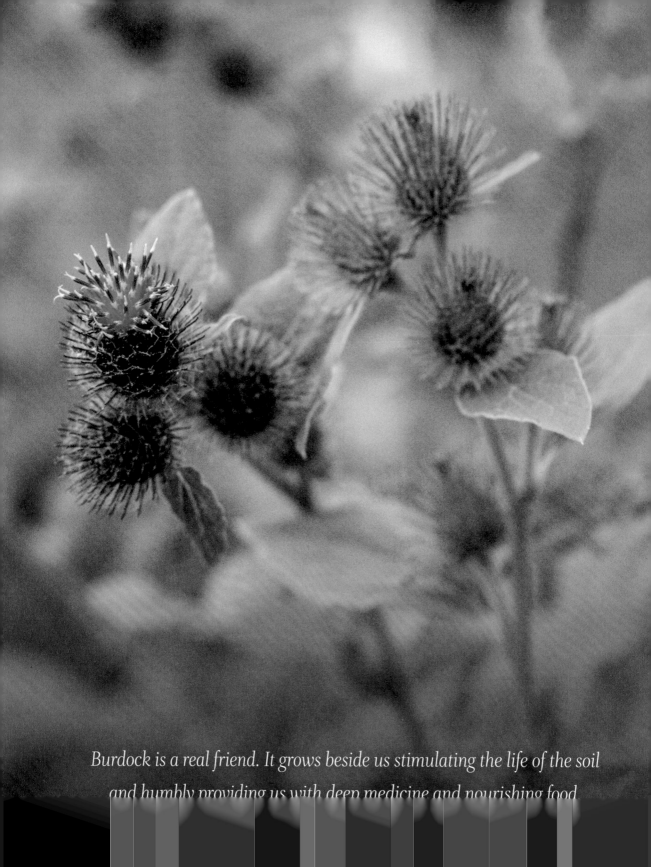

Burdock is a real friend. It grows beside us stimulating the life of the soil and humbly providing us with deep medicine and nourishing food.

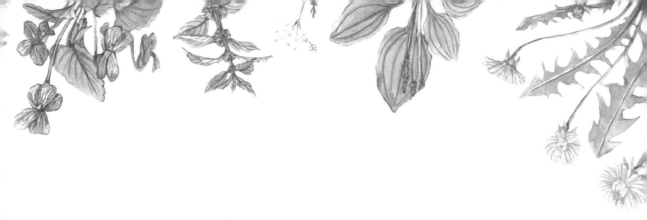

CHAPTER 25

BURDOCK

Burdock is a ubiquitous weed, a nourishing food, a powerful medicine, and a bane to long-haired animals all rolled up into one plant. It's both loved by herbalists and hated by ranchers. These many roles illustrate the nonduality of plants. So often the most despised weeds, like burdock, offer the most plentiful food and medicine. Burdock's deep taproots provide sustaining nourishment, its large leaves can be used to store food and as a cooling poultice, and the seeds offer potent medicine for acute symptoms.

Other common name: gobo
Botanical names: *Arctium lappa, A. minus*
Family: Asteraceae (aster)
Parts used: roots, seeds, leaves, stalks
Energetics: cooling, balancing dry and moist
Taste: bitter, sweet
Properties: alterative, diaphoretic (seeds), diuretic, hepatic, lymphatic, nutritive
Uses: food, move stagnant lymph, over- or underactive sebaceous glands, prebiotic, promoting healthy skin, fluid retention, supporting liver health
Preparations: decoction, food, tincture

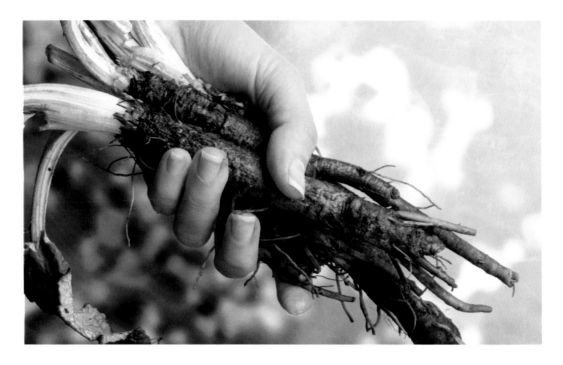

Burdock has been used as a food and medicine for thousands of years throughout Asia and Europe. Many ancient texts mention this plant, and given its pervasive growing habits, we can guess that it was used as a folk remedy. In addition to burdock's edible and medicinal benefits, its clingy, mature burrs can be used as makeshift buttons. However, these burrs weren't the inspiration for Velcro, as commonly claimed. That distinction goes to another burred plant, cocklebur (*Xanthium* spp.).

MEDICINAL PROPERTIES AND ENERGETICS

Burdock helps eliminate naturally occurring metabolic wastes. In other words, it helps support your natural detox system. To understand this, think of your body as a river. Ideally you want the water to be clear and moving along quickly. However, if your body's elimination systems slow down, your water can become a stagnant pond. For example, when lymph becomes stagnant, your lymph glands swell or you get lymphedema. If your liver is impaired, this can show up on the skin as rashes or acne, or it can be a contributing factor to hormone imbalances. When the colon isn't moving waste properly, you experience constipation. If your kidneys are sluggish, you may get edema. The examples go on and on.

Herbs that restore function to elimination organs are called alterative herbs. Essentially they break up stagnations to remove these metaphorical stagnant ponds and get your river running clear again. Alterative herbs often have an affinity for a particular organ system. In the case of burdock, both the root and seeds shine at improving metabolic function in a way that promotes healthy skin.

Burdock could also be considered a nutritive alterative. Taken over time, it provides nutrients as well as helps your body to better process nutrients, especially fat. It is often combined with dandelion root for this purpose.

PLANT GIFTS

Promotes Healthy Skin

Burdock can be used to address chronic and acute skin rashes ranging from eczema and psoriasis to acne and boils. What makes burdock so successful is that its underlying actions affect many different systems of the body, including the sebaceous glands, liver, lymph, and kidneys. When any of these become deficient or sluggish, it can result in problems on the skin.

Burdock promotes healthy sebaceous gland secretions. Sebaceous glands are tiny glands found in the skin. They excrete sebum, a waxy or oily substance that moisturizes your skin and hair. Sebum can also help to waterproof your skin, and it can insulate your skin to keep you warm. When sebaceous glands on the face over-secrete, sebum can block pores and make skin more prone to acne. When sebaceous glands are deficient, it can lead to dry, scaly skin. Burdock root and seed address both conditions by helping to keep your sebaceous glands working just right.

Relieves Arthritis

Herbalists have long reached for burdock to help ease the pain of arthritis, and new research illuminates some of the ways burdock does this. In one study, patients with osteoarthritis who drank burdock tea daily for 42 days had significant benefits, including a lowered C-reactive protein showing reduced inflammation. The researchers concluded, "The results suggested that *Arctium lappa* L. root tea improves inflammatory status and oxidative stress in patients with knee osteoarthritis."[1]

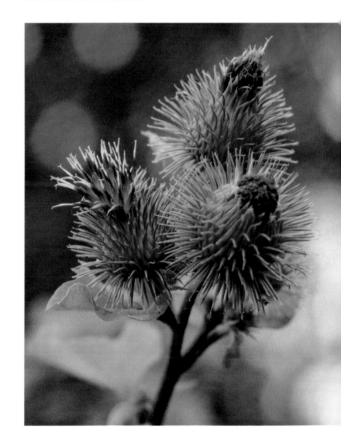

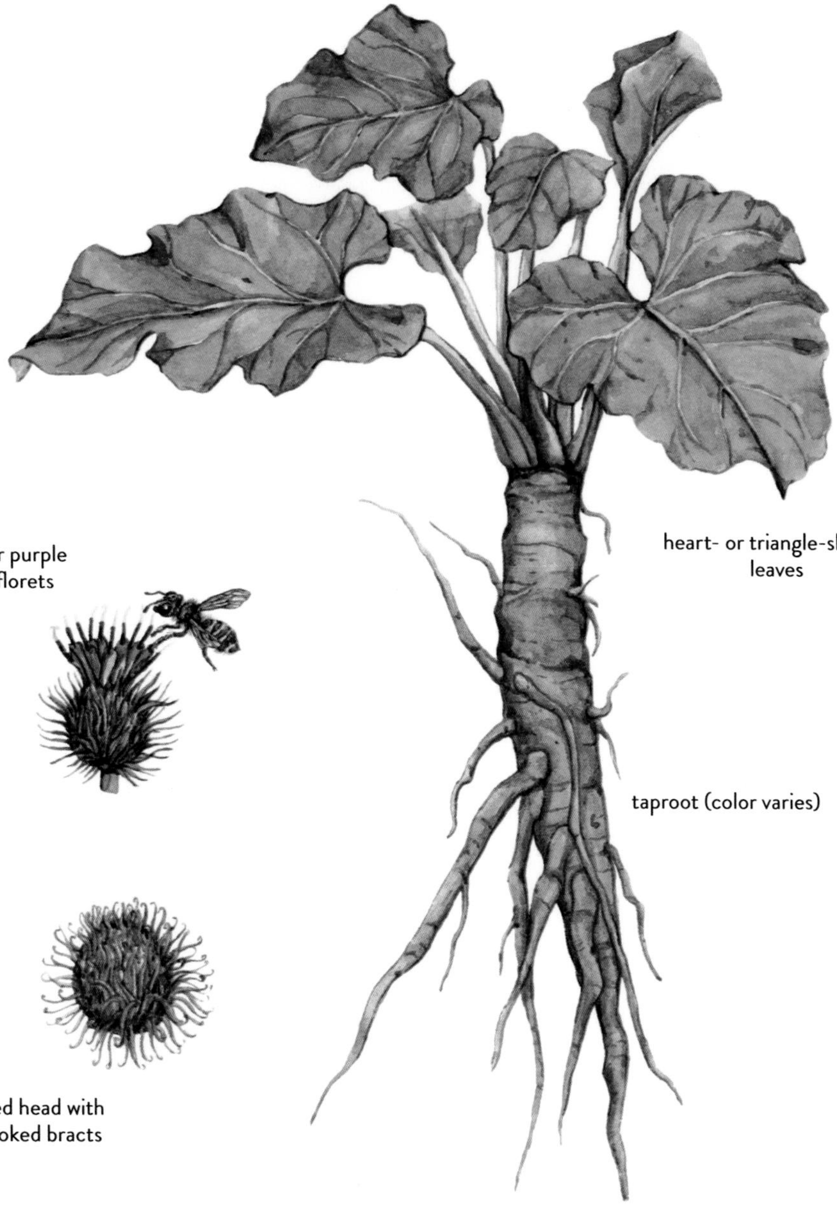

pink or purple
disk florets

heart- or triangle-shaped
leaves

taproot (color varies)

seed head with
hooked bracts

burdock (*Arctium minus*), shown with pugnacious leaf-cutter bee (*Megachile pugnata*)

Life cycle: herbaceous biennial, sometimes perennial
Reproduces by: seed
Growth habit: large basal rosette, erect flowering stalks, 2–9 feet tall
Habitat: abandoned fields, creek beds, disturbed areas, ditches, fencerows, meadows, pastures, railways, roadsides, stream banks, vacant lots, woodland edges
Sun: full sun to partial shade
Soil: variable; prefers damp and loamy
USDA Hardiness Zones: 3–9

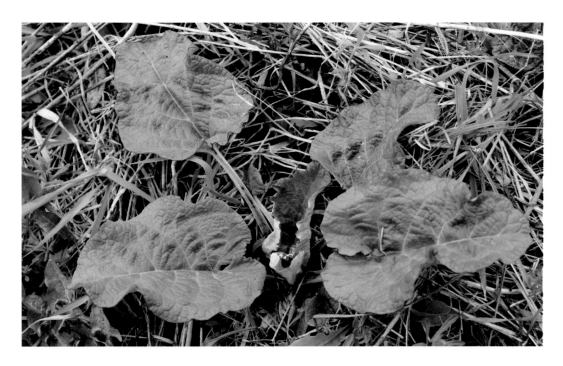

Supports the Urinary System

Both burdock root and seed are diuretics, although the seed has a stronger action. In addition to promoting diuresis, burdock can be used for urinary gravel and stones, painful urination, and involuntary urination. *King's American Dispensatory*, an Eclectic herbal text from 1898, refers to burdock seed as a urinary alterative and recommends taking it as an alcohol extract.

Provides Prebiotics

Burdock root contains a high percentage of inulin, with many sources citing as much as 45 to 50 percent in the fresh root. Inulin (not to be confused with insulin) is a starchy carbohydrate that is indigestible to humans but provides nutrients for the gut flora. Consuming prebiotic foods like burdock along with fermented foods or probiotics can more effectively support a diverse microbiome than probiotics alone. Burdock's ability to support healthy gut flora may be one reason it enhances nutrient absorption when used over a long period.

Addresses Cancer

Historically burdock has been used for people with cancer. It was a main herb in two famous cancer therapies from the 1920s: Essiac and the Hoxsey formula. To date there haven't been any human clinical trials using the whole herb, but there have been several in vitro studies using isolated extracts with promising results. One constituent, the lignan arctigenin, has been shown to induce apoptosis (cell death) in ovarian cancer cells and estrogen receptor–negative breast cancer.[2] Arctigenin and other lignans have also been shown to have positive effects against multidrug–resistant cancer cells.[3]

Leaves Provide Medicine and Tools

Burdock has large leaves that can be used as medicine or tools. A fresh poultice made from the leaves can be used topically to soothe burns and heal wounds or to draw out infections such as boils and abscesses. Before modern-day refrigeration, people used the leaves to wrap and preserve foods such as butter.

HOW TO IDENTIFY

In North America the burdock species commonly found growing in the wild is *Arctium* *minus*, and the cultivated burdock is *A. lappa*. The descriptions below can apply to both.

In its first year, the plant forms a low-growing basal rosette of large, coarse leaves. The leaves are alternate, either cordate or triangular, and may be toothed or ruffled. They can grow up to 2 feet long and 1.5 feet wide. The leaf stems of *A. minus* are hollow. The plant has a fleshy yellow, brown, or white taproot.

In the second year, the plant produces a sturdy, erect stalk up to 9 feet tall (typically taller in *A. lappa* and shorter in *A. minus*). The stalk may or may not be branched, and the leaves become progressively smaller up the stem.

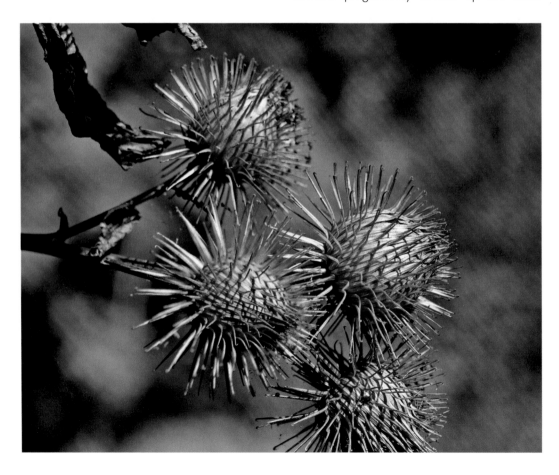

Prickly composite flower heads are arranged in panicles and consist of numerous pink or purple disk florets. (It has no ray florets.) Surrounding the florets are bracts with tiny hooks that curve inward. The round seed heads are light brown with short bristles. Although burdock is usually a biennial plant, it has been known to grow as a perennial, taking several years to flower and then dying after flowering.

ECOLOGICAL CONNECTIONS

Burdock's long taproot breaks up hard ground and pulls up minerals from deep below. Caterpillars of painted lady butterflies (*Vanessa cardui*) eat the foliage, and caterpillars of borer moths (*Papaipema* spp.) bore through the stems. The flowers are mainly pollinated by long-tongued bees, including bumblebees, honeybees, miner bees, and leaf-cutting bees, as well as butterflies and skippers. Birds may feed on the seeds and insects within the seed heads; however, birds can also become trapped in the burrs. The bristly fruits easily attach to mammals' fur and humans' clothing, transporting the seeds to new locations.

HOW TO HARVEST

Harvest burdock root in the autumn of the plant's first year or the spring of the second year, before it produces stalks. The taproot can grow up to 4 feet long and be very difficult to harvest. Dig wide and deep using a long shovel; it can be easier to dig after a rain when the soil is softer. Gather the leaves as needed, but it's best to cut them before the flowering stalks grow. Collect the seeds after the burrs have dried and turned brown. Place the burrs in a bag and whack them with a stick or rolling pin to break them open and release the seeds. Separating the seeds from the chaff can stir up tiny hairs, irritating the skin and respiratory system; consider wearing gloves or a mask.

Burdock reproduces by seed, and one plant can produce 15,000 of them! However, remember that when you harvest a root, the plant dies and can't make flowers and seeds the next year, so leave enough plants in the stand.

Harvesting Cautions

The edible leaves of bitter dock (*Rumex obtusifolius*) are sometimes mistaken for burdock. Be cautious of the poisonous leaves of rhubarb (*Rheum* spp.). While the underside of burdock leaves are woolly, the underside of rhubarb leaves are smooth. Cocklebur (*Xanthium* spp.) may also be mistaken for burdock; note its elliptic rather than round fruits or seed heads.

GARDENING TIPS

Because burdock is a biennial, consider creating a burdock garden bed to maintain an annual supply of fresh burdock roots. Burdock is easy to grow, but loose, loamy soil is needed to harvest fully developed roots. Adding composted manure will greatly improve root development. Plant seeds in early spring and plan to harvest some of the plants in their first year, allowing the rest to go to seed and self-sow in the second year. Burdock can easily become invasive and is classified as a "noxious" weed in several U.S. states.

USING BURDOCK IN YOUR LIFE

Burdock roots are commonly eaten as a vegetable in Chinese, Japanese, and Korean cuisines. They can be stir-fried, braised, roasted, added to stews, and pickled. People have also used the roots in recipes for beer and soda. While the wild *A. minus* roots are undoubtedly strong medicine and probably higher in nutrients, the *A. lappa* roots found in gardens and East Asian and natural grocery stores are a lot easier to harvest. We often reserve the wild roots for medicinal applications and use the cultivated roots for food.

The roots, leaves, and seeds are all used as medicine. The roots can be eaten (food as medicine!), dried and used as a decoction, or made into an alcohol or vinegar extract. The roots are often used for chronic issues and are best when taken daily for weeks or months at a time. The leaves can be used as a fresh poultice. They can also be used in bitters blends or made into a bitter tea to stimulate digestion. The seeds are often made into an alcohol extract and are typically used for more acute issues such as sties or urinary tract infections or as a diaphoretic to support the fever process.

Recommended Amounts

- *Decoction (root):* 15 to 30 grams

- *Seeds:* 3 to 10 grams

- *Tincture (seeds):* 1:5, 50% alcohol; 2 to 4 ml, 3 times daily

Special Considerations

- Burdock root is a common vegetable and is considered to be safe for most people.

- As with many alteratives, people with skin conditions may experience an increase in symptoms when they start to take burdock. To decrease this effect, try combining it with more eliminating herbs as well as starting with a lower dose and slowly increasing it.

- There have been a few reports of burdock having adverse effects in people allergic to Asteraceae family plants.

- Safety of the seed has not been conclusively established in pregnancy and lactation.

BURDOCK AND GINGER SODA

People have long used burdock root to flavor sodas and root beers. Classic springtime brews include burdock with dandelion and nettle. For autumn (or any time of year, really!), we like pairing burdock with warming ginger, allspice, cardamom, and star anise. The result is lightly spicy and very refreshing.

Yield: About 6 drinks

¼ cup (1 ounce) scrubbed, thinly sliced fresh burdock root, or 2 tablespoons (¼ ounce) dried burdock root

¼ cup (1 ounce) peeled, thinly sliced fresh ginger, or 2 tablespoons (¼ ounce) dried ginger

1½ cups water

1 lemon, sliced into rounds

4 whole allspice berries

1 whole star anise pod

1 green cardamom pod, cracked

¾ cup mild-flavored honey, or to taste

Chilled seltzer or club soda, for serving

1. Combine the burdock, ginger, and water in a saucepan. Bring to a boil over high heat. Cover the pan, reduce the heat to low, and simmer for 30 minutes.

2. Remove from the heat and stir in the lemon slices, allspice, star anise, cardamom, and honey. Let cool completely.

3. Strain the syrup through a fine-mesh strainer, then transfer to a clean jar or bottle. It can be stored in the refrigerator for up to 1 week.

4. To make a soda, mix 1 part syrup with 4 parts seltzer; taste, and adjust quantities as desired.

Variation: If you are accustomed to making fermented sodas using a ginger bug, you can mix this syrup with water to make your wort. Instead of ginger, you can also make a burdock bug with foraged or homegrown burdock root (store-bought burdock doesn't always ferment reliably).

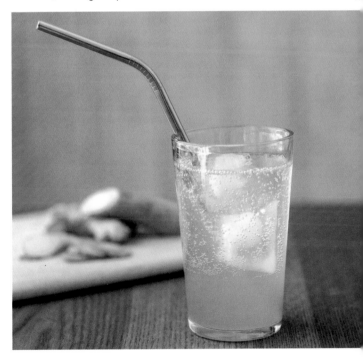

BRAISED BURDOCK ROOT

Burdock root may look intimidating, but it's easy to cook once you learn a few cleaning and cutting techniques. The flavors in this braised burdock dish were inspired by Emily's mother-in-law, whose Korean-style burdock (called gobo or ueong) is mildly earthy, salty, and sweet. It can be served as a side dish or prepared as a lightly crunchy filling for seaweed rolls (page 290). This recipe calls for ½ pound of burdock root, which you'll get from about 1½ feet of root, but this will vary according to the thickness of the root.

Yield: 4 servings

½ pound burdock root (about 4 cups julienned; see step 2 for instructions)

1 tablespoon neutral-tasting oil for sautéing

¼ cup water, plus large bowl of water for soaking in step 2

1½ tablespoons soy sauce

1 tablespoon brown rice syrup or honey

1 tablespoon mirim (sweet Korean rice wine) or mirin (sweet Japanese rice wine)

½ teaspoon toasted sesame oil

1 teaspoon toasted sesame seeds

1. Scrub the burdock root with a vegetable scrubber or scouring pad to remove the dirt, and rinse it well. (You can peel the root if you wish, but we like to leave as much nutritious peel as possible.)

2. Have a large bowl of water near your cutting area. Tough and fibrous, burdock root is easiest to cut on the bias. Use a sharp knife to cut the root on the diagonal to produce oval slices about 2 inches long and ⅛ inch thick. Stack a few of the slices at a time and cut them into thin matchsticks. As you work, soak the cut pieces in the bowl of water, which helps prevent oxidation and removes some of the bitterness. When finished cutting, drain and rinse the burdock. Pat dry with a clean towel.

3. Heat 1 tablespoon of neutral oil in a large skillet over medium heat. Add the burdock and cook, stirring frequently, until crisp-tender and lightly browned, about 6 minutes. Add ¼ cup of water and the soy sauce, brown rice syrup, and mirim. Continue to cook, stirring occasionally, until the liquid is absorbed, about 8 minutes. Stir in the sesame oil and sesame seeds.

4. Serve hot or at room temperature. This dish can be stored in an airtight container in the refrigerator for 1 week.

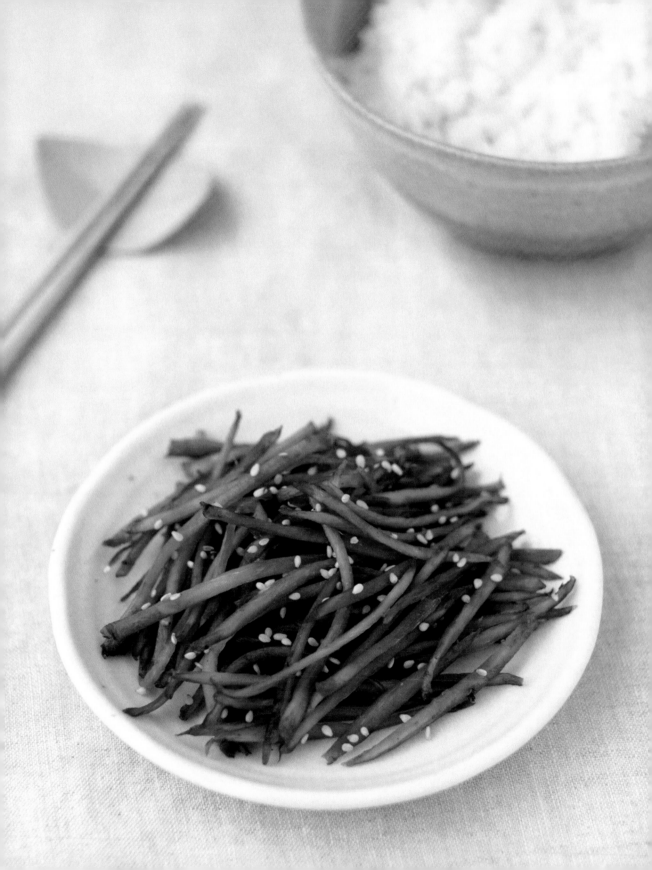

SEAWEED ROLLS WITH BURDOCK

Braised burdock root makes a great filling for gimbap, or Korean-style seaweed rolls. We enjoy packing these bite-size snacks for lunches, picnics, and potlucks. Although the recipe includes suggested fillings, these rolls are a great vehicle for any leftover grains, vegetables, and various odds and ends you have in the fridge. You'll need a bamboo mat to make these, or you can improvise with a kitchen towel. (For instructions, search online for "How to make sushi without a mat.")

Yield: About 32 pieces

---

3 cups cooked short-grain white rice

2 tablespoons toasted sesame oil, divided

½ teaspoon kosher salt, divided

1 pound spinach (about 4 cups)

1½ teaspoons toasted sesame seeds, divided

1 carrot, cut into matchsticks (about 1 cup)

2 large eggs

4 sheets roasted seaweed (also called gim, nori, or laver)

4 pencil-size strips danmuji (pickled daikon) or cucumber

1 cup braised burdock root (page 288)

½ cup warm water

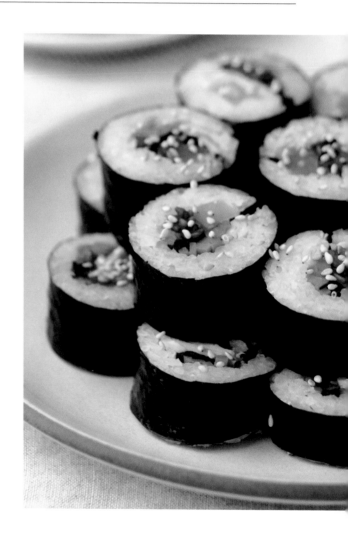

1. Season the rice: Using a rice paddle or wooden spoon, mix the rice with 2 teaspoons of the sesame oil and ¼ teaspoon salt. Set aside. If the rice is still warm, let it cool to room temperature before making the rolls.

2. Blanch the spinach: Bring a large pot of water to a boil. Add the spinach and boil until it is bright green, about 1 minute. Drain and rinse under cold running water. Squeeze out all the liquid. Using your hands, mix the spinach with ½ teaspoon of the sesame seeds and ⅛ teaspoon salt. Set aside.

3. Cook the carrot: Heat 1 teaspoon sesame oil in a medium skillet over medium heat. Add the carrot and cook, stirring, until crisp-tender, about 2 minutes. Remove from the pan and set aside.

4. Make an egg omelet: Whisk the eggs with ⅛ teaspoon salt. Heat 1 teaspoon sesame oil in the same skillet over medium heat. Pour the egg into the skillet and swirl it so the egg covers the entire surface. Cook for about 2 minutes, until the bottom is set, then flip it over and cook for about 1 minute on the other side. Transfer the omelet to a cutting board and cut it into ½-inch-wide strips.

5. Set up your work area: Lay out a bamboo rolling mat, the seaweed sheets, fillings (rice, pickled daikon or cucumber, burdock, spinach, carrot, egg), a small bowl of warm water, the remaining 2 teaspoons sesame oil, and a platter for finished rolls.

6. Assemble the rolls: Position the bamboo rolling mat with a long side nearest you; the bamboo sticks should be horizontal. With dry hands, place one sheet of seaweed on the bamboo mat with the shiny side down. Lightly moisten your hands with water and evenly spread a quarter of the rice on the lower two-thirds of the seaweed. (If the rice sticks to your fingers, lightly dip them in water.) About an inch up from the bottom of the rice, arrange the fillings in neat, horizontal rows.

7. Starting from the side nearest you, roll the bamboo mat up and over the fillings, using firm but gentle pressure to hold the ingredients in place. As you roll forward, pull the mat up and out so it doesn't get caught in the roll. Keep rolling and releasing the mat until you form a compact cylinder. Dip a finger in the water and moisten the edge of the seaweed to seal the roll. Using your fingers, lightly rub sesame oil on the outside of the roll. Transfer the roll to the platter.

8. Repeat to make the rest of the rolls. When all four rolls are complete, slice each one into bite-size rounds (about 8 pieces each) using a knife coated in a thin layer of sesame oil.

9. Sprinkle the remaining 1 teaspoon sesame seeds over the cut rolls and serve.

Variation: Strips of baked tofu, avocado, bulgogi (Korean grilled beef), or eomuk (Korean fish cake) can be substituted for the egg.

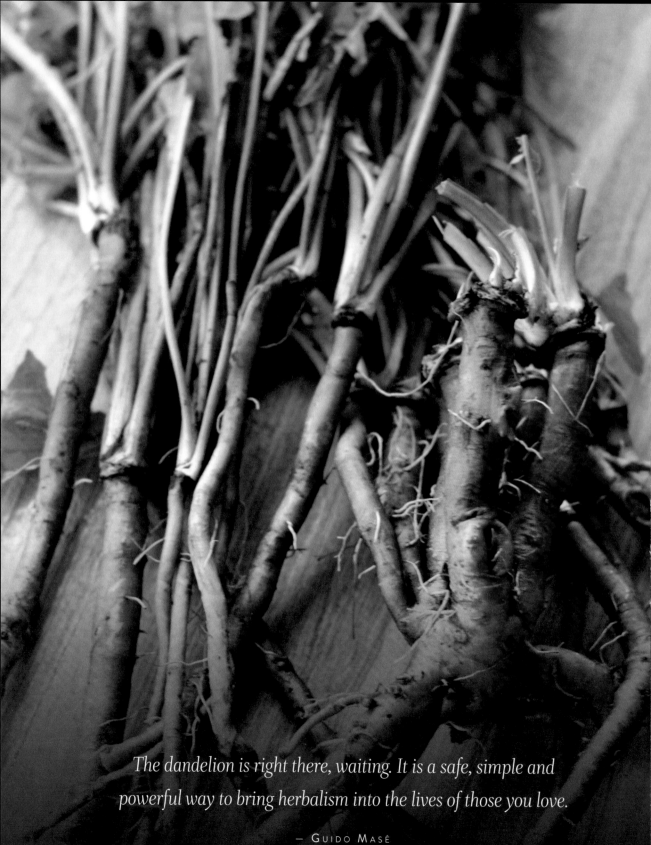

The dandelion is right there, waiting. It is a safe, simple and powerful way to bring herbalism into the lives of those you love.

— GUIDO MASÉ

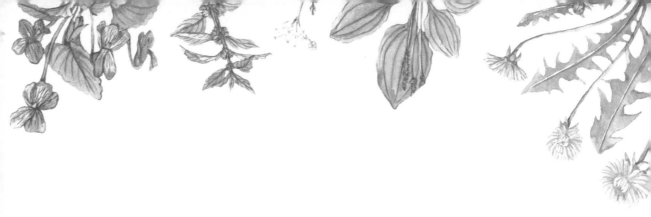

CHAPTER 26

DANDELION ROOT

Dandelion root reaches down into the earth, pulling up vitamins and minerals
that nourish the surrounding soil, the plant itself, and those who eat it. Have you
dug dandelion roots? If so, you know they don't give up their home easily. If you pull
too hard or don't loosen the soil enough, the crown of the plant will pop off. Even
with intentional digging, it's common for parts of the root to remain in the soil.
Dandelion's tenacious ability to hold back a bit for itself is effective! If enough root
remains in the ground, it will continue to live and more dandelions will grow. While this
ingenious self-preservation method is frustrating to those who want to eradicate the
plant, it's a blessing to those of us enchanted with the charm and medicine of dandelion.

Botanical name: *Taraxacum officinale*
Family: Asteraceae (aster)
Parts used: roots, leaves and flowers (see Chapter 9), sap, seeds
Energetics: cooling, drying
Taste: bitter, sweet, salty
Properties: alterative, mild diuretic, mild laxative, nutritive, stimulates bile
Uses: food, healthy liver stagnation, poor digestion, skin eruptions
Preparations: decoction, food, tincture, vinegar

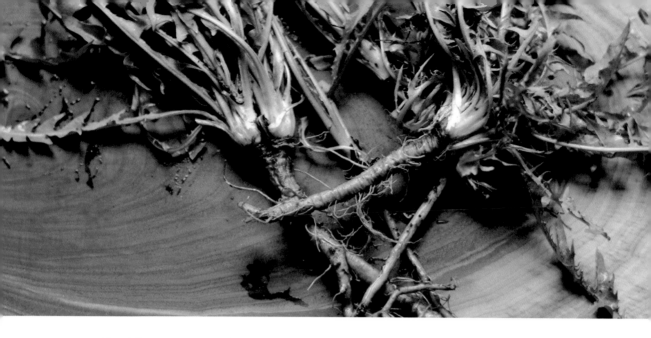

Dandelion root is used as medicine by Western herbalists, in Chinese medicine, and in Ayurveda. Interestingly, the first mention of dandelion root that we know of in Western literature didn't appear until 1539 in a work by German botanist Hieronymus Bock. Herbalist Peter Holmes surmises that Bock may have learned about the uses of dandelion from wise women practitioners and helped to popularize it with physicians at the time.[1] It's probably a safe bet that people have relied on dandelion as a traditional remedy for thousands of years. Dandelion root was in the *United States Pharmacopoeia* from 1831 to 1926. It remains in the pharmacopoeias of Austria, Hungary, and Poland.[2]

MEDICINAL PROPERTIES AND ENERGETICS

Dandelion root has a somewhat bitter taste and a strong affinity for the liver. It is loaded with vitamins and minerals, including potassium, calcium, phosphorus, and magnesium.[3] The bitterness of dandelion root is milder than that of many other bitters such as gentian root, artichoke leaf, or even a mature dandelion leaf,

and it also has a sweeter taste. Herbalist jim mcdonald aptly refers to dandelion root as a nutritive bitter.

PLANT GIFTS

Supports the Liver

Many herbalists reach for dandelion root to address a wide range of liver complaints, especially liver stagnation. Symptoms of a stagnant liver might include poor digestion (especially poor fat digestion or absorption), sour belching, estrogen dominance, and excessive premenstrual syndrome (PMS) symptoms, including bloating, clots, cramping, irregular bowel movements, and emotional dysregulation. Herbalists often consider eruptive skin conditions to have their roots in poor liver function. Dandelion root can be paired with other alterative herbs such as burdock root and red clover to address skin conditions like acne, boils, and rashes.

Your liver is a powerful organ that plays an important role in detoxification. Supporting your body's ability to eliminate naturally occurring wastes day in and day out is the best detox you can do. Dandelion root is the perfect example of how useful, practical, and sustainable herbalism can be. Instead of buying expensive and harsh detox kits from the store, consider dandelion. Although they don't have fancy marketing, the dandelion roots growing in your yard can be a safer and more effective way to support your systems of elimination.

Promotes Digestion

As dandelion root supports liver health, it also promotes healthy digestion. That bitter taste helps to stimulate bile flow in the liver and gallbladder, helping to digest fats. The root is also a mild laxative. When you eat roots harvested in the autumn, you are also getting lots of inulin, a prebiotic that feeds healthy gut flora. For more information on inulin, see Provides Prebiotics on page 283.

Addresses Cancer

Dandelion root has a history of use to support people with cancer. This traditional use has piqued interest in modern times, and multiple in vitro studies have looked at how dandelion root acts against cancer cells. Studies have shown positive results in using dandelion root against various cancer cells, including breast, prostate, lung, gastric, and colorectal.[4] In vitro studies are a first step in learning more about how dandelion root can address cancer. Future human clinical trials are needed for a better understanding of dandelion's gifts in supporting people with cancer.

HOW TO IDENTIFY

For a general description of the dandelion plant, including leaves and flowers, see page 94.

Dandelions have a whitish taproot, typically 6 to 24 inches long, although the roots have been known to grow to 15 feet! Dandelions grown in dry, rocky soils tend to have smaller roots, and those grown in moist, fertile soils have larger ones.

ECOLOGICAL CONNECTIONS

Dandelion roots can deeply penetrate soils, benefiting other plants and the soil itself. In the book *Invasive Plant Medicine*, Timothy Lee Scott writes that dandelion "is considered an excellent dynamic accumulator of potassium, phosphorus, calcium, copper, and iron, bringing these subsurface minerals to the topsoil and thereby providing fertilizer that benefits the surrounding plants." Scott also reports that in phytoremediation programs, dandelion has rid soils of heavy metals like copper, zinc, manganese, lead, and cadmium.[5]

HOW TO GATHER

Dandelion roots can be harvested in autumn or early spring. Roots harvested in autumn will have a sweeter taste and may be more pleasant as food. Spring roots often have a stronger bitter flavor, and some herbalists prefer spring roots for supporting liver health specifically. The ease or difficulty of digging the roots can depend on the soil they grow in. A *hori hori* is particularly useful for digging dandelion roots.

Dandelions tend to grow without our help, but you can help keep a stand going by leaving part of the taproot in the soil. Just an inch-long piece of root can regrow. Dandelions can also be propagated by seed.

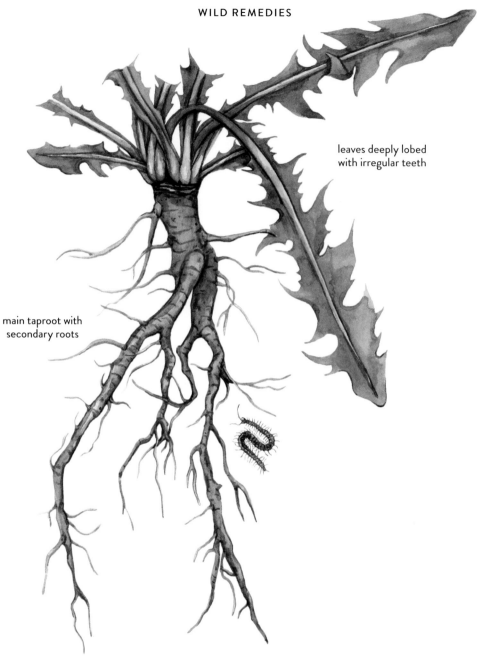

leaves deeply lobed
with irregular teeth

main taproot with
secondary roots

dandelion (*Taraxacum officinale*), shown with soil centipede (*Geophilus flavus*)

Life cycle: herbaceous perennial
Reproduces by: seed, root
Growth habit: basal leaf rosette with upright stem, 2–12 inches tall
Habitat: disturbed areas, fields, lawns, meadows, pastures, roadsides, sidewalk cracks
Sun: full sun to partial shade
Soil: prefers loamy, moist
USDA Hardiness Zones: 5–9

Harvesting Cautions

Every year billions of dollars are spent on herbicides by those wishing to eradicate the dandelion. Harvest dandelions in an area that hasn't been poisoned for at least three years and is free of heavy metals.

Potential look-alike plants include cat's ear (*Hypochaeris radicata*), hawkweed (*Hieracium pilosella*), sow thistle (*Sonchus* spp.), chicory (*Cichorium intybus*), and young wild lettuce (*Lactuca* spp.) plants. Fortunately, none of these are poisonous.

GARDENING TIPS

See Dandelion Leaf and Flower, Chapter 9.

USING DANDELION ROOT IN YOUR LIFE

Dandelion root, mildly bitter and full of nutrients, is a wonderful way to use food as your medicine. When eaten regularly, the nourishing roots can support digestion, liver health, and a diverse gut microbiome. They can be eaten as you would any other root vegetable. While they can be eaten raw, they are more easily digested after they've been cooked. The bitterness of dandelion roots can vary with the season as well as growing conditions. For those with sensitive palates, marinating the roots can be one way to offset the bitter flavor.

Dandelion root can be extracted into alcohol or vinegar. To make dandelion vinegar, follow the Chickweed Vinegar process on page 85, using 1½ cups chopped fresh dandelion root (or ¾ cup dried) and infusing for 1 to 2 weeks.

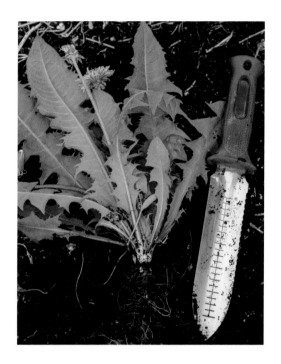

Dandelion root can also be dried and made into a decoction. Roasting before simmering gives it a rich flavor (although it may decrease the inulin content). Roast chopped, dried roots in a dry cast-iron pan over medium-high heat, stirring frequently, until they have a rich, aromatic smell.

Recommended Amounts

- *Decoction or powder (dried root):* 3 to 15 grams

- *Tincture (fresh root):* 1:2, 30% alcohol; 4 to 5 ml, 3 times daily

Special Considerations

Some people are sensitive to plants in the Asteraceae family, which can result in a rare and usually mild reaction to dandelion.

ROASTED ROOTS BREW

Grab your favorite sweater and a cozy blanket and curl up with this deeply nourishing brew on a crisp autumn day. We also love it served with dessert after a holiday meal; the slight bitterness pairs well with sweets and promotes digestion.

Yield: 1¼ cups (1 serving)

1 teaspoon finely chopped roasted dandelion root

1 teaspoon finely chopped roasted chicory root

1 teaspoon finely chopped dried burdock root

1½ cups water

Milk and honey (optional)

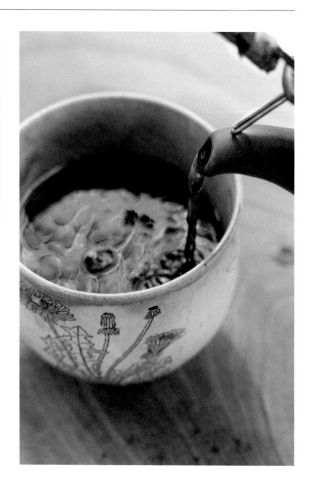

1. Place all the herbs in a small saucepan. Add the water and bring to a boil, then reduce the heat and simmer for 30 minutes, covered.

2. Strain. Add milk and honey, if desired. Consume within 24 hours.

DANDELION ROOT STIR-FRY

The bitterness of the dandelion root is tempered in this sweet and salty stir-fry. This is an easy meal to whip up on a weeknight—we suggest making larger batches so you'll have leftovers. The nutty taste of tempeh gives additional depth to this recipe, but if that's not your thing, you can use sliced chicken breast or sliced beef flank steak instead. Serve on rice, if desired.

Yield: 4 servings

2 garlic cloves, minced

1 teaspoon minced fresh gingerroot

½ cup tamari or soy sauce

½ cup water

⅓ cup honey

8 ounces tempeh cut into pieces 1 inch long and ½ inch thick

½ cup dandelion root cut into 1-inch-long matchsticks (3 to 5 dandelion roots)

2 tablespoons olive oil

½ cup carrots cut into 1-inch-long matchsticks (1 to 2 medium carrots)

6 cups chopped broccoli florets and stems

3 to 5 green onions cut into 1-inch-long pieces, with a few pieces minced for garnish

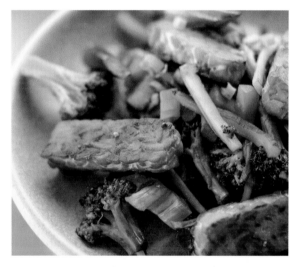

1. Combine the garlic, ginger, tamari or soy sauce, honey, and water in a large baking dish. Add the tempeh and dandelion root and marinate for 20 minutes to 1 hour.

2. Heat the olive oil in a large skillet over medium-high heat. Remove the tempeh from the marinade, add it to the skillet, and cook until golden brown on each side, about 2 minutes. Remove the tempeh from the skillet and place it on a plate.

3. Increase the heat to high, and add the carrots, broccoli, dandelion roots, and marinade to the skillet. Sauté until the vegetables are tender but still crisp, 4 to 5 minutes. Stir in the green onions and tempeh to reheat briefly.

4. Serve warm, garnished with minced green onions.

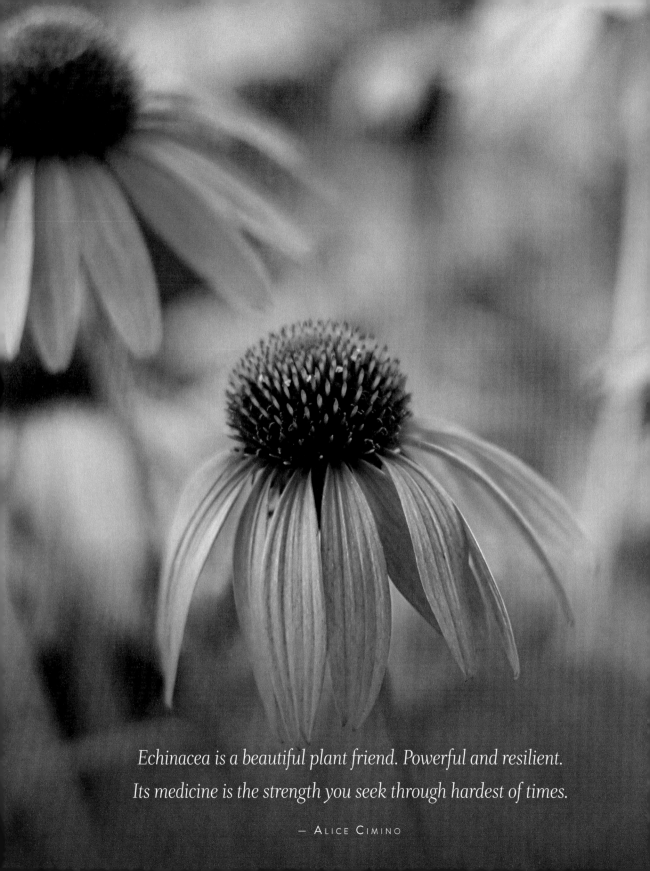

Echinacea is a beautiful plant friend. Powerful and resilient.
Its medicine is the strength you seek through hardest of times.

— ALICE CIMINO

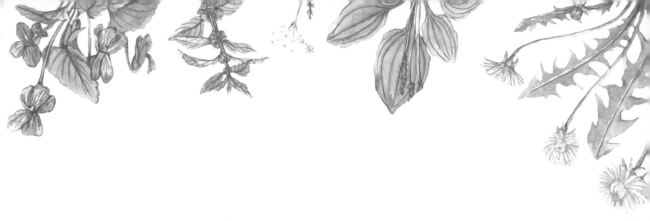

CHAPTER 27

ECHINACEA

Echinacea's strong, gorgeous flowers and pink hues attract humans and pollinators alike. Their prickly blooms are reminiscent of a hedgehog, which is another common name for the plant as well as the basis (in Greek) of the word *echinacea*. This is powerful medicine. Echinacea modulates the immune system and can dramatically address venomous bites and stings. But it is also cautionary medicine. Its presence in the wild has been greatly diminished, a tragic example of a taker's approach to wildcrafting.

Other common names: hedgehog coneflower, purple coneflower
Botanical names: *Echinacea angustifolia, E. purpurea, E. pallida*
Family: Asteraceae (aster)
Parts used: whole plant, flowers, roots, leaves (cultivated sources only)
Energetics: cooling, drying
Taste: pungent, acrid
Properties: alterative, antimicrobial, immunomodulator, inflammatory modulator, lymphagogue, sialagogue, vulnerary
Uses: abscesses, acne, boils, colds and flu, fevers, infected wounds, mouth infections, septicemia, venomous bites, warts
Preparations: decoction, mixed with clay, mouthwash, poultice, tea, tincture

Echinacea is endemic to North America and once grew abundantly throughout the eastern and central areas of the continent. Many different First Nations peoples have known it and used it as medicine. In the late 1800s, it became popular among the Eclectic physicians, who considered it one of their most important remedies. Echinacea's popularity has risen faster than an awareness of the need to protect this sensitive plant. As a result, it has been tragically overharvested from the wild. Many consider echinacea to be a poster child for Western herbalism. But what does it say about our approach when we destroy native plant communities and then turn their flowers into our logos?

MEDICINAL PROPERTIES AND ENERGETICS

As with all medicinal plants, you won't really understand echinacea until you taste it. And does it have a surprise in store for you! Echinacea zings. It pricks your taste buds, stimulates saliva, and then leaves a slight numbness in its wake. If you aren't prepared for this, it can be quite alarming. Echinacea stimulates the immune system and moves stagnant and swollen lymph. While it is currently popular for its ability to help ward off a cold or flu, this plant has many powerful gifts.

PLANT GIFTS

Heals Infections

Echinacea shines in its ability to help the body deal with infections. It works in both acute and chronic situations. It is a reliable herb for addressing recurring boils, acne, and other types of chronic skin abscesses. It can also be used on infected wounds, cuts, and scratches. For best results, it can be taken internally, or it

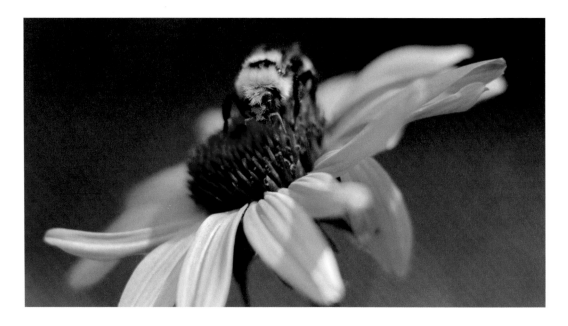

can be used externally as a tea wash or diluted tincture wash.

Long employed as a toothache plant, echinacea can be used as a mouthwash to address tooth infections, bleeding gums, and ulcerations of the oral mucous membranes. A pilot study showed that an oral patch containing *Echinacea purpurea*, gotu kola (*Centella asiatica*), and elderberry (*Sambucus nigra*) was effective in reducing inflammation associated with gingivitis in patients diagnosed with periodontitis.[1]

Soothes Venomous Bites and Stings

While often simply thought of as a "cold and flu herb," echinacea has some real superpowers. It can inhibit hyaluronidase, the tissue-destroying enzyme found in venomous bites and stings from rattlesnakes, lizards, scorpions, bees, caterpillars, and spiders. While antivenom medicines may be necessary for things like rattlesnake bites, taking echinacea while on your way to the hospital isn't a bad idea. In this situation, taking a liberal amount of tincture or glycerite, around 1 to 2 ounces, is recommended.

The first popularized use of echinacea by the Eclectic herbalists was for rattlesnake bites. We can trace this story back to H. C. F. Meyer. Historical references say that the self-described doctor learned about using echinacea for snake bites from a Native American woman. He then experimented with it for a number of years. In 1919, Eclectic physician Finley Ellingwood reported that Meyer willingly injected himself with rattlesnake venom on his right hand. After six hours, significant swelling had reached his elbow. He then dosed himself with his blend of herbs, which included echinacea, taking them both internally and externally, went to sleep, and woke up four hours later to find the pain and swelling were gone.[2]

Stimulates the Immune System

In recent years echinacea has been popularized for helping ward off a cold or flu. Interestingly, this is a relatively new use for this plant. Many ethnobotanical references cite it for other things such as toothaches, infections, and venomous bites. It was used extensively for sore throats, and in vitro studies have shown that *Echinacea purpurea* is active against the bacteria that cause strep throat (*Streptococcus pyogenes*).[3]

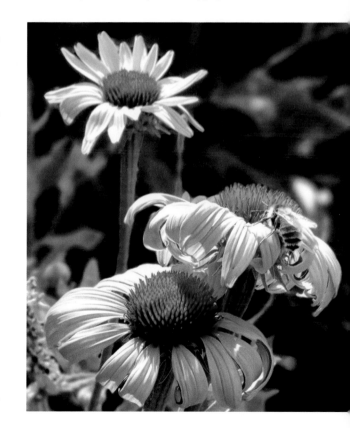

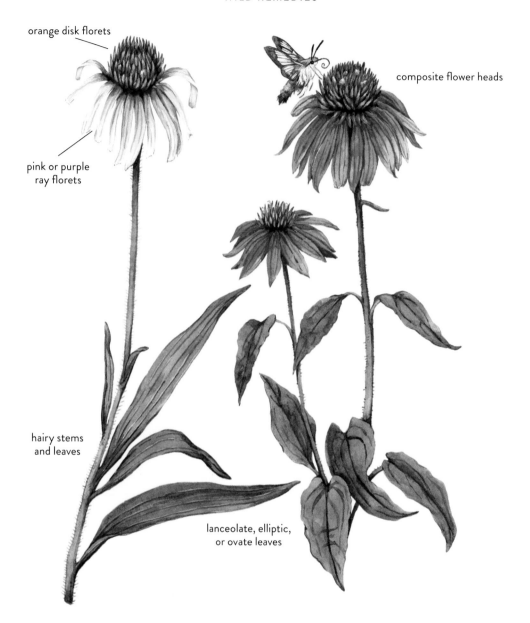

orange disk florets

pink or purple
ray florets

composite flower heads

hairy stems
and leaves

lanceolate, elliptic,
or ovate leaves

left: echinacea (*Echinacea angustifolia*) and right: echinacea (*Echinacea purpurea*),
shown with hummingbird clearwing moth (*Hemaris thysbe*)

Life cycle: herbaceous perennial
Reproduces by: seed
Growth habit: upright, 1–5 feet tall
Habitat: gardens, meadows, open woodlands, prairies
Sun: full sun to partial shade
Soil: dry to medium moisture, well drained
USDA Hardiness Zones: 3–9, depending on species

Numerous studies have looked at echinacea's ability to stop a cold or flu, and the results have been mixed. A deeper look at the negative results often reveals a problem with the design of the study, such as incorrect dosage or incorrect frequency of dosage. Like many herbal medicines, echinacea must be taken frequently and in adequate amounts to help with acute conditions like the onset of a cold or the flu. One meta-analysis of several studies concluded that "evidence indicates that echinacea potently lowers the risk of recurrent respiratory infections and complications thereof. Immune modulatory, antiviral, and anti-inflammatory effects might contribute to the observed clinical benefits, which appear strongest in susceptible individuals."[4] Another study found that "echinacea preparations can alleviate 'cold and flu' symptoms, and possibly other respiratory disorders, by inhibiting viral growth and the secretion of pro-inflammatory cytokines."[5]

A recent study found a formulation of echinacea and elderberry was just as effective as taking the commonly prescribed influenza pharmaceutical drug oseltamivir. There was one big difference between the two therapies, however: the echinacea drink was found to have fewer negative effects. The researchers wrote, "It appears to be an attractive treatment option, particularly suitable for self-care."[6]

Echinacea promotes immune system functions, notably phagocytosis (your body's cleanup system that envelops and eliminates pathogens and old cells). As a result, it is often classified as an immune stimulant, something used in the short term to quickly boost your immune system functions. But, as we learn more about how echinacea works, we are seeing that it doesn't fit well into a small box. One researcher found that in addition to echinacea's antiviral and antimicrobial activities, it also displays many immune modulating activities that involve the upregulation or downregulation of relevant genes and their transcription factors.[7] It may be that echinacea's effects also depend on *who* is using it. Herbalist Kevin Spelman, Ph.D., who has studied echinacea vigorously, says, "Intriguingly, *E. purpurea* extracts appear to function differently in a healthy individual's system than in an ill individual's system."[8]

Eclectic physicians used echinacea extensively, including for syphilis, chronic leg ulcers, gonorrhea, rabies, fevers, and septicemia (blood infection).[9] Above all, they thought of echinacea as an alterative herb with specific effects on the lymphatic system. It is commonly used today to address swollen lymph glands, especially in the throat.

HOW TO IDENTIFY

There are at least 12 species of echinacea. Each has its own identifying characteristics, and you should consult a local field guide or gardening reference for specific details. Generally speaking, these plants have stout, upright stems and lanceolate, elliptic, or ovate leaves. The stems and leaves are hairy and rough to the touch. Echinacea's showy composite flower heads are 2 to 5 inches wide and composed of disk florets and ray florets. The disk florets are orange-brown and form a central disk or cone. The outer ray florets range in color from pink to purple.

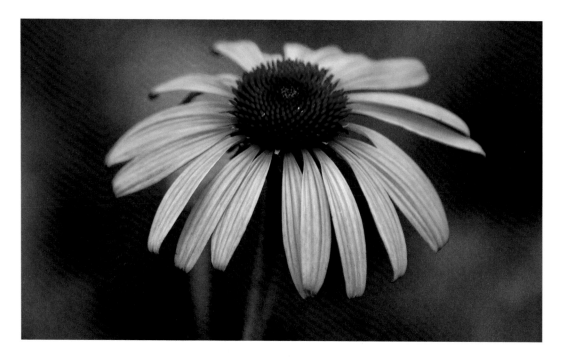

ECOLOGICAL CONNECTIONS

Filled with nectar and pollen, echinacea's flowers entice insects from butterflies and skippers to sphinx moths, honeybees, sweat bees, bumblebees, bee flies, and hoverflies. They also attract hummingbirds, not so much for the nectar but to feast on the insects. Birds, particularly finches, visit the flower heads through the winter to eat the seeds. Gophers eat the roots.

HOW TO HARVEST

Never harvest or purchase wild echinacea. United Plant Savers has placed echinacea on its "At Risk" list, due to major habitat loss as well as overharvesting. Please only grow echinacea yourself, trade with another gardener, or buy from cultivated sources.

If you live in echinacea's native area, consider planting seeds and supporting habitat preservation efforts. And when you do encounter this stunning flower in the wild, offer your attention and gratitude.

If you have access to cultivated echinacea in a garden, you can harvest the entire plant throughout the growing season. Clip the aboveground parts (stems, leaves, flowers) with pruning shears. Dig the roots with a shovel or garden fork, preferably in the autumn. (Most echinacea species have a long taproot, while *E. purpurea* has a fibrous root mass.)

GARDENING TIPS

Echinacea is easy to grow, tolerates most soil conditions, and is suitable for containers. Most species benefit from stratification for at least 90 days. In cold-winter regions, the seed can be sown directly in late autumn, allowing weather to naturally stratify. Echinacea needs regular watering until well established. As a mature perennial, it's drought tolerant. After year three, divide plant clumps to produce additional plants.

The two easiest species to find from cultivated sources are *Echinacea purpurea* and *E. angustifolia*. *E. purpurea* is easiest to grow and tends to be cheaper to buy. Medicine makers use the entire plant, including flowers, stems, leaves, and roots. *E. angustifolia* is harder to grow and is therefore often more expensive to buy. Medicine makers generally use only the roots of the plant. Some herbalists maintain that *E. angustifolia* root is the best material to make echinacea products from. We feel that perspective is overly simplified and that both plants can be made into powerful herbal medicines.

Recently echinacea plants have been hybridized into cultivars. These plants often have larger flowers with vibrant blooms that vary in color. For medicinal purposes, seek out *E. purpurea*, *E. angustifolia*, or *E. pallida* and avoid the hybrids. See the Recommended Resources on page 377 for seed and plant sources.

USING ECHINACEA IN YOUR LIFE

Echinacea can be made into a tea (decoction), tincture, or glycerite. Echinacea contains many important constituents, some of them better extracted in alcohol (e.g., alkylamides) and others better extracted with water (e.g., polysaccharides). Herbalists often recommend both preparations at the same time to get a wide range of benefits. With *E. purpurea*, the whole fresh plant is used, including the roots, leaves, flowers, and seeds. With *E. angustifolia*, the roots are used either fresh or dry.

Recommended Amounts

- *Tincture (fresh plant):* 1:2, 50% alcohol; 3 to 5 ml, 3 times daily, or smaller doses more frequently for acute situations

- *Tea or powder:* Up to 3 grams daily

Special Considerations

- Avoid using echinacea to prop up a weakened immune system. Instead, consider therapies to build up the health of the immune system, such as rest, a nutrient-dense diet, regular exercise, joyful experiences, and tonic immune-building herbs like *Astragalus* or medicinal mushrooms.

- There is conflicting evidence that echinacea may adversely affect people with autoimmune conditions. If you have an autoimmune condition, it will be safest to avoid this herb or to consult an herbalist to assess your individual needs.

ECHINACEA GLYCERITE

While echinacea works great as an alcohol extract (tincture), it also can be effectively extracted with vegetable glycerine, making a convenient alcohol-free remedy. We recommend *Echinacea angustifolia* for this recipe, either grown by you or bought from a cultivated source. Take this at the first sign of a cold or flu, for a sore throat, and as a preventive measure just before and during travel.

Yield: 1¼ cups

---

75 grams (about ¾ cup) finely cut dried *Echinacea angustifolia* roots

1 cup vegetable glycerin

⅔ cup water

1. Place the echinacea roots in a pint jar.

2. Whisk together the glycerin and the water in a medium mixing bowl with a spout.

3. Add the liquid to the jar, filling to ½ inch below the rim. Reserve any extra liquid. Tightly cover the jar and label it.

4. Store the jar in a cool, dark place for 4 weeks. Shake the jar daily for the first week. If necessary, as the dried root soaks up the liquid, add some of the reserved liquid to keep the jar full.

5. Strain the mixture through cheesecloth, squeezing it well to extract all the liquid.

6. Use a funnel to pour the tincture into clean dropper bottles. Label and store in a cool, dark place. Use within 2 years.

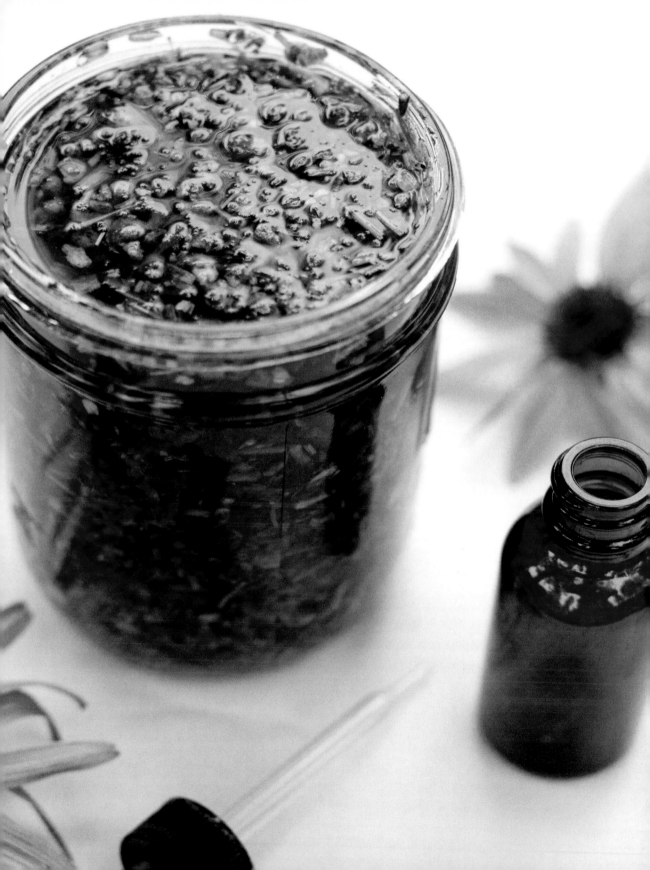

ECHINACEA AND PEPPERMINT MOUTHWASH

Zippity zing! Use this mouthwash regularly to restore or maintain gum health. The tingly powers of echinacea combine with the wound-healing gifts of calendula and plantain; fresh peppermint gives a nice flavor without being overpowering. (To learn more about calendula, download the bonus chapter at wildremediesbook.com/adventures.) To use this, place 20 drops in 1 tablespoon of water. Swish for at least 30 seconds, up to 20 minutes, at least once a day.

Yield: 1 ½ cups

⅔ cup (60 grams) finely chopped fresh *Echinacea purpurea* flowers

⅔ cup (25 grams) finely chopped fresh peppermint leaves

⅓ cup (20 grams) finely chopped fresh calendula flowers (or self-heal flowers)

⅓ cup (20 grams) finely chopped fresh plantain leaves

Up to 2 cups (100-proof) grain alcohol (or substitute 80-proof vodka)

1. Place the herbs in a pint jar.

2. Pour in enough alcohol to fill the jar and submerge the herbs completely. (You might not use the entire 2 cups.) Tightly cover the jar and label it.

3. Store the jar in a cool, dark place for 4 weeks. Shake the jar daily for the first week, and make sure the plant material stays submerged for the entire macerating time, adding more alcohol as needed.

4. Strain the mixture through cheesecloth, squeezing it well to extract all the liquid.

5. Use a funnel to pour the mouthwash into clean dropper bottles. Label and store in a cool, dark place. Best if used within 2 years.

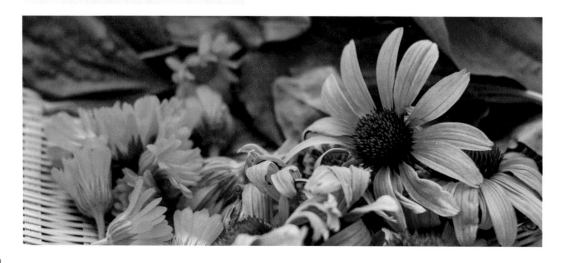

FLOWER POWER THROAT SPRAY

This blend of beautiful flowers packs a powerful punch for soothing sore throats. (To learn more about self-heal, download the bonus chapter at wildremediesbook.com/adventures.) For best results, take at the onset of a sore throat or as needed during a cold or flu. We recommend putting it in a small spray bottle, but you can also simply take it by the teaspoonful.

Yield: 1½ cups

5 fresh *Echinacea purpurea* flowers, chopped

½ cup fresh self-heal flowers and leaves, chopped

⅓ cup fresh yarrow flowers

¼ cup honey

1½ cups vodka or brandy

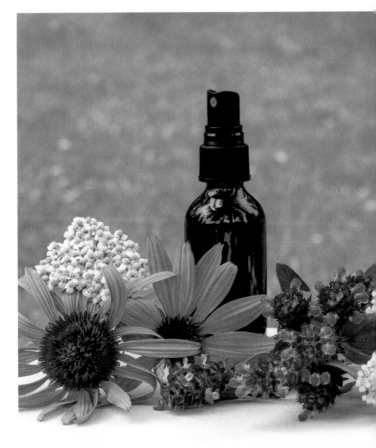

1. Place the flowers and honey in a pint jar.

2. Pour in enough alcohol to fill the jar and submerge the flowers completely. (You might not use the entire 1½ cups.) Tightly cover the jar and label it.

3. Store the jar in a cool, dark place for 4 weeks. Shake the jar daily for the first week, and make sure the plant material stays submerged for the entire macerating time.

4. Strain the tincture through cheesecloth, squeezing it well to extract all the liquid.

5. Use a funnel to pour the mixture into clean dropper bottles or spray bottles. Store in a cool, dark place. Best if used within 2 years.

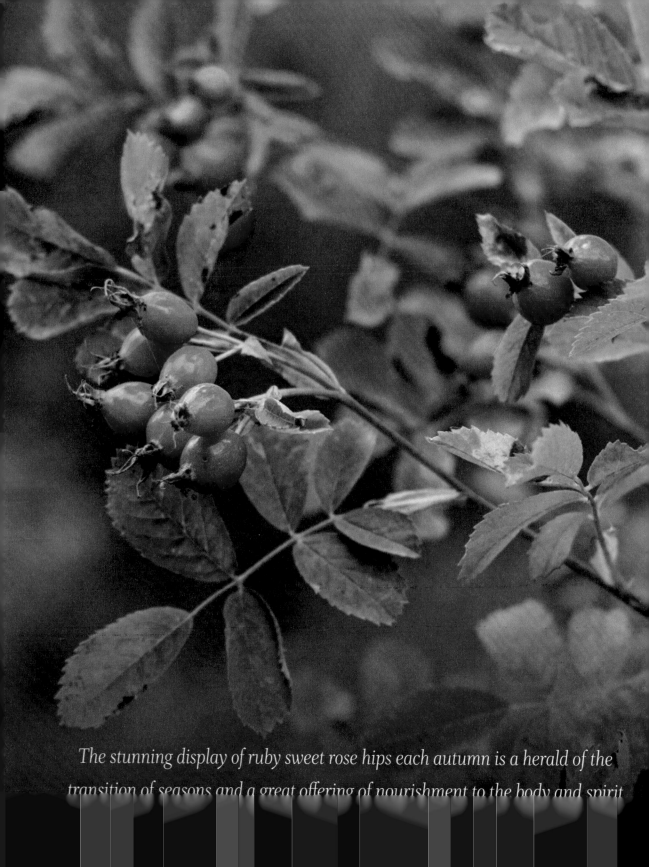

*The stunning display of ruby sweet rose hips each autumn is a herald of the
transition of seasons and a great offering of nourishment to the body and spirit.*

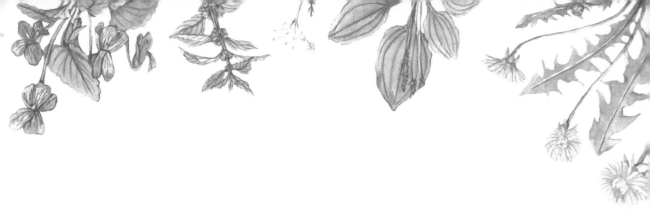

CHAPTER 28

ROSE HIP

After successful pollination of the summer's aromatic flowers, the fruit of the rose slowly begins to develop. Over the next months, it will change from something that looks like a small green pea to a richly colored, small, fleshy fruit or hip. Rose hips vary widely in flavor, color, and size, and the only way to assess your local hips is by taste! Go ahead and nibble a few, but be careful to avoid the inner seeds and irritating hairs. Is the rose hip plump and fleshy? Or tight and dry? Is it sweet or tart? Bitter or bland? With regular tastings, you'll soon find your favorite patch.

Botanical names: *Rosa* spp. (including *R. canina*, *R. multiflora*, *R. nutkana*, *R. palustris*, *R. rugosa*, *R. woodsii*, and many other species)

Family: Rosaceae (rose)

Parts used: fruits (hips), leaves, petals

Energetics: cooling, moistening

Taste: sour

Properties: analgesic, antioxidant, astringent, demulcent, inflammatory modulator, nutritive

Uses: colds and flu, food, inflammation, pain, wounds

Preparations: food, honey, syrup, tea, tincture, vinegar

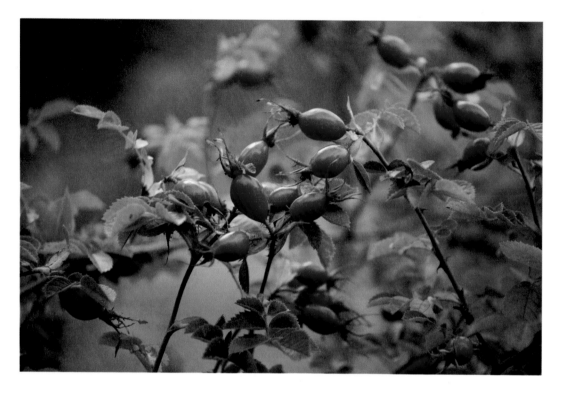

Rose hips have been eaten and used as medicine by many people throughout the world, including Native Americans, Europeans, and Asians. In the United Kingdom during World War II, fresh fruits and vegetables were scarce in the winter months, and the health department recommended that people supplement with rose hip syrup. Women and children harvested hundreds of tons of rose hips. This bounty was boiled down into a "vitamin syrup" notably high in vitamin C.[1] Newspapers all over the country regularly boasted how big their local harvest was. The campaign was so successful that the British even sent syrup to neighboring countries. One newspaper article published in 1945 said that more than 1,000 gallons of rose hip syrup went to Polish children who had been living in a war camp in France.[2]

MEDICINAL PROPERTIES AND ENERGETICS

The fruit or hip of the rose is both astringent and demulcent because it contains both tannins and pectins. The fleshy part of the hip can be used to tighten and tone tissues as well as soothe and protect.

Rich in bioflavonoids, rose hips are the perfect example of food as medicine. Eating them regularly can decrease oxidative stress, which is thought to be the underlying cause of many chronic inflammatory diseases, including arthritis, heart disease, diabetes, and cancer. Studies have repeatedly shown that supplements containing antioxidants are not nearly as helpful at decreasing oxidative stress as eating whole, nutrient-dense foods like rose hips.

PLANT GIFTS

Relieves Inflammation and Pain

Filled with a wide range of phytonutrients, rose hips modulate inflammation, therefore decreasing inflammatory pain. Rose hips can be enjoyed regularly as part of a wellness anti-inflammatory diet. Studies have even shown that regularly eating rose hips can decrease the pain and inflammation associated with osteoarthritis and rheumatoid arthritis.[3] One review of the literature stated that because of rose hips' analgesic, antiarthritic, anti-inflammatory, antioxidative, and bone-preserving activities, "the *Rosa* genus is a treasure waiting for further exploration by researchers interested in the development of safe and effective anti-arthritic agents."[4]

Supports Heart Health

Many of the heart health problems we commonly experience today are rooted in inflammation. When taken daily in large amounts (40 grams per day), rose hip powder has been shown to improve blood pressure and plasma cholesterol, thus reducing cardiovascular risk factors.[5]

Provides Nutrition

Rose hips are high in phytochemicals as well as many vitamins and minerals, including vitamin C, calcium, magnesium, potassium, beta-carotene, quercetin, tocopherols, and lycopene.[6] The amount of nutrients in rose hips varies widely among species and growing conditions, including altitude.[7] Rose hips are famously high in vitamin C. When fresh off the bush, they often have more vitamin C per weight than an orange. However, vitamin C is a delicate constituent that begins to decrease quickly after picking and is further degraded by drying or heat. The best way to get lots of vitamin C from rose hips is to eat them just after they've been picked. However, contrary to popular belief, a decreased amount of vitamin C doesn't make dried or heated rose hips useless. These are still rich in nutrients and bioflavonoids.

To learn about using rose petals for food and medicine, download a bonus chapter at wildremediesbook.com/adventures.

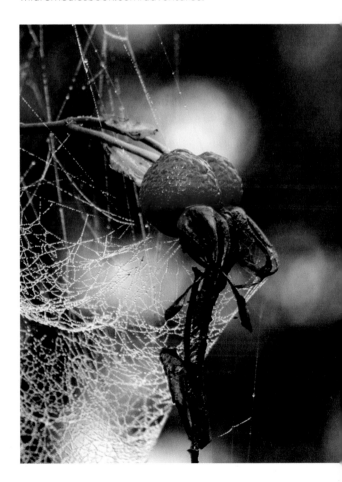

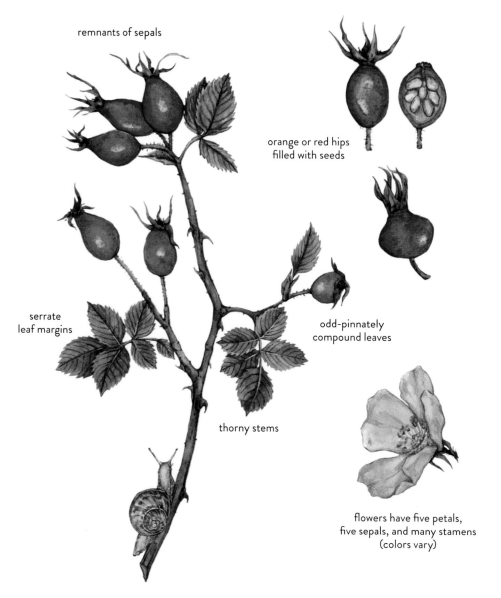

remnants of sepals

orange or red hips
filled with seeds

serrate
leaf margins

odd-pinnately
compound leaves

thorny stems

flowers have five petals,
five sepals, and many stamens
(colors vary)

rose (*Rosa* spp.), shown with garden snail (*Cornu aspersum*)

Life cycle: deciduous or evergreen woody perennial
Reproduces by: seed, rhizome
Growth habit: thorny shrub, 1–15 feet tall
Habitat: coastal areas, dry slopes, fields, forest understories, hedgerows, lakeshores, marshes, meadows, pastures, riparian areas, roadsides, sand dunes, stream banks, woodland edges
Sun: full sun to partial shade
Soil: dry to moist, well drained
USDA Hardiness Zones: 3–9, depending on variety

HOW TO IDENTIFY

It can be hard to tell one *Rosa* species from another, and they also hybridize. However, any and all wild and cultivated roses can make fine food and medicine if the petals smell fragrant and the hips taste good.

Wild rose stalks are covered in thorns and may be upright, climbing, trailing, or growing in dense thickets. Unlike the multi-petalled roses that you may find at the florist or in a garden, wild roses have only five petals, along with five sepals and many stamens. They grow in varying shades of white, pink, scarlet, and yellow. The leaves are pinnately compound with an odd number (usually three to nine) of leaflets. The leaflets have serrate margins.

The hips are aggregate fruits that start out green and hard. As they ripen, they soften and turn orange or red. Some are as small as a pea, while others are the size of a large grape. Their shapes vary, too, from elliptic to pear-shaped to round. Remnants of the sepals may be seen at the tops of the hips. Inside the hips are many tiny achenes, or fruits, which contain the seeds.

ECOLOGICAL CONNECTIONS

Wild rose thickets provide nesting sites for birds and shelter for small mammals like rabbits and mice. Various animals eat the twigs and foliage, and insects such as bees, flies, and beetles gather the flower pollen and nectar. Rose hips are an important source of winter nutrition for animals, including bears, rabbits, mice, beavers, skunks, coyotes, and fruit-eating birds like waxwings, robins, and grouse. Some small mammals, such as voles, eat only the flesh and leave the seeds behind. Meanwhile, birds like finches prefer the seeds and poke holes through the flesh to reach them. These animals can help to spread the roses' seeds through their droppings.

The rugosa rose (*R. rugosa*) can tolerate salt spray and forms large stands in many coastal regions. Though often considered invasive, it can also help control erosion and stabilize sand dunes.

HOW TO HARVEST

Rose hips generally ripen from summer to autumn and may persist on the plant through the winter. Pluck them individually by hand. Gloves are usually not necessary unless you're harvesting from a dense, thorny thicket. It's commonly recommended to gather rose hips after the first frost, which can make them softer and sweeter. However, studies have shown that while a frost can concentrate some constituents like lycopene and beta-carotene, it can also decrease other constituents like vitamin C.[8] Rose hips harvested after multiple frosts were shown to have lower antioxidant capacities.[9]

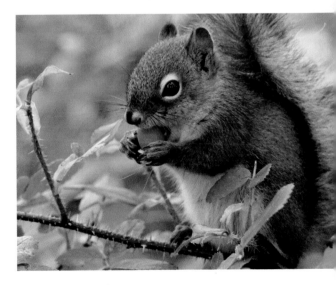

Roses reproduce by seeds and rhizomes. Leave enough hips on the plant so it can reseed and also feed wildlife. If you've scraped out the seeds while processing rose hips, you might consider planting them.

Harvesting Cautions

Roses do not have any poisonous look-alikes. However, some plants, like rock rose (*Cistus* spp.), are commonly called roses when they are not actually in the *Rosa* genus. That's why knowing the Latin botanical name can be useful!

GARDENING TIPS

For best success and easy maintenance, select a rose variety that is native to your region. Either purchase native rose plants or gently remove new suckers from existing plants and transplant. Know that propagation by seed and cuttings takes months, sometimes years.

Permanent homes are necessary for roses as they are not easy to relocate. Allow space for their sprawling and large size, ideally with a little bit of afternoon shade. Limited space requires harsh pruning, which is not human-friendly. Prepare a loose and humus-rich soil, and fertilize with composted manure. Water regularly and prune out dead branches to maintain air flow.

Wildlife may browse roses, and a unique rose cane gall may appear on older bushes. The galls are created by the tiny cynipid wasp, which lays eggs in the leaf nodes. When the larvae hatch, they begin to eat the plant's tissue, and the rose responds by generating excessive stem cell growth to cover the larvae, creating large, round masses that are often covered in mosslike growths. The galls can be removed by cutting off the branch, or they can simply be observed as they do not cause any problems for the rose.

USING ROSE HIP IN YOUR LIFE

The flesh of the rose hip can be eaten fresh, used to make a syrup or vinegar, or dried for later use. Rose hips can also be incorporated in fruit leather, jam, sauces, and compotes. Rose hip soup is traditional in Sweden. To make removing the seeds easier, fresh rose hips can be frozen and then cut open to remove the seeds. Rose hips can also be dried whole and used whenever you are making a preparation that will be strained to remove the irritating hairs.

Rose hips are food as medicine. As a result, generally larger amounts are used.

Recommended Amounts

- Rose hips are considered to be food and can be safely taken in large amounts.

- *Tea or powder:* 5 to 45 grams daily

Special Considerations

- Avoid roses that have been sprayed with pesticides, especially those that come from florists.

- Rose seed hairs can irritate the mouth and digestive tract. Be sure to remove the seeds or filter out the hairs before ingesting rose hips.

RASPBERRY– ROSE HIP SAUCE

Drizzle this bright, tangy sauce on ice cream, or splash some in sparkling water.

This recipe is from *The Sioux Chef's Indigenous Kitchen* by Sean Sherman with Beth Dooley.[10] The Sioux Chef is a team of Anishinaabe, Mdewakanton Dakota, Navajo, Northern Cheyenne, Oglala Lakota, and Wahpeton-Sisseton Dakota, and ever-growing chefs, ethnobotanists, food preservationists, adventurers, foragers, caterers, event planners, artists, musicians, food truckers, and food lovers. They are committed to revitalizing Native American cuisine, while reidentifying North American cuisine and reclaiming an important culinary culture. Find more of their offerings at sioux-chef.com.

Yield: 1 cup

---

1 cup raspberries

½ cup fresh rose hips or ¼ cup dried rose hips

½ cup water or more as needed

Splash of maple syrup, to taste

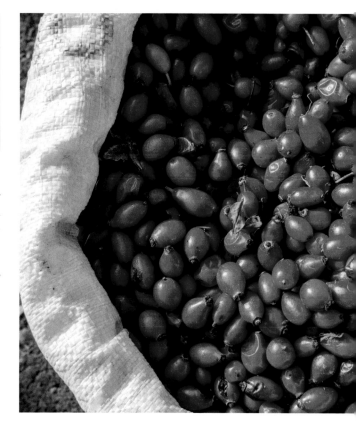

1. Combine the raspberries, rose hips, and water in a small saucepan, and set over medium heat. Bring to a simmer and cook until the raspberries have collapsed and the rose hips are soft.

2. Strain through a fine-mesh strainer, pressing out as much of the pulp as possible.

3. Sweeten to taste with the maple syrup.

SAFFRON RICE WITH ROSE HIPS AND CRISPY SHALLOTS

Inspired by Persian-style rice, this fragrant and colorful dish is flecked with dried fruits (in this case rose hips), herbs, and a medley of savory, sweet, and sour flavors. True Persian rice (*polow*) is a labor of love to cook; for this simplified version, we adapted techniques from chefs Louisa Shafia and Yotam Otto-lenghi. This rice makes a wonderful accompaniment to slow-cooked meats, grilled chicken or salmon, or stewed lentils.

Yield: 6 to 8 servings

---

3 cups water (plus more for cleaning and soaking the rice)

2 cups basmati rice

Salt

Neutral-tasting oil, for frying

1½ cups thinly sliced shallots (about 6 medium shallots)

⅓ cup cut and sifted dried rose hips

2 tablespoons unsalted butter or olive oil

⅓ cup chopped fresh dill

½ teaspoon saffron threads, finely ground and dissolved in 2 tablespoons hot water

2 tablespoons dried rose petals (optional)

1. Clean the rice by placing it in a large bowl and cover it with plenty of water. Swish the rice around with your hand until the water turns cloudy, then pour off the water. Repeat this process several times until the water is almost clear. Cover the rice with cold water and a generous pinch of salt. Let soak for 1 hour.

2. Meanwhile, pour about ½ inch of oil into a medium saucepan. Add the shallots and place the pan over high heat. Cook, stirring frequently, until the shallots start to bubble. Lower the heat to medium and continue to cook, stirring frequently, until the shallots are light golden brown. Use a slotted spoon to transfer the shallots to a strainer to drain. Blot with towels and set aside. (The leftover oil can be used for stir-fries and other dishes.)

3. Bring 3 cups of water to a boil in a medium saucepan. Drain the rice in a sieve or strainer and add it to the pan along with a generous pinch of salt. Return to a boil, then reduce the heat to very low. Cover and cook until the water is absorbed and the rice is tender, about 20 minutes. Remove from the heat. Lift the lid, lay a clean, dry kitchen towel over the pot, and replace the lid. Let stand while the rose hips are rehydrating in the next step.

4. While the rice is resting, put the rose hips in a small bowl with just enough lukewarm water to cover. They should take about 10 to 15 minutes to rehydrate. As soon as the rose hips are soft enough to eat, drain off any excess water.

5. Add the butter to the rice and fluff with a fork. Transfer three-quarters of the rice to a large bowl or serving dish. Gently mix in the rose hips and dill. Depending on the size and shape of your rose hips, they might have clumped together when rehydrated. That's okay; simply drop small clumps of the rose hips into the rice and gently mix to distribute them.

6. Pour the saffron and its soaking water over the remaining rice in the pot, and fluff it with a fork. Gently fold the saffron rice into the rose hip rice without overmixing; you want to have a medley of colors. Taste and season with salt.

7. Scatter the shallots and rose petals, if using, over the rice. Serve warm or at room temperature.

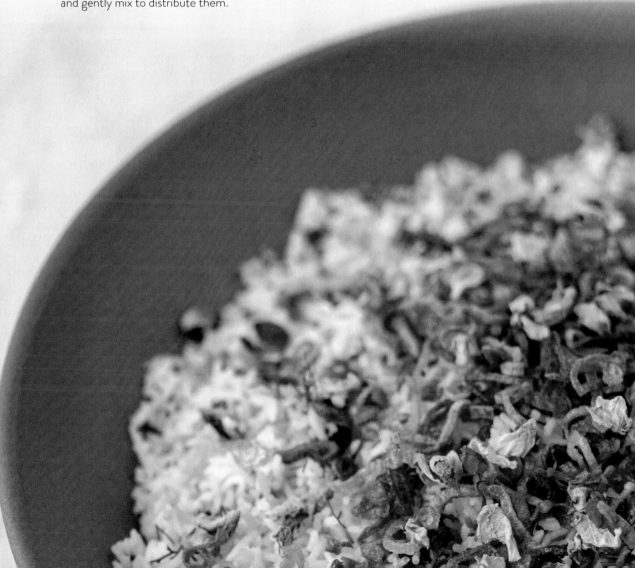

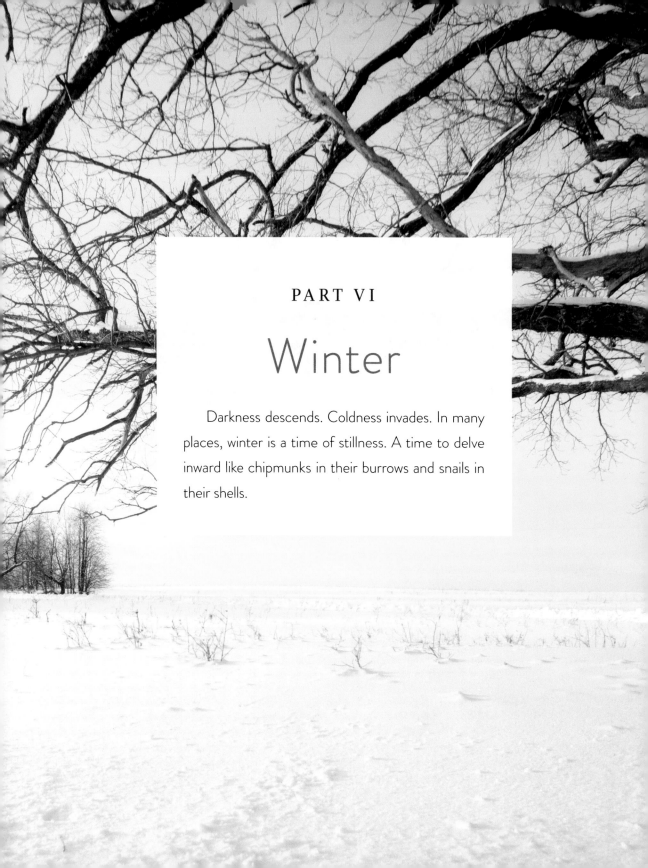

PART VI

Winter

Darkness descends. Coldness invades. In many places, winter is a time of stillness. A time to delve inward like chipmunks in their burrows and snails in their shells.

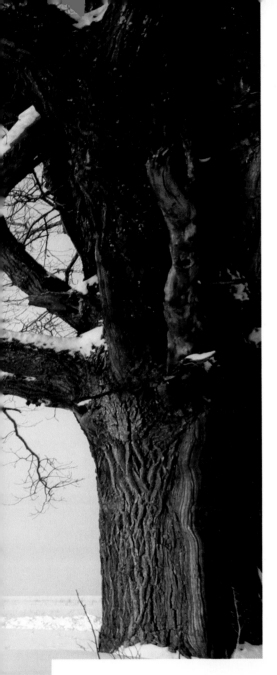

Busyness has been laid to rest, and you are invited to lose yourself by gazing at the hearth's fire. Snuggle with your favorite blankets, people, and furry friends. Savor each cup of steaming tea, reminiscing about the adventures that brought it to your apothecary: the bright days with full baskets, soil-scrubbed hands, and a sun-kissed face. In warm locales, winter may contain the dual possibilities of indoor restoration and outdoor activity. As cooler, wetter weather awakens plant growth, hiking shoes and harvesting baskets reappear.

The longest night of the year has traditionally been one of celebration around the world, for with it comes the dawn of a longer day and a promise that the sun will return. Perhaps in an effort to ward off a fear of darkness or a fear of turning inward, many people in modern society have forgotten how to settle into the quiet of winter. Instead of resting and reflecting, people exhaust themselves in a frenzy of rampant consumerism and stress-filled feasts. But we don't have to buy in to that. Celebrations can be more meaningful when simplified. Gifts made with your hands, curated from the earth's natural bounty, are priceless.

While much of the earth slumbers, one can still find life stirring in tucked-away spaces. Evergreen trees gracefully hold snow. As the distant sun shines low on the horizon, birds and mammals scurry to find morsels to eat. Rose hips, the hardy fruits of seasons past, cling to their branches and offer sweet, red jewels for the adventurous gatherer. Meanwhile, dormant deciduous trees patiently wait, their buds growing slowly with the returning light.

Winter Activities

- Gaze at the stars
- Look for birds' nests in leafless trees
- Make a nature arrangement
- Go snowshoeing or sledding
- Cozy up with your favorite book

- Reflect on your year
- Sip warm beverages
- Draw twigs and buds
- Make herbal gifts for family and friends
- Keep a journal (see Chapter 7)

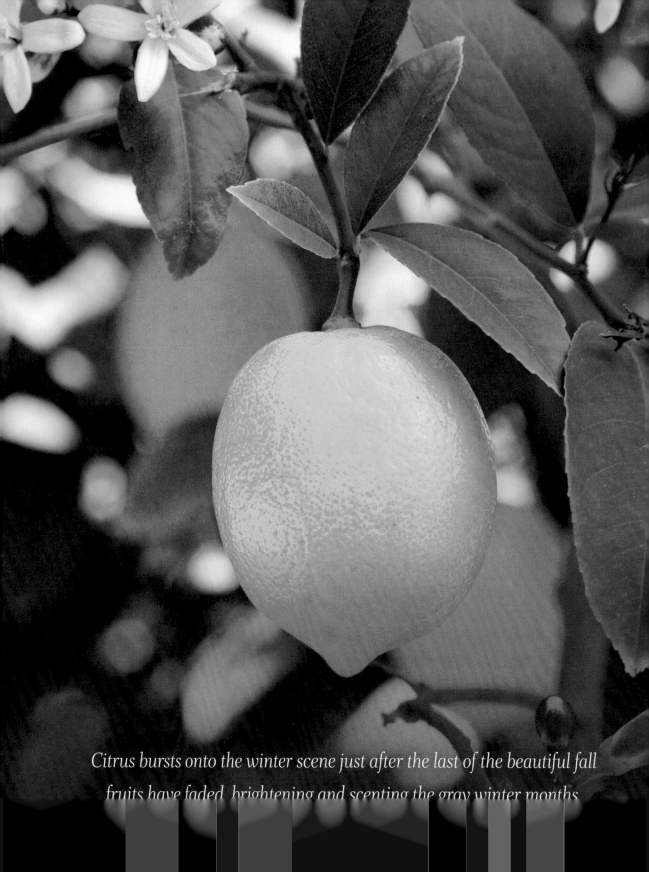

Citrus bursts onto the winter scene just after the last of the beautiful fall fruits have faded, brightening and scenting the gray winter months.

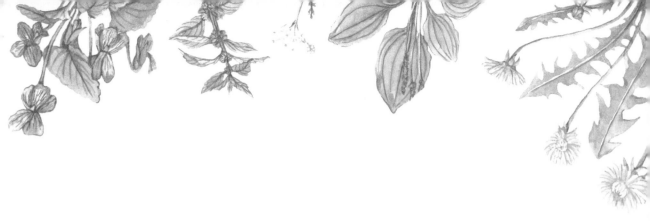

CHAPTER 29

CITRUS

For most people a citrus fruit consists of two parts: the part you peel away and toss, and the part you eat or juice. What a shame to miss out on citrus peel's gifts! While the pulp of oranges and other citrus fruits is undoubtedly wonderful, those in the know hang on to the peels for food and medicine. And if you have the good fortune of living near citrus trees, you can also experience a third gift: their heavenly scented flowers.

Botanical names: *Citrus* spp., including *C.* x *aurantium* (bitter/sour orange), *C. limon* (lemon), *C.* x *paradisi* (grapefruit), *C. reticulata* (mandarin orange), *C.* x *sinensis* (sweet orange), and other species

Family: Rutaceae (rue or citrus)

Parts used: peel, fruit, leaves, flowers, seeds

Energetics: peel: warming, drying; fruit: cooling

Taste: bitter, sour

Properties: antimicrobial, antispasmodic, carminative, circulatory stimulant, inflammatory modulator, relaxing nervine, stimulating expectorant

Uses: bloating, chest congestion, cough, flatulence, food, heartburn, indigestion, poor nutrition

Preparations: essential oil, food, hydrosol, juice, liqueur, tea, tincture

Citrus has a long and winding lineage. Recent genetic research suggests that citrus originated in the southeast foothills of the Himalayas some eight million years ago. Four million years later, it dispersed through Asia and Australia.[1] The ancient Chinese text *Yu Gong* (ca. 8th century B.C.E.) mentions kumquats, mandarins, and pomelos. To this day, oranges and pomelos symbolize good fortune in Chinese culture; they are included in food offerings to ancestors and given as gifts at the new year. The Arabs spread citrus cultivation to Spain, Sicily, and North Africa by the 10th century C.E. Spanish and Portuguese colonizers then brought citrus to America in the 15th century.[2] In addition to its use as food, citrus has a history of use in Chinese medicine, Ayurveda, and Western medicine.

MEDICINAL PROPERTIES AND ENERGETICS

Almost all citrus can hybridize, and they are prone to genetic mutation. Through wild crossing and selective breeding, we have ended up with an impressive array, from bitter orange to sweet orange, lemon, lime, citron, and grapefruit. The peels of bitter orange (*Citrus x aurantium*) and mandarin orange (*C. reticulata*) have been the most widely used for medicine, but many citrus species can be used similarly. Citrus peels can help get stagnant things moving, from digestion to chest congestion.

PLANT GIFTS

Stimulates Digestion

The bitter-tasting peels of all citrus fruits, but especially the bitter orange (*Citrus x aurantium*),

can aid the body's digestive process by stimulating bile flow and digestive enzymes. The peel is also carminative and can be used to move stagnant digestion and address gas and bloating. In both cases, the peel can be taken as an alcohol extract (tincture or bitters), in an infusion, or in a whole food form like powder. Tisanes (herbal teas) made with fresh or dried orange blossoms or a few drops of orange flower water (hydrosol) also have some carminative action as well as a mild sedative effect, not to mention a delightful aroma.

Relieves Chest Congestion

As a stimulating expectorant, orange peel can promote expectoration, relieving the upper respiratory tract of congested phlegm. Note that orange peel is drying, so it should be used in the case of wet coughs rather than dry coughs or dry mucous membranes. In addition to preparations taken internally (teas, tinctures), the peels can be used in a steam inhalation to help loosen phlegm. As a bonus, the smell of citrus has been shown to reduce anxiety.

Provides Vitamin C

In the 18th century, citrus was prescribed for sailors on long sea voyages in order to prevent scurvy, or vitamin C deficiency. Citrus fruits have varying amounts of vitamin C (ascorbic acid), which is an essential vitamin for healthy blood vessels, bones, gums, and teeth. Vitamin C also helps the body absorb iron from plant-based foods and is an antioxidant that can neutralize free radicals. (There is conflicting evidence on whether vitamin C can prevent colds.) Of all the citrus fruits, orange is the best source of vitamin C, followed by grapefruit and then lemon.[3] Because vitamin C is easily destroyed during storage, preparation, and cooking, it's best to get it from recently harvested fruits.

HOW TO IDENTIFY

Each species has its own identifying characteristics, and you should consult a horticultural guide for specific information. Generally speaking, citrus trees have alternately arranged, ovate, glossy leaves with smooth margins. Some species have thorns on the stems. The fragrant flowers are typically white (sometimes with some pink or red) and have five petals and numerous stamens. They may be solitary or in corymbs. Citrus fruits have a leathery peel pocked with oil glands, and flesh that is divided into segments filled with pulp.

ECOLOGICAL CONNECTIONS

Although most citrus trees self-pollinate, insects are attracted to their nectar and pollen. Honeybees are the best-known pollinators. Ants are often found on citrus trees doing their own foraging—they collect nectar as well as the sugary honeydew excreted by sap-feeding insects like aphids and scale. Weaver ants (*Oecophylla* spp.) have an especially long relationship with humans and citrus. For at least 1,700 years, farmers in China have relied on the ants to keep citrus groves healthy by preying on unwanted insects. Citrus trees can also provide perching and nesting areas for birds.

The Asian citrus psyllid (*Diaphorina citri*) is a tiny insect that originated in Asia and has spread around the world. It feeds on the leaves of citrus trees and can transmit the bacteria that cause Huanglongbing (HLB) disease (aka citrus greening), which can kill citrus trees. To help prevent the spread of the disease, avoid transporting citrus plants or plant material out of your area.

HOW TO HARVEST

Citrus flowers and leaves may be gathered by hand, typically in spring. The fruits ripen at various times of year depending on the variety and climate, but most commonly they are a winter harvest. Pick them when ripe, as they do not continue to ripen off the tree. Ripe fruits will often fall from the tree. These can be collected as long as they are free of cracks, bruises, and mold. To pick a fruit from the tree, use your hand to gently twist it off, or use a fruit picker for fruits out of reach.

In most places, citrus trees aren't vital to their ecosystem, so simply harvest with gratitude. Though the trees usually produce plenty of flowers, make sure not to take too many—for the benefit of the insects and for your future fruit harvest.

GARDENING TIPS

Citrus trees prefer heat to cold and do not tolerate winter frost. Optimistic gardeners in colder climates try to move citrus north by adapting them. Some semi-hardy varieties can be grown in USDA Zones 7 and 8—but not without significant protection and considerable angst during the colder months. Dwarf citrus can be grown in containers and brought indoors for winter protection.

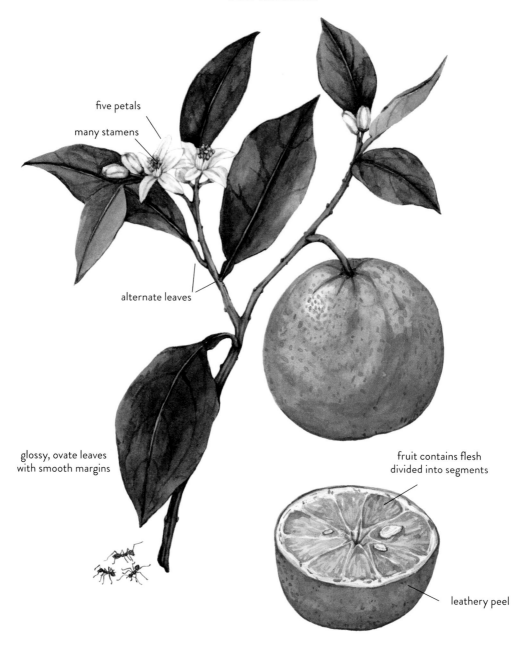

five petals

many stamens

alternate leaves

glossy, ovate leaves
with smooth margins

fruit contains flesh
divided into segments

leathery peel

bitter orange (*Citrus* x *aurantium*), shown with green weaver ants (*Oecophylla smaragdina*)

Life cycle: evergreen woody perennial
Reproduces by: seed
Growth habit: tree or shrub, 10–40 feet tall
Habitat: old groves, parks, roadsides, yards
Sun: full sun
Soil: fertile, well drained
USDA Hardiness Zones: 9–11

USING CITRUS IN YOUR LIFE

Every part of the fruit can be used for food. Grate the peels and use them in baked goods, gremolata, and vinaigrette. Squeeze the aromatic oil from the peels into a cocktail glass. Freeze the zest so you always have some on hand. Juice the pulp or eat it any way you like. Make limoncello. Preserve whole fruits in salt (see Preserved Lemons recipe on page 332). Use the seeds to make homemade pectin, and then make marmalade.

Fresh or dried citrus peels can be used to make digestive bitters. Dried peels can be used in teas and powdered for use in pastilles (lozenges). To dry the peels, mince them finely and use a dehydrator or oven on the lowest possible setting. Leave the slightly bitter white pith on the underside of the peel intact, as this is an important part of the medicine.

Fresh or dried leaves and flowers can be used in infusions. The flowers can also be distilled to make hydrosol.

Recommended Amounts

Citrus sinensis tea: 2 grams of cut peel in 150 ml boiled water, 3 times daily[4]

Special Considerations

• The *Botanical Safety Handbook* gives its highest safety rating to *Citrus* x *aurantium* fruit and peel, *Citrus bergamia* peel, *Citrus* x *limon* peel, and *Citrus reticulata* peel.[5]

• When using citrus peels, avoid fruits that have been sprayed with pesticides or coated in synthetic dyes or synthetic waxes.

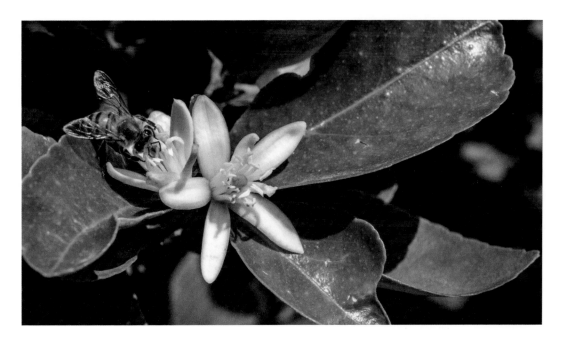

MANDARIN AND DOUGLAS-FIR BITTERS

Citrus and evergreens are sure signs of winter! This festive bitters blend is the perfect remedy to support healthy digestion during a time when we are most likely to be eating the heavier foods of winter. Although the recipe calls for Douglas-fir, you can use any evergreen that is tasty and edible.

Yield: 5 cups

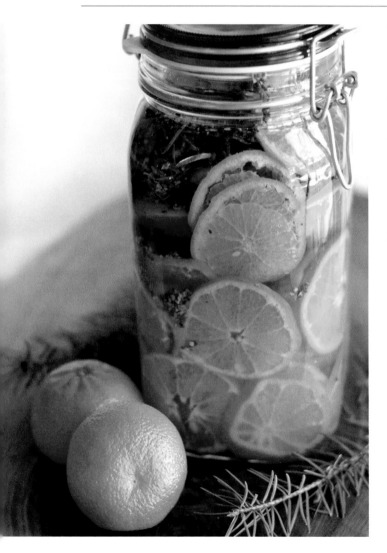

5 mandarins, thinly sliced (peels included)

½ cup (20 grams) fresh Douglas-fir needles

¼ cup (30 grams) dried roasted dandelion root

1 teaspoon (1 gram) dried artichoke leaves

¼ cup honey, or to taste

4 cups vodka or brandy

1. Put the mandarins and herbs in a 1.5-liter or half-gallon jar.

2. Add the honey. Fill the jar with the vodka or brandy. Stir well. Tightly cover the jar and label it.

3. Shake the jar daily. After 3 days, taste the mixture daily. When the flavors have infused to your liking, strain off the herbs, reserving the alcohol. (We like it infused for about 7 to 10 days.)

4. Store in a dark bottle or dark location. Use within 1 year.

CITRUS PEEL CLEANER

Have you ever noticed how the smell of citrus can make you feel energized? Scientists have found that lemon, orange, and grapefruit scents reduce stress and boost alertness. Here's an easy way to turn leftover citrus peels into an effective multipurpose cleaner that can freshen your spirits and your home. Besides being less expensive than store-bought household cleaners, it's much healthier for our bodies and the environment.

Yield: Variable

Citrus peels to half-fill a jar of your choosing

Distilled white vinegar

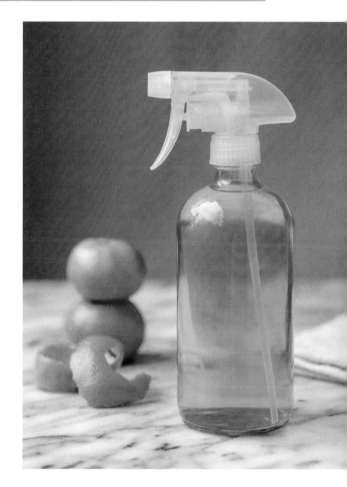

1. Put the citrus peels in a glass jar. They should more or less fill the jar halfway. (*Tip:* If you don't have enough citrus peels ready at once, collect them in a jar in the refrigerator.)

2. Fill the jar with vinegar. Cover the jar, preferably with a glass or plastic lid. If using a metal lid, place parchment paper between the lid and the jar (vinegar will corrode metal). Label the jar.

3. Let the jar sit at room temperature, out of direct sunlight, for about 2 weeks, shaking it every few days.

4. Strain the vinegar into a clean jar and label it.

5. Combine 1 part citrus vinegar with 1 part water in a spray bottle or cleaning bucket. Use to disinfect, deodorize, and degrease countertops, floors, windows, mirrors, and more. It is not recommended for use on porous surfaces like marble, stone, and hardwood.

PRESERVED LEMONS

While fresh lemons are bracingly tart, salt-cured lemons have a savory, umami quality. Finely chop the soft peels and use them to add a rich, citrusy punch to grain bowls, pasta dishes, roasted potatoes or chicken, salad dressings, pesto, and more. For example, you might try preserved lemon in chermoula (page 110) or pesto (page 86). In Vietnam and China, salt-cured citrus fruits are used in beverages like salty lemonade and sore throat–soothing tea.

To put your own spin on these, try tucking some spices into the jar—a bay leaf, cinnamon stick, dried chile pepper, or pinch of coriander seeds all make tasty additions. You can also preserve other types of citrus like Meyer lemons, blood oranges, and kumquats; just top them off with lemon juice to ensure the brine is properly acidic.

Yield: 1 quart

½ to 1 cup kosher salt (see note below)

5 to 8 lemons, depending on size

Freshly squeezed lemon juice, if needed

Note: Use salt that is free of iodine and anticaking agents, which can inhibit fermentation. Other additive-free salts may be used in place of kosher salt.

1. Put 2 tablespoons of the salt into a quart jar.

2. Scrub and dry the lemons.

3. Cut a lemon lengthwise into quarters, without cutting all the way through, so it remains intact at one end. Working over the jar, gently open up the lemon and pour about 1 tablespoon of salt into the fruit, making sure all the cut surfaces are coated. Put the lemon into the jar.

4. Repeat this process with as many lemons as you need to tightly pack the jar, pressing down on the fruits to release their juice. A pestle or wooden spoon works well for this. Once all of the lemons are in the jar, they should be completely covered with liquid. If needed, add more freshly squeezed lemon juice to the jar.

5. Tightly cover the jar and label it.

6. Let the jar sit at room temperature, out of direct sunlight, for 1 week, shaking it daily. Make sure the lemons stay submerged in the brine; if necessary, press down on the fruit with a clean spoon or add more freshly squeezed lemon juice.

7. Transfer the jar to the refrigerator and let the lemons cure for about 3 weeks before using. Preserved lemons will last up to 1 year in the refrigerator.

8. To use preserved lemons, remove a piece from the jar, scrape out and discard the pulp, and rinse the peel to remove excess salt before using.

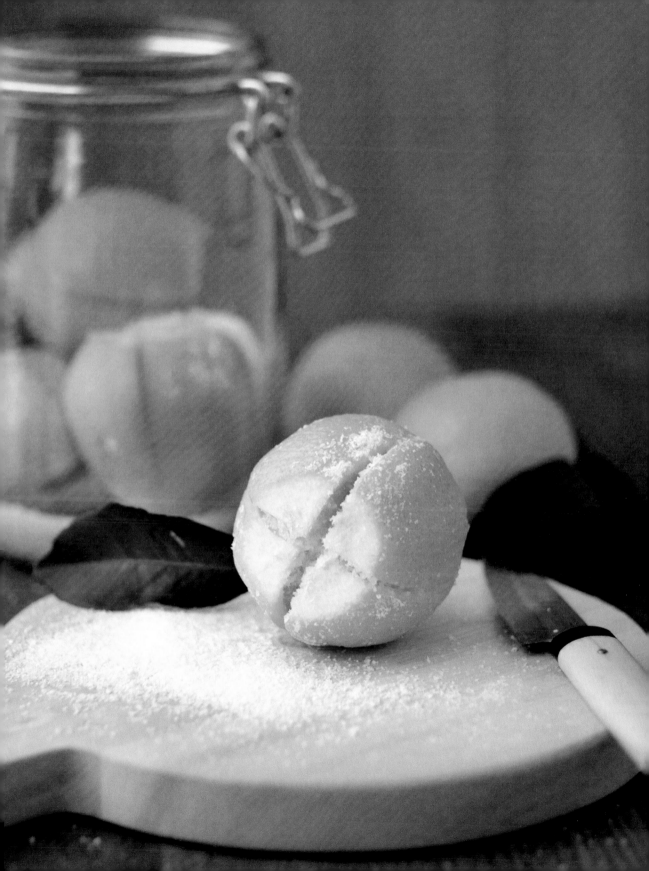

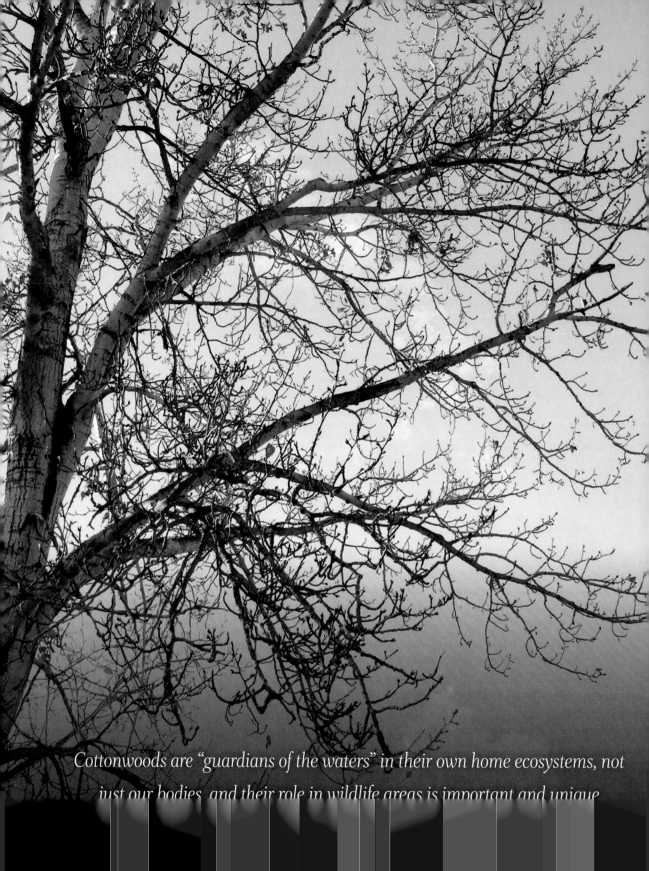

Cottonwoods are "guardians of the waters" in their own home ecosystems, not just our bodies, and their role in wildlife areas is important and unique.

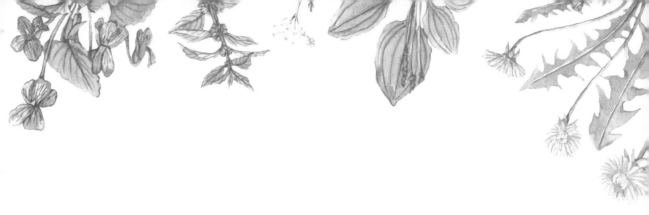

CHAPTER 30

COTTONWOOD

Starting as fluffy encased seeds, cottonwoods quickly grow along riverbeds, forming a canopy of fluttering leaves while their roots fasten themselves to the soil. If you spend much time with cottonwood, you may find yourself swooning. Its handsome stature, graceful canopy, and evocative scent are cherished by many. Bees gather the resins for their hives, fish spawn among river drift logs, and deer forage the buds eagerly on the winter landscape.

Other common name: balm of Gilead resin (not to be confused with several unrelated tree resins of the same common name)

Botanical names: *Populus alba, P. angustifolia, P. balsamifera, P. deltoides, P. fremontii, P. heterophylla, P. nigra, P. trichocarpa,* and other species

Family: Salicaceae (willow)

Parts used: buds, bark

Energetics: cooling, drying

Taste: bitter, astringent, resinous

Properties: antimicrobial, antioxidant, inflammatory modulator, stimulating expectorant

Uses: congested coughs, fevers, infections, pain, preservative, supporting skin health

Preparations: decoction, infused oil, poultice, salve, tea, tincture

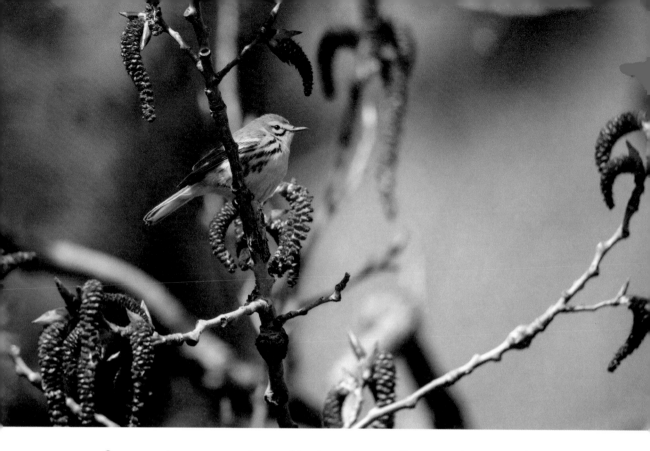

Cottonwood trees are native to North America and an important plant for many different Native American peoples. It is used extensively as medicine as well as to make tools, homes, and canoes. It's a preferred wood for making a bow-drill or friction fire. Native *Populus* species can also be found in many other parts of the world.

MEDICINAL PROPERTIES AND ENERGETICS

The sticky, resinous buds of the cottonwood make a powerful medicine that smells so heady it could become your favorite perfume. Those resins protect the buds from insects that would like to pilfer their inner sweet treats. With their strong antimicrobial action, the resins also form a sticky barrier against bacteria and fungus. Cottonwood trees are high in salicylates, chemicals that decrease pain (and are a main ingredient in aspirin).

PLANT GIFTS

Heals Wounds and Relieves Pain

Cottonwood makes an ideal all-purpose salve for healing cuts, scrapes, and scratches. Its resin's antimicrobial properties inhibit infection and also relieve pain. Cottonwood also modulates inflammation and can quicken the healing of a variety of skin rashes and minor burns. One time Rosalee used a resinous bud directly on a blood blister on her thumb. She was amazed at how it relieved the pain within moments and made the red blister disappear within hours. Overworked muscles and even chronic joint pain can be diminished by cottonwood-infused oil or salve. The bark can also be used as a bath herb for general rheumatic pains. See Willow Leaf Bath on page 367 for a bath with similar effects.

Soothes Upper Respiratory Infections

Cottonwood has several applications for a cold or flu. Its resins act as a stimulating expectorant, encouraging stuck or stagnant mucus to move out of the lungs. Herbalist Michael Moore recommended a tincture of the buds as "an excellent expectorant for thick, intractable mucus from bronchitis and bronchorrhea, as it has both expectorant aromatics and analgesic salicylates."[1] The astringent, antimicrobial, and anodyne qualities make it a wonderful herb for soothing a sore throat. It both tightens and tones swollen tissues, is broadly antimicrobial, and relieves pain. You can make a potent antimicrobial and pain-relieving throat syrup by combining equal parts of cottonwood tincture and honey.

Supports Skin Health

Cottonwood has been shown to be beneficial for the skin in some interesting ways. One study showed that *Populus euphratica* was far better at both treating warts and stopping recurring warts than cryotherapy (freezing). Intriguingly, the treatment was smoke from burning the leaves.[2] An in vitro study analyzed the phenolic content of *Populus nigra* and found that it supported antioxidant defenses, inflammatory response, and cell renewal. From this researchers concluded that it had potential for use in cosmetic products.[3]

HOW TO IDENTIFY

Moisture-loving cottonwoods can be found near waterways from rivers to swamps, depending on your local species. Each *Populus* species has its own identifying characteristics, and you should consult a local guide for specific information. (It's also not uncommon for species to hybridize.) Generally speaking, cottonwoods are fast-growing, deciduous trees with deeply furrowed bark at maturity. Their leaf buds are pointed and sticky with resin. Drooping catkins appear before the leaves develop. The leaves are alternately arranged and may be deltoid, cordate, lanceolate, or ovate with varying leaf margins. Fertilized catkins develop fluffy, cottonlike seeds that give the tree its common name.

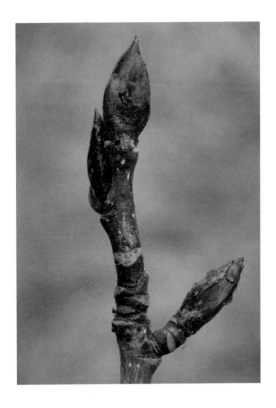

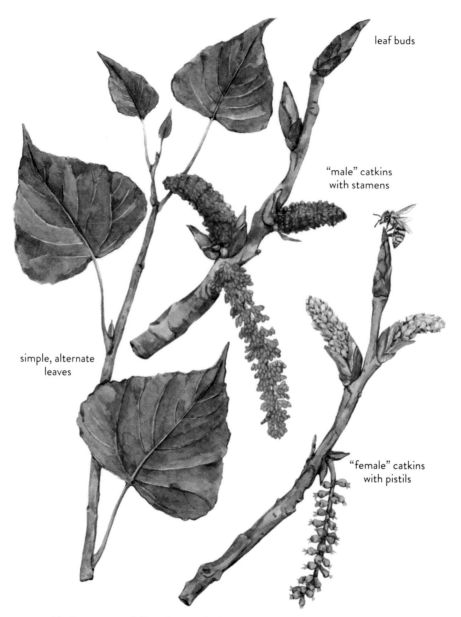

leaf buds

"male" catkins
with stamens

simple, alternate
leaves

"female" catkins
with pistils

black cottonwood (*Populus nigra*), shown with western honey bee (*Apis mellifera*)

Life cycle: deciduous woody perennial
Reproduces by: seed, sucker
Growth habit: tree, 20–160 feet tall
Habitat: floodplains, irrigated fields, lowland areas, pond margins, riparian
areas, riverbanks, wetlands, wet forest edges
Sun: full sun to partial shade
Soil: moist, well drained, sandy or loamy
USDA Hardiness Zones: 3–9

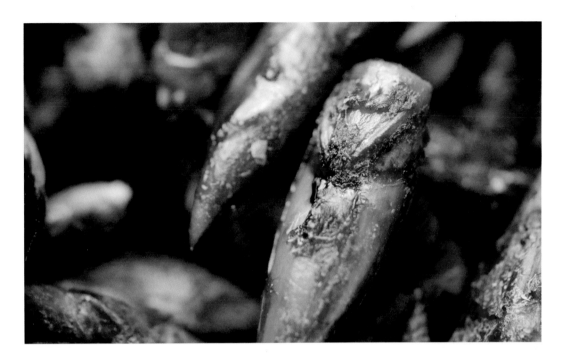

ECOLOGICAL CONNECTIONS

Cottonwood is a pioneer species, often being one of the first plants to grow along a waterway. These trees can create good habitats for fish as their roots stabilize soils on riverbanks; their canopies create a shaded, cool microclimate; and their decomposing leaves provide nutrients for aquatic insect larvae, which in turn become fish food. Many birds roost and nest in cottonwood trees. Woodpeckers and other birds drill into the soft bark to hunt for insects. Rabbits, field mice, and deer eat the young leaves and bark. Beavers use the wood to build dams, and bees collect the bud resin to seal holes in their hives. (This resin is a major component of propolis.) When a cottonwood tree dies, it can host fungi like oyster mushrooms.

There have been numerous studies to determine various *Populus* species' ability to clean contaminated soil as well as to increase CO_2 sequestration (reducing excess atmospheric carbon that contributes to climate change). Not only does cottonwood remove many contaminants from the soil, it continues to metabolize them into less toxic compounds within the tree.[4]

HOW TO HARVEST

Pick cottonwood buds when they are resinous and before they open, from winter to early spring. Whenever possible, gather the buds from downed branches, which are common due to the tree's weak wood. Only a small number of buds (if any) should be gathered from a live tree. Avoid harvesting the terminal buds. As you gather, your fingers will become sticky with resin—enjoy the heady scent! To clean the resin off your hands, olive oil or another oil will do the trick.

Harvest carefully to ensure the health of the tree and other creatures in the ecosystem. The trees can be propagated from cuttings, but as these can grow into significant trees, learn about the needs of the ecosystem before indiscriminately planting.

Harvesting Cautions

It may be possible to mistake willow (*Salix* spp.) flowers for cottonwood catkins, but the plants are not similar in appearance otherwise.

GARDENING TIPS

The hardest part of growing members of the *Populus* genus is keeping them under control. Several of the species form a clonal root system, pushing up invasive suckers in lawns and gardens, and can damage pavement, septic systems, and irrigation systems. Other species will eventually become too big for small yards. If space permits, select a native *Populus* species that will survive in your climate and designated habitat. Water regularly and cover with metal protection to prevent deer from browsing.

USING COTTONWOOD IN YOUR LIFE

Many parts of the tree are used as medicine, but the buds are by far the most popular with Western herbalists. Those resinous buds infuse well into oil or into high-proof alcohol (75 to 95 percent). Cottonwood is a strong preservative and can prolong the shelf life of salves and oils. We recommend including a bit of cottonwood-infused oil in your oil-based preparations.

Recommended Amounts

- *Tincture of buds:* 1:2, 75% to 95% alcohol; 15 to 30 drops (⅛ to ¼ teaspoon) taken frequently for acute situations

- *Bark decoction:* 2 to 4 ounces, up to 4 times daily for acute conditions[5]

Special Considerations

- Those who are sensitive or allergic to aspirin should avoid cottonwood.

- Very few people actually have hay fever due to cottonwoods; they are more likely reacting to grass pollen.[6]

- There have been reports of rare occurrences of contact dermatitis due to *Populus tremula*.[7]

COTTONWOOD SALVE

Cottonwood salve is an all-purpose first-aid ointment. It has the same attributes as cottonwood oil but is hardened with beeswax, making it easier to use. Apply it to clean cuts, scrapes, and minor burns to prevent infection and reduce pain. You can also rub it on sore muscles or soft tissue injuries such as bruises and sprains. Once you experience how wonderfully this works, you'll want some at home, at the office, in the car, in your travel first-aid kit, and anywhere else you can think of!

Yield: 8 ounces

---

1 ounce (28 grams) beeswax

1 cup Cottonwood Oil (page 342)

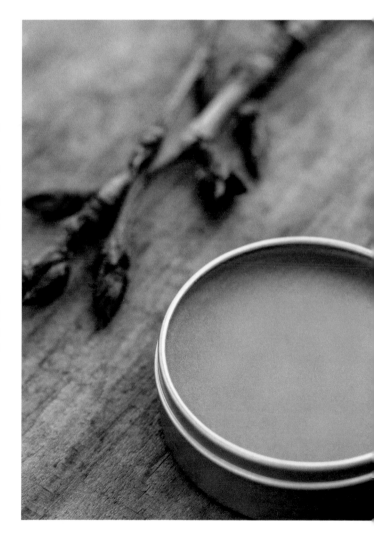

1. Melt the beeswax in the top of a double boiler or a saucepan over very low heat.

2. Once the beeswax is melted, add the cottonwood bud oil. Stir well to combine, using as little heat as possible to keep the mixture liquid. (*Note:* It's normal for the beeswax to harden slightly when you add the oil. Allow it to melt again.)

3. Immediately pour into tins or glass jars.

4. Let the salve sit until it hardens. Label and store in a cool place. This salve will last for 2 years, possibly longer. If it starts to smell rancid (like crayons), it's time for a new batch.

COTTONWOOD OIL

Making cottonwood-infused oil is a favorite tradition for many herbalists. The oil captures cottonwood's alluring scent and is a powerful healing remedy that can be used topically to heal wounds, such as scrapes or burns, as well as relieve the pain and tension of sore muscles. You can even use it as a moisturizing oil to protect and soothe your skin.

Yield: About 2 cups

1½ cups fresh cottonwood buds

Up to 2 cups olive oil (or carrier oil of your choice)

1. Place the cottonwood buds in a pint jar.

2. Pour in enough oil to fill the jar and submerge the herbs completely. (You might not use the entire 2 cups.)

3. Using a clean instrument, stir well and end by pushing the buds under the oil. Tightly cover the jar and label it. Place the jar on a plate and keep it on the counter so you can easily keep an eye on it.

4. Infuse the oil for at least 4 weeks. (Many herbalists infuse it for a year, as the potency gets stronger with time.) During the first few weeks, open the jar daily and stir it well. Fresh cottonwood buds may ferment a bit, and if this happens, some oil may escape the jar. That's okay! Prepare for this by keeping a plate underneath the jar.

5. Strain the oil through a fine-mesh strainer or cheesecloth. Squeeze well to extract the oil from the buds.

6. Store in a cool, dark place. Use within 2 years.

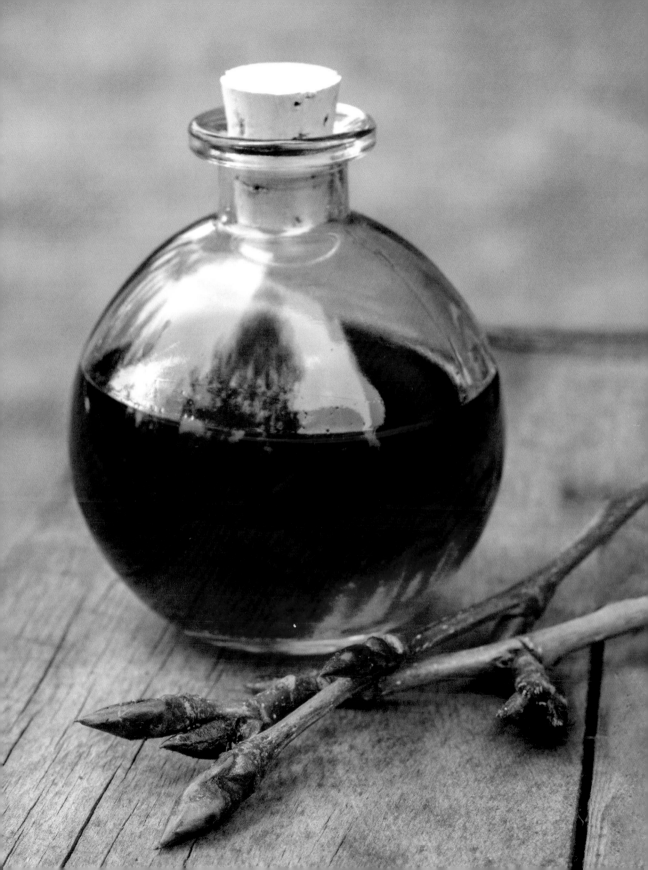

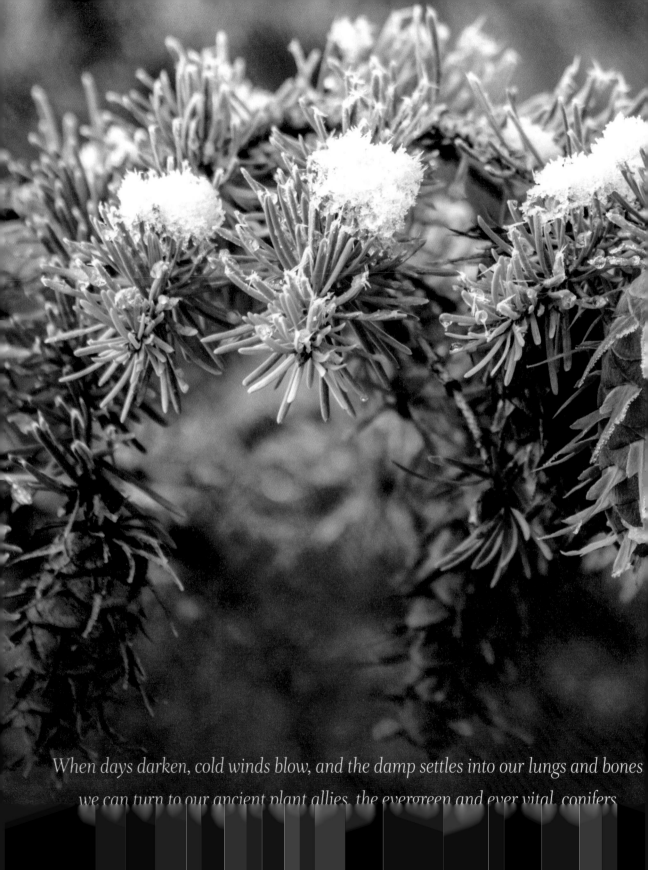

When days darken, cold winds blow, and the damp settles into our lungs and bones
we can turn to our ancient plant allies, the evergreen and ever vital, conifers.

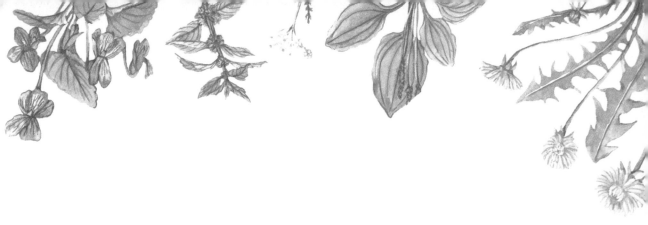

CHAPTER 31

EVERGREEN CONIFERS

As winter approaches, trees in the pine family generously share their gifts. They provide shelter to many animals and insects, including humans. Pinewood may be found in the foundation of many houses and is often burned for heating. The trees themselves lift our spirits and are a part of many traditional holiday celebrations. Their aromatic resin and vitamin C–rich needles offer us many medicines during the cold, dark months of the year.

Other common names: Douglas-fir, fir, hemlock, pine, piñon, pinyon, spruce
Botanical names: *Abies* spp., *Picea* spp., *Pinus* spp., *Pseudotsuga* spp., *Tsuga* spp.
Family: Pinaceae (pine)
Parts used: bark, needles (leaves), resin, pollen, seeds
Energetics: warming, drying
Taste: pungent, bitter, sour
Properties: antimicrobial, diuretic, inflammatory modulator, nutritive, stimulating diaphoretic, stimulating expectorant, vulnerary
Uses: cold and flu, food, rheumatism, splinters, wounds
Preparations: decoction, food, liqueur, oil, salve, tea

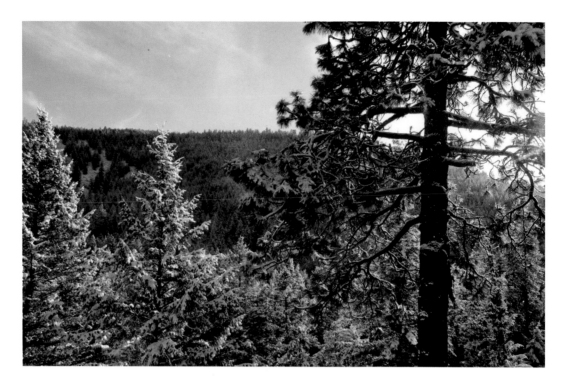

Trees of the Pinaceae or pine family are among the oldest and largest plants used in herbal medicine. They can live for hundreds or even thousands of years. One of the world's oldest living organisms is a bristlecone pine tree (*Pinus longaeva*) called Methuselah that is at least 4,600 years old. Ancient cousins of the modern-day species lived as many as 300,000 years ago and grew alongside dinosaurs. Over hundreds of thousands of years, evergreen conifer trees have developed many mechanisms for living in a variety of climates and fending off pathogens and herbivores. Those same defense mechanisms give us a wide range of medicines. People have used pine tar, a substance obtained from the carbonization of pinewood, as medicine for more than 2,000 years.[1]

MEDICINAL PROPERTIES AND ENERGETICS

The Pinaceae family contains 11 genera and more than 220 species. If you live in the Northern Hemisphere, then chances are you have some kind of pine-family tree growing near you. While each genus and species has its unique gifts, many of these trees can be used similarly. You may need to research the specific trees found near you for more information on their gifts.

Almost every part of an evergreen conifer tree has some medicinal virtues. A big part of their medicine is the aromatic resin that they exude when injured. This resin forms a protective layer across the bark, helps to repel or trap boring insects, and is also antimicrobial, thus further protecting the tree from pathogens.

PLANT GIFTS

Relieves Pain

Various pine (*Pinus*) resin products have a history of use for decreasing arthritic and muscular pains, especially those that get worse with cold and damp. One way it may work is by helping to stimulate circulation. Resin can be used as a topical cream or salve or as a bath herb.

Provides Vitamin C

Nibbling on an evergreen conifer needle gives an explosion of taste. Depending on the particular species, it most likely has some combination of a resinous and bitter flavor, but often the most notable taste is sourness or tartness, indicating the plant is high in ascorbic acid or vitamin C. One study showed that the ascorbic acid content was higher in pine (*Pinus*) needles gathered in the winter than in needles gathered in warmer months. Scientists hypothesize that the ascorbic acid may protect the tree in some way against the cold.[2] Scientists have identified 39 different flavor profiles in pine needle tea, so tasting the varieties that grow near you will unveil a complex local flavor.[3]

Relieves Coughs, Congestion, and Fevers

The pungent and aromatic qualities of evergreen resin or pitch can stimulate mucus production, helping to both thin and expectorate congestion in the lungs and sinuses and thereby relieve coughing. Herbalist Michael Moore recommends chewing a pea-size piece of pitch to swiftly encourage "strong, fruitful expectoration and a general softening of bronchial mucus."[4] A strong decoction of the needles can do this as well. Some herbalists prefer rubbing an infused oil or salve over the chest and back.

A hot tea of the needles can support the fever process by helping you to warm up. Sip the tea when you are feeling chilled, especially at the onset of a cold or flu. A dollop of honey added to the tea will smooth out the flavor while providing a perfect blend for soothing a sore throat.

Heals the Skin and Infections

Pine (*Pinus*) resins modulate inflammation, increase circulation, and are widely antimicrobial, making pine one of our best vulnerary or wound-healing herbs. Herbalists commonly use the resin as a salve for this. Think of it as your local and sustainable Neosporin. Pine tar has been used in medicine since the age of Hippocrates as a topical treatment for itchy, inflamed, and dry rashes, including eczema, psoriasis, and dandruff.[5] Katja Swift, coauthor of *Herbal Medicine for Beginners*, says that pine is the herb she uses most frequently . She loves white pine "for almost any kind of skin issue, from wounds to eczema, especially if there is any risk of infection."[6]

Provides the Benefits of Forest Bathing

While powerful healing herbal potions can be made from evergreen conifer trees, some of the best medicine is simply spending time with them in the forest. The Japanese practice of *shinrin-yoku*, or "forest bathing," was developed by the Japanese government in 1982 and inspired by ancient Shinto and Buddhist beliefs.

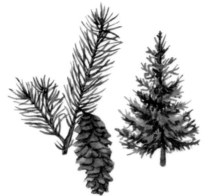

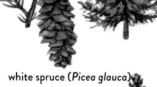

white spruce (*Picea glauca*)

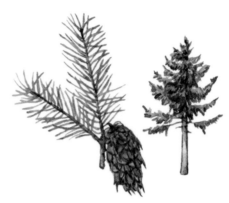

Douglas-fir (*Pseudotsuga menziesii*)

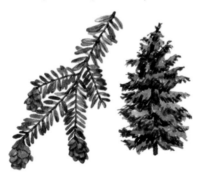

ponderosa pine (*Pinus ponderosa*)

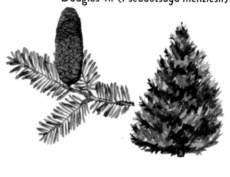

balsam fir (*Abies balsamea*)

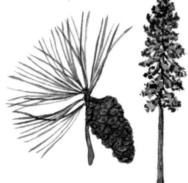

eastern hemlock (*Tsuga canadensis*)

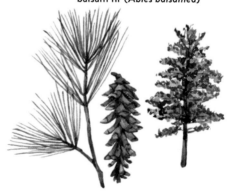

eastern white pine (*Pinus strobus*)

Life cycle: evergreen perennial
Reproduces by: seed
Growth habit: tree, varying heights
Habitat: coastal areas, forests, mountain slopes, parks, stream banks
Sun: full sun to partial shade
Soil: variable
USDA Hardiness Zones: 3–10

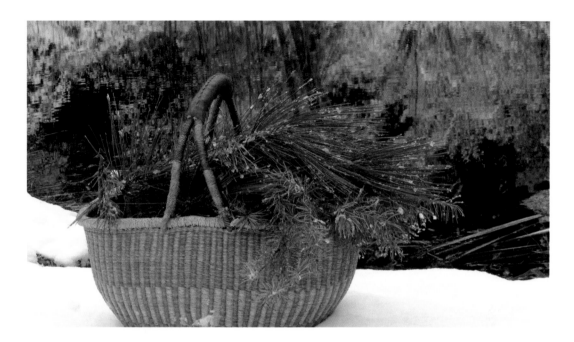

Part of this practice involves using all five senses while immersed in nature.[7] Forest bathing took off in the 1990s, and since then numerous studies have shown that spending time in forests has significant benefits, decreasing stress and improving immunity.[8]

HOW TO IDENTIFY

Trees in the Pinaceae family have learned to adapt to a variety of environments and as a result are among the most common trees in the Northern Hemisphere. They can be found in the desert as well as the boreal forest. Cultivated trees (such as Christmas trees) can be used if they are aromatic and organically grown. Each species has its own identifying characteristics, and you should consult a local guide for specific information. Here is a brief look at some major types of trees and their distinguishing traits:

- Douglas-fir (*Pseudotsuga* spp.) trees have flat needles attached to the branch with stalks. Their cones hang downward and have three-pointed bracts between the cone scales. Some describe these as looking like mouse tails or snake tongues.

- Fir (*Abies* spp.) trees have soft, flat needles attached to the branch with a base that looks like a suction cup. Their cones stand upright on the branches

- Hemlock (*Tsuga* spp.) trees have flat needles attached to the branch with slender stalks. Their cones are small and ovoid, about 1 to 3 inches long. This genus is not to be confused with poison

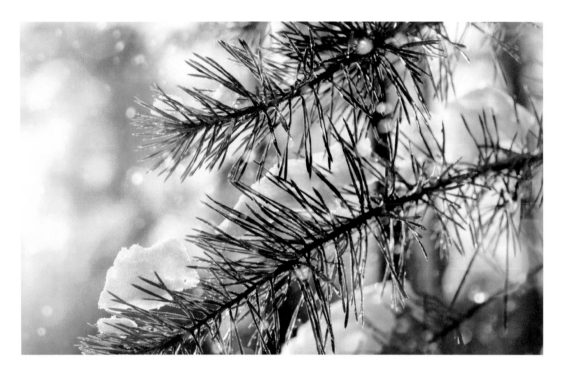

hemlock (*Conium maculatum*) or water hemlock (*Cicuta* spp.).

- Pine (*Pinus* spp.) trees have 1 to 5 long, slender needles bundled in a small, papery sheath at the base.

- Spruce (*Picea* spp.) trees have sharp needles that are often square in cross-section; you can feel this by rolling one around between your fingers. Their cones are narrow and flexible and hang downward.

ECOLOGICAL CONNECTIONS

Evergreen conifers provide nesting places for owls and other birds, bedding for deer, and habitats for invertebrates. Bears, squirrels, chipmunks, mice, birds, and other animals eat their seeds and frequently depend on them for winter survival. It can be a mutually beneficial relationship when the animals bury seeds and forget about them, effectively planting trees in new locations. These trees often have extensive mycorrhizae (symbiotic relationships with fungi) and provide places for lichens to grow.

Interestingly, pine pollen may play an important role in the functioning of food webs. Each year, a massive quantity of pollen falls to the ground and enriches the soil, feeding soil microbes and small creatures like worms with all the nutrition that the tree embodies. How wonderful to think of these towering trees circling around to feed the smallest microbes growing at their feet!

HOW TO HARVEST

Leaves (needles) may be harvested throughout the year; however, the taste, texture, and vitamin C content can vary. Whenever possible, gather them from recently fallen branches. Otherwise, pick them by hand or use pruning shears to make a clean cut from the newer growth at the tips of the branches. (Avoid cutting the top of the tree, which can leave it vulnerable to decay and disease.) Move around so you don't harvest too much from any one tree.

The cones open and drop their seeds in autumn. To harvest the seeds, gather the cones when they are still closed, or just barely open, and store them in a warm, dry place until they open. Or, if the tree has open cones on its branches, you can lay a tarp under the tree, shake the branches, and catch the seeds as they fall. Either way, you will need to shell the individual seeds before eating them.

The resin may be gathered year-round, whenever it is available. Bring a dedicated butter knife (or similar tool) and a jar to carry the sticky resin. Ideally, collect it from fallen branches or from the ground near the tree. Remember that trees make resin to protect and heal wounds. Never remove resin from a wound; however, if resin has dripped down below the wound, you can gently scrape it off the bark with a knife or directly into your container of choice. If possible, we recommend harvesting the resin when it is below freezing for a less messy process.

For the benefit of local wildlife and plant reproduction, avoid harvesting too many cones. Consider planting seedlings and participating in efforts to protect and restore habitats.

Harvesting Cautions

Although most Pinaceae plants are safe, avoid the potentially deadly yew (*Taxus* spp.), which has single, flat needles and distinctive red berries. And though it is not truly a pine, the so-called Norfolk Island pine (*Araucaria*

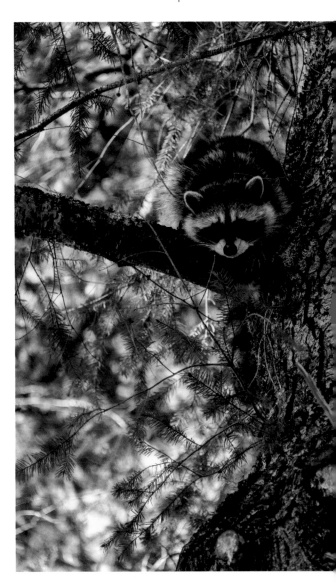

heterophylla) can cause gastrointestinal upset and dermatitis.

Some pine-family trees are endangered, threatened, or under stress from drought, fire, or pine beetles. Learn about your area's particular species and ecosystem before harvesting.

GARDENING TIPS

Coniferous evergreens offer an array of species and sizes, grow in differing climates and habitats, and are easy to grow once established. The key to growing evergreens is *location*. Select a species that grows easily in your region and then consider its size at maturity. Plant it away from structures, pavement, and utility wires. Some species drop many needles, cones, and pitch each year and may require pruning as they grow. Dwarf pine cultivars are well suited to smaller spaces and containers.

USING EVERGREENS IN YOUR LIFE

Tea or food made with local evergreen conifer needles gives you a definite terroir, or taste of the land. To get the most vitamin C from the needles, eat them raw or infuse them into honey or cold water. Making a hot tea from the needles decreases the amount of vitamin C, but some remains in the warm brew. Older needles may have higher amounts of vitamin C than younger needles.[9] Simmer the needles for enhanced expectorant qualities. The needles can also be used in syrups and baked goods

and extracted into vinegar, high-proof alcohol, oil, or honey.

The seeds, especially of certain species like pinyon pine (*Pinus cembroides*), are important foods to wildlife and humans. (All pine trees form seeds, but many are too small for human consumption.) These seeds are commonly called pine nuts or piñons.

The sticky resin can be eaten or infused into oil or high-proof alcohol. A simple salve can be made by warming and mixing a blend of half resin and half beeswax, then allowing it to cool in the final container.

Recommended Amounts

There is no minimum or upper limit for the therapeutic use of evergreen conifers.

Special Considerations

- On rare occasions, resins can cause dermatitis. If you tend to have sensitive skin, use a small amount on your skin at first to ensure there isn't a reaction.

- Cattle eating insanely large amounts of ponderosa pine (*Pinus ponderosa*) needles aborted their fetuses. This effect hasn't been seen in humans, but it is frequently recommended that people avoid eating the needles or tea during pregnancy and breastfeeding.

EVERGREEN SEASONING SALT

A sprinkle of evergreen-infused salt can turn a simple plate of roasted vegetables, salmon, popcorn, or even shortbread cookies into something truly unique. Depending on the particular tree, your salt may be more woodsy, citrusy, subtle, or strong. For this reason, it can be fun to make small batches, comparing the fragrances and flavors of various trees and times of year. You might also find that you prefer a different ratio of salt to evergreen, or that you'd like to enhance the blend with a garlic clove, some lemon zest, or a dried porcini mushroom. Experiment to find your perfect blend.

Yield: About ½ cup

¼ cup coarsely chopped fresh evergreen conifer needles (no stems)

½ cup kosher salt or flaky sea salt

1. Combine the evergreen conifer needles and salt in the bowl of a food processor. Pulse until the mixture is the texture of coarse sand. (Alternatively, you can use a knife to mince the needles. Then combine the needles and salt on the cutting board and continue chopping until they are well blended.)

2. Spread the mixture on a parchment paper–lined baking sheet to dry. It may take anywhere from a couple of hours to a couple of days. (Alternatively, you can dry the salt in a low-temperature oven and cool before storing.)

3. Store in an airtight container. The intensity of flavor will diminish over time, but it can last for up to 1 year.

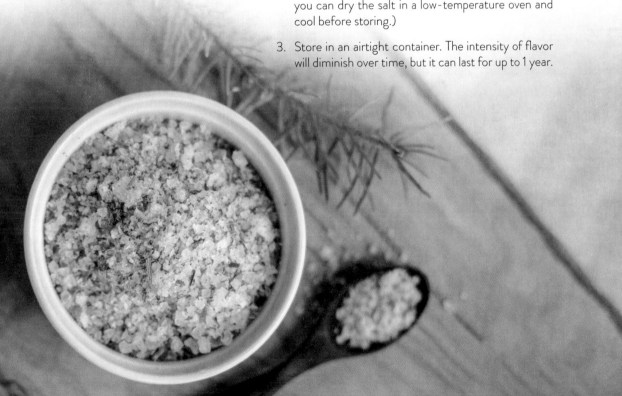

EVERGREEN OXYMEL

This oxymel can play the dual roles of powerful medicine *and* delicious drink. For a wet cough, you can take a spoonful as a stimulating expectorant. Or you can add a splash to a glass of sparkling water to make a zingy beverage. Follow your palate when making this oxymel. Some people will want to add more honey, while others will prefer less.

Yield: About 2 cups

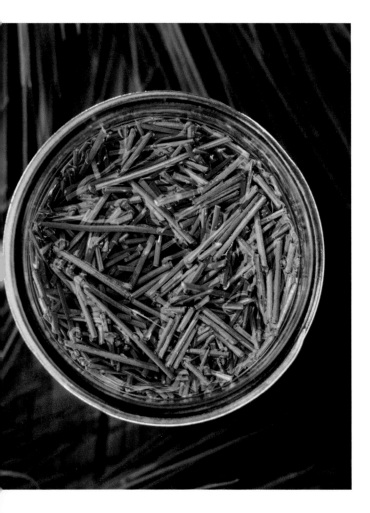

1 cup coarsely chopped fresh evergreen conifer needles

1 cup apple cider vinegar (at least 5% acidity)

1 cup honey, or to taste

1. Put the evergreen conifer needles in a pint jar. Pour the vinegar over them.

2. Cover the jar, preferably with a glass or plastic lid. If using a metal lid, place parchment paper between the lid and the jar (vinegar will corrode metal). Label the jar.

3. Let the jar sit at room temperature, out of direct sunlight, for 4 weeks, shaking it every few days.

4. Strain the vinegar into a clean jar. (This evergreen vinegar is tasty in its own right. You may wish to reserve some to use in salad dressings and other dishes.)

5. To make the oxymel, add honey to taste and stir to combine. Cover with a nonreactive lid and label it. Store in the refrigerator and use within 1 year.

SPICED EVERGREEN LIQUEUR

We are grateful to Rebecca Altman for sharing this delicious treat with us. Rebecca is an herbalist who connects people to the earth through her herbal products, writing, and healing work. You can learn more at wonderbotanica.com. Here's what Rebecca says about this recipe: "Evergreen liqueur is a beautiful way to capture the essence of the conifer forests in a bottle. It has the added benefit of aiding digestion and lifting the spirits due to its aromatic properties. To process the needles, strip them off the twigs they're attached to, because the twigs will make the liqueur more bitter."

Yield: About 1 quart

2 cups fresh evergreen
conifer needles

1 cup sugar

3 whole allspice berries

2 green cardamom pods

1 whole clove

¼ cinnamon stick

About 3 cups vodka

1. Place the evergreen conifer needles into a quart jar with an airtight lid. Add the sugar and spices, then pour in the vodka until it's ¼ inch shy of the rim.

2. Tightly cover the jar and give it a good shake. Label the jar. Place it in a cool, dark place for 3 weeks, shaking it every few days.

3. Strain out the needles and spices. Pour the resulting liquid into a bottle, seal tightly, and label it.

4. Now the hard part: set it aside for a year in a cool, dark place. Aging the liqueur takes off the harsh edges. In a year you can break it open and serve over ice, add it to cocktails, or drink with soda water as an aperitif.

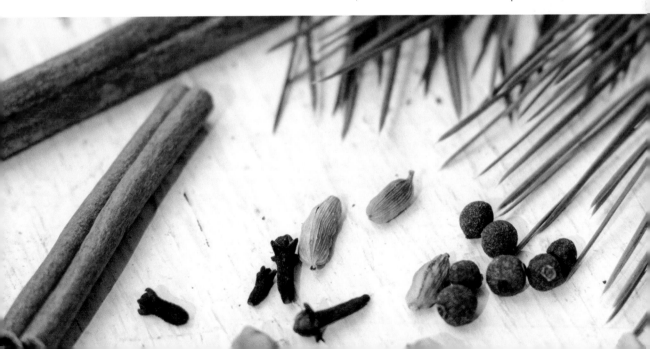

EVERGREEN OIL

The resinous needles of many evergreens can be infused into oil, resulting in an antioxidant-rich oil that smells like a deep conifer forest. We especially love using Douglas-fir. This recipe can be used as a massage oil, or simply slather it on your skin after a hot shower. It can also be used to make Evergreen Lip Balm (page 357) or Forest Facial Cream (page 358). We recommend extra-virgin olive oil for the lip balm and a lighter carrier oil like jojoba, grapeseed, or apricot kernel for the face cream.

Yield: 1¼ cups

1½ cups carrier oil

1½ cups fresh evergreen conifer needles, minced

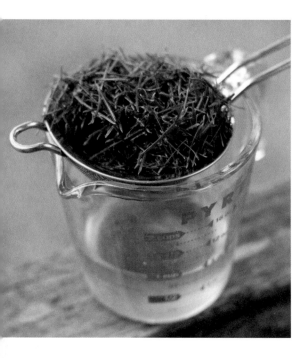

1. Place the oil in the top part of a double boiler, or in a bowl resting on top of a pan that has 2 inches of water in it (the water should not touch the bottom of the bowl). Add the evergreen conifer needles and stir well.

2. Bring the water to a boil and then reduce to a simmer. Gently heat the oil until it is fairly warm to the touch, about 100°F. Remove from the heat and allow the mixture to sit for several hours. Repeat this process (reheating and allowing to cool) 3 to 5 times per day for 3 to 5 days. (Alternatively, you can put this in a modified slow cooker or yogurt incubator, as long as the temperature of the oil doesn't exceed 110°F.)

3. When the needles have infused well with the oil, the oil should be green and fragrant.

4. Strain through a double layer of cheesecloth, reserving the oil.

5. Store the oil in a cool place and use within 1 year.

EVERGREEN LIP BALM

Treat your lips right with this delicious and all-natural lip balm. It's the perfect blend of oils, herbs, and beeswax to protect your lips from the elements, whether it's the harsh cold of winter or the blazing summer sun. This makes a wonderful gift, too!

Yield: 20 small (.15-ounce) lip balm tubes

---

15 grams beeswax

¼ cup Evergreen Oil (page 356)

20 drops peppermint essential oil (optional)

20 lip balm tubes (or an assortment of small jars)

1. Melt the beeswax in a double boiler or a saucepan over very low heat.

2. Once the beeswax is liquid, add the Evergreen Oil. Stir well to combine. (*Note:* It's normal for the beeswax to harden slightly when you add the oil. Keep stirring until it melts again and the mixture is clear.)

3. Remove from the heat and add the peppermint essential oil, if using. Stir well.

4. Immediately pour the mixture into a container with a spout (such as a glass measuring cup), and then carefully pour it into the lip balm tubes.

5. Let the tubes stand, undisturbed, until they are cool and solid. Then put on the caps and label. Use within 1 year.

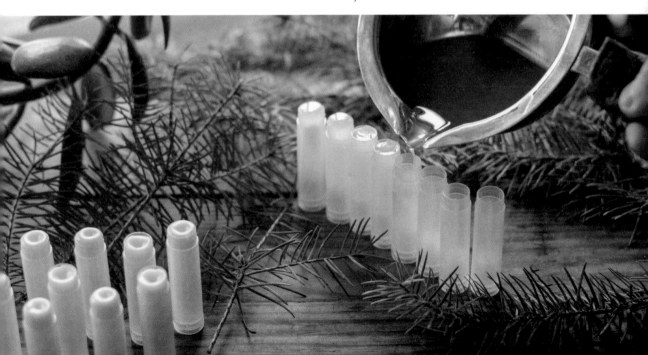

FOREST FACIAL CREAM

Homemade facial creams are a luxurious gift, either to yourself or to loved ones. Herbal creams can be a bit intimidating to make; however, once you get this down, you'll find it's worth the extra time and care.

This recipe doesn't include any harsh preservatives, so cleanliness is extra important. Make sure all instruments are very clean and dry; any water can increase the likelihood of spoilage. After many years of making this recipe, we've rarely had a batch spoil. You can tell a batch has spoiled if you see mold growing on the cream.

The optional soy lecithin, rosemary antioxidant, and lavender essential oil help to preserve and stabilize the cream. Rosemary antioxidant also has protective qualities for the skin. Many thanks to Leslie Lekos of Wild Root Botanicals for helping us out with this recipe.

Yield: About 2 cups

1 ounce (28 grams) beeswax

1¼ cups Evergreen Oil (page 356)

1 teaspoon soy lecithin liquid (optional)

1 cup hydrosol, such as lavender, rose, or calendula (or distilled water)

1 teaspoon rosemary antioxidant (optional)

30 to 50 drops lavender (*Lavandula angustifolia*) essential oil (optional)

1. Melt the beeswax in a double boiler or a saucepan over very low heat.

2. Once the beeswax is liquid, add the Evergreen Oil and the soy lecithin liquid, if using. (*Note:* It's normal for the beeswax to harden slightly when you add the oil. Keep stirring until it melts again and the mixture is clear.)

3. Pour the warm mixture into a food processor or blender. Let cool just until solid. This may take a couple of hours.

4. Mix the hydrosol with the rosemary antioxidant and lavender essential oil, if using. Turn on the food processor or blender and slowly drizzle in the hydrosol mixture. Continue to blend until combined to form a thick cream. Do not overblend. If necessary, use a spatula to scrape down the sides and around the blade and then blend again.

5. Spoon the cream into containers. Store in a cool, dark place or the refrigerator for up to 6 months.

6. To use, massage a tiny amount of cream into your face and neck just after washing with warm water. It may feel thick for a few minutes but will soon be absorbed, leaving your skin feeling silky and smooth.

Cleanup tip: Use a paper towel to wipe out any container that held oil. Remove as much as possible, then wash with hot, soapy water.

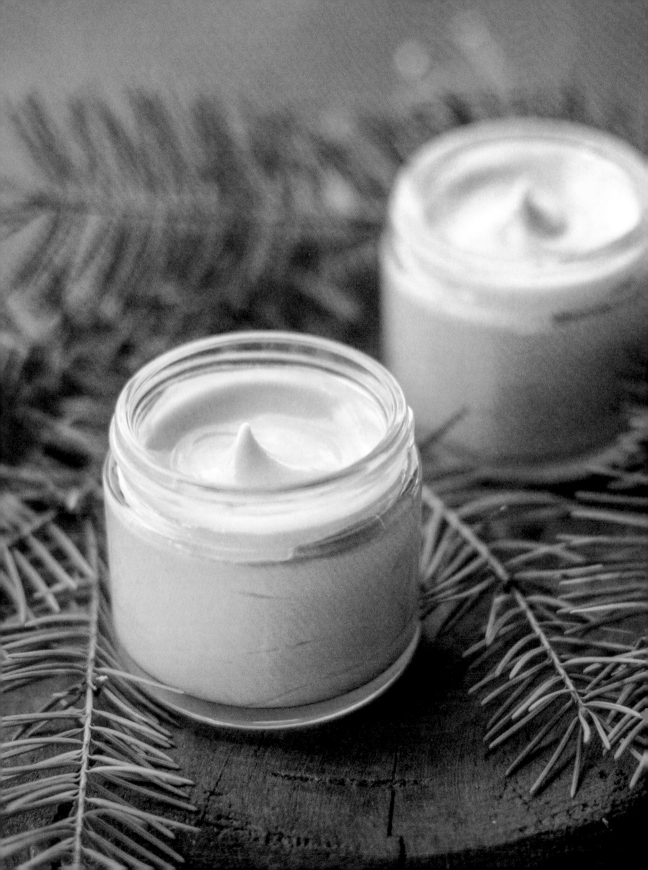

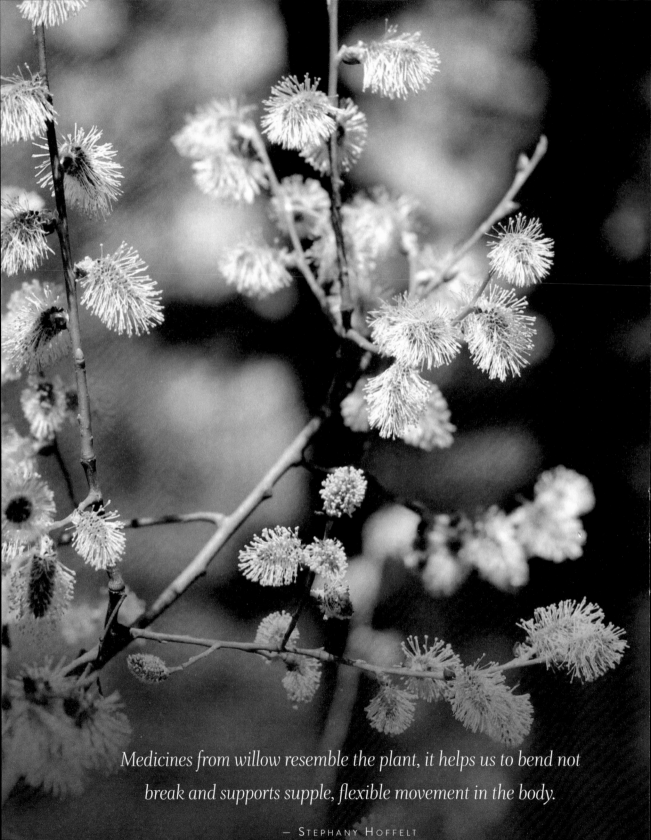

Medicines from willow resemble the plant, it helps us to bend not break and supports supple, flexible movement in the body.

— STEPHANY HOFFELT

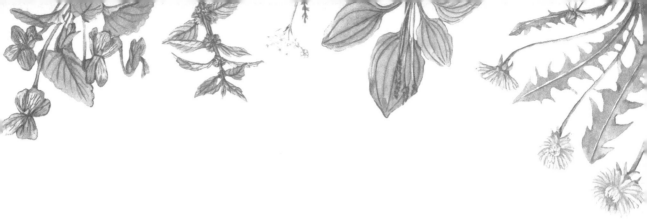

CHAPTER 32

WILLOW

Down by the creek or riverbed, beside the flowing current, you'll often find willow bracing the bank, deliciously soaking up lots of fresh water. In late winter to early spring, its catkins are among the first flowers to emerge, giving sweet nectar to pollinators. This is also the best time to harvest willow for its medicinal bark. As the willow leafs out, its canopy offers a cool shelter from the sun, making it the perfect spot to enjoy your next picnic.

Botanical names: *Salix* spp. (including *S. alba, S. nigra, S. purpurea,* and many other species)
Family: Salicaceae (willow)
Parts used: bark, leaves, catkins
Energetics: cooling, drying
Taste: bitter
Properties: anodyne, astringent, febrifuge, inflammatory modulator
Uses: fevers, inflammation, lax tissues, pain, strengthening transplanted plants
Preparations: decoction, powder, tea, tincture

When it comes to medicine, willow may win the popularity contest. Everywhere willow grows, it has played an important role in medicine and toolmaking. Archaeologists have found that people in Finland were making nets from willow at least 9,000 years ago![1] Our oldest written herbals from China, Assyria, Egypt, and Europe all mention willow, and many Native American people use it extensively. A variety of willow species grow commonly all over the Northern Hemisphere, making this a generous plant of the people.

The analgesic constituent salicin was isolated from willow in 1828, which led to further studies until aspirin, the pharmaceutical, was created and patented in 1899 (the final product was derived from another plant with similar constituents, meadowsweet). More than 100 years later, aspirin remains one of the most popular over-the-counter drugs.

MEDICINAL PROPERTIES AND ENERGETICS

Willow is a cooling and drying medicine used to relieve pain and stop excess discharges. Don't think of willow as a weaker form of aspirin! Its gifts are broader and different from this synthetic, isolated pharmaceutical. In many ways willow is safer than aspirin, and it is most likely conveniently growing somewhere near you.

PLANT GIFTS

Relieves Pain and Inflammation

Willow can relieve many types of pain, including headaches, arthritis, low back pain,

osteoarthritis, and muscular soreness. Scientists have studied how exactly willow works. Interestingly, it has very little salicin, and researchers surmise that its pain-relieving effects are due to many constituents such as flavonoids and polyphenols. One study reviewing the differences in action between willow and aspirin stated, "The multi-component active principle of willow bark provides a broader mechanism of action than aspirin and is devoid of serious adverse events. In contrast to synthetic aspirin, willow bark does not damage the gastrointestinal mucosa."[2]

Aspirin is known to reduce pain, inflammation, and fever through blocking the COX-1 and COX-2 enzymes. But as Kerry Bone and Simon Mills point out in *Principles and Practice of Phytotherapy*, it is unlikely that willow works in the same way.[3] Many herbalists consider willow to be a safer choice than aspirin, especially in regard to pain, inflammation, and fevers. Human clinical trials have shown willow bark extracts to be safe and effective at relieving low back pain and osteoarthritis.[4]

Acts as an Astringent and Antiseptic

As an astringent plant, willow bark tightens and tones lax tissues. It is most often used for mouth sores and diarrhea. Black willow (see more below) has been used specifically to curb excessive discharges relating to sexual function, including nocturnal emissions, spermatorrhea, leukorrhea, and premature ejaculation. It works especially well as a wash for wounds, due to its ability to pull tissues together, lessen pain, and prevent infection.

Curbs Excess Sex Hormones

Herbalists have long used fresh catkins from black willow (*S. nigra*) as an anaphrodisiac to address sexual overstimulation. Herbalist and author Henriette Kress recommends them "for teens (whose hormones rule them instead of them ruling their hormones), for menopausal people, and for anybody else who suffers from their hormones being utterly out of whack."[5] *King's American Dispensatory*, published in 1898, gives a wide range of uses for black willow, including "to moderate sexual erethism, irritability, and passion; lascivious dreams; libidinous thoughts; nocturnal emissions; nymphomania and satyriasis; cystitis, urethral irritation, prostatitis, ovaritis, and other sexual disorders arising from sexual abuse or excesses."[6] The traditional preparation for this is fresh catkins in a decoction or alcohol extract (tincture).

Relieves Cold and Flu Symptoms

Willow has been used extensively for lowering a person's temperature during a fever, but whether willow is the best choice for fevers has become a bit of a controversy. There is a growing appreciation for letting fevers run their course, as they are an important part of the immune system. Artificially lowering a fever prematurely weakens the body's vital defenses and could give a pathogen an open door to wreak more havoc. Many herbalists recommend using willow for this purpose only if there is danger associated with a prolonged high fever. Willow's analgesic qualities can also help to relieve the aches and pains associated with fevers.

HOW TO IDENTIFY

Look for water-loving willows near streams and other places with damp soils. Willows often hybridize, and it can be hard to identify the exact species. That is okay for medicine-making purposes, as the most important thing is the taste of the bark (see Using Willow in Your Life on page 366).

Willows grow in many forms, from tall trees to stemmy shrubs to dwarf willows that spread across the ground. The bark may be gray, brown, yellowish, or blackish. The twigs are usually slender and flexible. Alternately growing leaves are typically narrow and lanceolate, but some species have more rounded leaves. The leaves may have smooth or serrate margins. In late winter or early spring, willows produce yellow-green flower spikes called catkins. These may droop or stand upright. Willows are dioecious, meaning each plant has either all-"male" or all-"female" catkins.

ECOLOGICAL CONNECTIONS

Birds, rodents, and insects find shelter among willow trees. When the catkins appear in late winter or early spring, willows are often the first plants to provide nectar and pollen to bees. Animals such as beavers, elk, and deer browse willow leaves in summer and twigs in winter. The young willow shoots are food for beavers and rabbits. Willows also serve as host plants for willow gall sawflies (*Euura* and *Pontania* spp.), midges, moths, and butterflies.

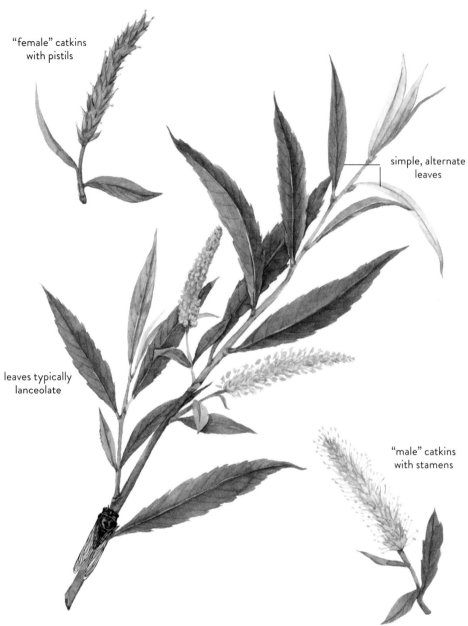

"female" catkins
with pistils

simple, alternate
leaves

leaves typically
lanceolate

"male" catkins
with stamens

white willow (*Salix alba*), shown with Linne's cicada (*Neotibicen linnei*)

Life cycle: woody perennial, mostly deciduous
Reproduces by: seed, sucker
Growth habit: small shrub to tree, up to 30 feet tall
Habitat: ditches, lakeshores, parks, ravines, riparian areas, riverbanks, stream banks
Sun: full sun
Soil: moist or wet
USDA Hardiness Zones: 3–11, depending on species

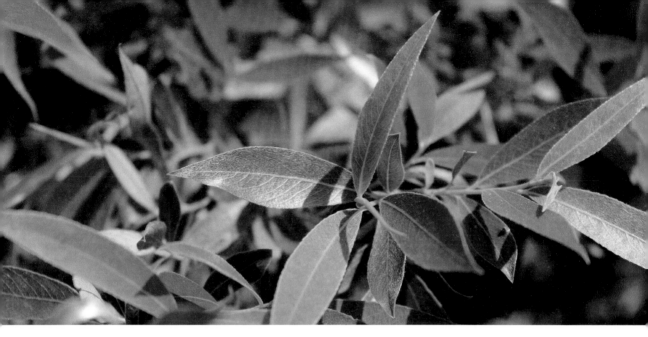

Willows are a pioneer species and have extensive fibrous roots that can stabilize stream banks and riverbanks and hold soil on slopes, preventing erosion. For this reason they are often used in land reclamation projects. They have also been used for phytoremediation of contaminated soils and to filter contaminants from wastewater.

HOW TO HARVEST

Harvest the leaves and bark whenever they are needed. However, it is easiest to work with the bark in late winter to early spring. Later in the season, it may be easier to harvest twigs. For medicine making, we use the inner bark. Do not peel this directly from the trunk, which can hurt or kill the tree. Instead, cut individual young branches or twigs with sharp clippers or a handsaw. Using a knife, peel the bark from the cut branches in strips and chop it into smaller lengths for immediate use or to dry for later. Leaves can be harvested by hand or with pruning shears.

As you will not be harvesting the entire tree or shrub, simply ensure that you harvest the bark in a respectful way and do not take too many branches or leaves from a single plant. Most willows easily grow from cuttings or broken branches, which you can root in water or plant directly in the ground. Willows also reproduce by seed but have very specific requirements for germination.

Harvesting Cautions

Though it may be possible to mistake *Populus* flowers for willow catkins, there are no strong look-alikes.

GARDENING TIPS

Willows are incredibly easy to propagate and maintain if you plant species native to your region or species with a similar preferred habitat. Propagate when the warmth of spring has arrived (such as when daffodils are blooming) by cutting a 10- to 20-inch hard branch that has bud growth and inserting it halfway down, cut end first, into weed-free soil. Lightly tamp soil around the stick. Soil should be loose rather than compacted as too much moisture can rot the sticks. Water and weed regularly during the first year. Many willows prefer moist conditions and will die quickly if not consistently watered. Avoid planting willow close to foundations and septic systems to avoid damage from their water-seeking roots.

USING WILLOW IN YOUR LIFE

Clinical herbalists often prefer standardized extracts of willow bark due to the large variation of constituents found in willows across the

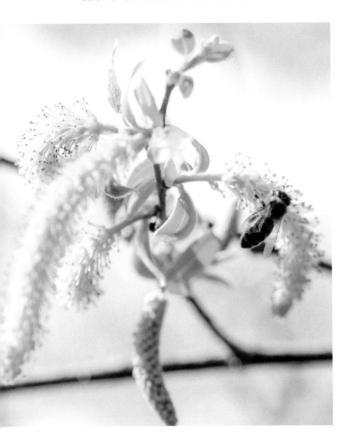

world. However, it is well worth getting to know your local species to determine how effective it can be. Herbalist Darcy Williamson says she likes to bite into willow barks to find out how bitter they are; she considers the most bitter-tasting willows to be the best ones for medicine. Willow leaves can be used fresh or dried for decoctions, washes, baths, and poultices.

Recommended Amounts

- *Decoction (bark):* 2 to 10 grams daily

- *Powder (bark):* 1 to 3 grams daily

- *Tincture (dried bark):* 1:4, 40% alcohol; 3 to 5 ml, 3 to 5 times daily

Special Considerations

- Those who are sensitive or allergic to aspirin should avoid willow.

- People who are breastfeeding should avoid willow bark as salicylates can be transferred into breast milk and cause hypersensitivity in the baby.

- No case studies or reports have shown that willow causes Reye's syndrome in children, but it is advised to avoid use in children.

- Willow bark may have a very mild effect on platelets and could add to the action of anticoagulant drugs.

WILLOW LEAF BATH

A willow bath can ease aching muscles and painful joints associated with sports injuries, arthritis, and other inflammations. Making a willow leaf tea produces a stronger effect than simply adding the leaves to your bath. However, we do like scattering some extra willow leaves in the tub, so we can imagine that we're relaxing in a willow tree–lined stream! You can also use this as a footbath or hand bath.

Yield: 1½ quarts, enough for 1 bath

2 quarts water

3 cups dried willow leaves or 4 cups fresh willow leaves, lightly crushed

1. Bring the water to a boil in a large saucepan.

2. Turn off the heat and add the willow leaves. Stir well to ensure they are submerged. Cover with a lid and let stand for 20 minutes.

3. Carefully pour the mixture through a large fine-mesh strainer. Compost the herbs and add the liquid to a full bath or use in a hand or footbath. Use within 1 day.

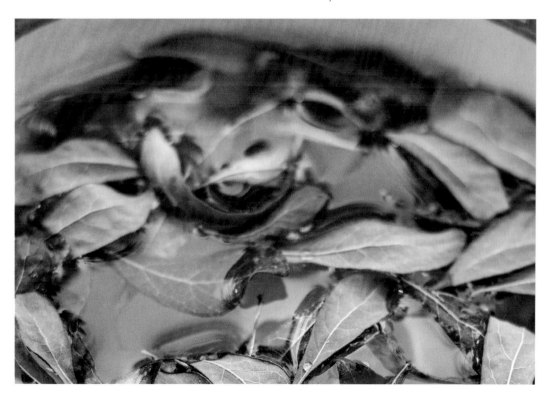

WILLOW DECOCTION

This versatile willow bark decoction can be consumed as a tea for inflammatory pain and gut conditions (warning: it's terribly bitter) and gargled to relieve sore gums and throat. Externally it can be added to bathwater or used as a wash to soothe itchy skin conditions like eczema and poison ivy or oak rashes. By soaking a cloth in the decoction, you can make a fomentation for musculoskeletal pain.

Yield: About 1 cup

1 ounce dried willow bark or twigs (about ½ cup)

2 cups cold water

1. Place the willow and the water in a saucepan. Cover and bring to a boil. Reduce the heat to low and simmer for 20 minutes.

2. Strain out the herbs and use the liquid as desired. If not using right away, let cool and refrigerate for up to 24 hours.

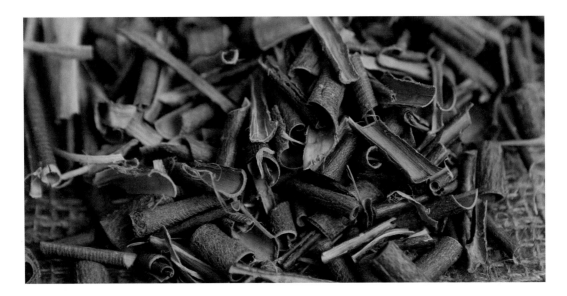

To make a fomentation: Let the liquid cool until it is comfortable enough to touch but still warm. Soak a cloth in the liquid, wring it out, and apply it to the affected area of the body. If heat feels good, apply a hot water bottle over the cloth. Or, if desired, cool the liquid before applying the cloth. Keep the cloth on for 20 minutes or as desired.

WILLOW TINCTURE

Willow Decoction (page 368) is quite bitter to drink, so for internal use a tincture is often preferable. It's also easy to carry when traveling. Willow tincture can be used to modulate inflammation and relieve pain for both acute and chronic conditions. This is a 1:5 tincture with about 10 percent glycerin in the menstruum. Willow is high in tannins, which can bind with other constituents and reduce a tincture's effectiveness. Adding glycerin helps to prevent this.

Yield: 2 cups

---

60 grams dried willow bark or twigs

270 ml 80-proof grain alcohol or vodka

30 ml vegetable glycerin

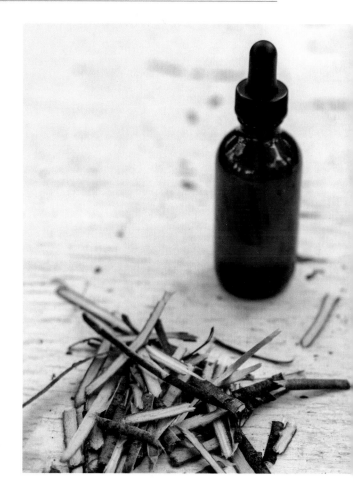

1. Place the willow bark or twigs in a pint jar.

2. Whisk the alcohol and glycerin to combine.

3. Pour the liquid over the herb and stir to release any air bubbles. Tightly cover the jar and label it.

4. Store the jar in a cool, dark place for 6 weeks. Shake the jar daily for the first week, and make sure the plant material stays submerged in the alcohol for the entire macerating time.

5. Strain the tincture through cheesecloth, squeezing it well to extract all the liquid.

6. Use a funnel to pour the tincture into clean dropper bottles. Label and store in a cool, dark place. This will keep indefinitely.

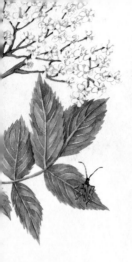

AFTERWORD

What if Everyone Wildcrafted?

When talking about harvesting wild plants, inevitably someone will ask, "But what if everyone wildcrafted?" In their mind's eye, they see bare hillsides stripped of plants and sensitive plant species wiped out. Undoubtedly if droves of people headed to wild places with the intention of taking more than they gave, we would have a disaster.

However, we ask the question, "What if everyone wildcrafted?" with hope. We imagine all the ways people would lead more joyful and enriched lives and what beautiful and resilient places they would leave behind.

Indeed, we wrote this book to help you heal and strengthen your connection to our earth. Gathering plants and making recipes that heal and nourish you, your family, and the world is a powerful way to do that. By weaving the Wild Remedies Ideals throughout your life, you will begin to improve your own health as well as the community around you. In other words, it's not just what you do, but how you do it.

What if everyone could regularly visit green spaces and forge a deep connection to the world around them? How much happier would everyone be if we all were rooted in presence?

How would everyone live their lives differently if they recognized interdependence? What kind of relationships would bloom if we all engaged in reciprocity with plants? Imagine a world where people gave to plants as much as we receive . . .

If everyone was empowered to make their own nourishing foods and herbal remedies, how much stronger and healthier would we be?

What if everyone deeply cared for the land around them? Forests would flourish, meadows would blossom, and wetlands would vibrate with the songs of migratory birds.

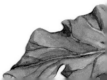

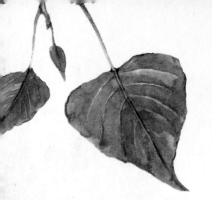
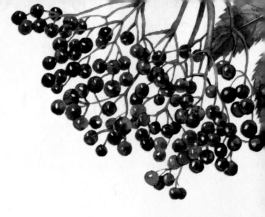

What if everyone worked together to build healthier communities? What if more of us relied on locally foraged foods and medicines with environmental justice and the health of our ecosystems as our highest priorities?

In any case, the reality is that not everyone will wildcraft. As you know by now, foraging is not as simple as snipping local plants with your scissors and filling your basket. Wildcrafting is transformative, empowering, and awe inspiring . . . but it's still work. It's continually observing and getting to know the place where you live. It's learning the many ways to caretake the lands where you harvest. It's knowing how to find plants, correctly identify them, gather them at the right time, and process them after the harvest.

If you have made it to the end of this book, then no doubt the green world has inspired you. You feel that itch to plunge your hands into the soil, to form relationships with plants, and to craft your own herbal foods and remedies. The possibilities are endless. Let's see what kind of wildcrafting world we can co-create.

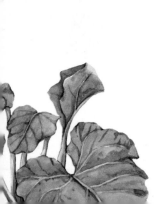
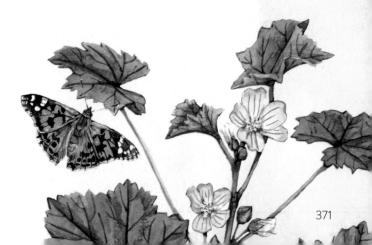

METRIC CONVERSION CHART

Standard Cup	Fine Powder (e.g., flour)	Grain (e.g., rice)	Granular (e.g., sugar)	Liquid Solids (e.g., butter)	Liquid (e.g., milk)
1	140 g	150 g	190 g	200 g	240 ml
¾	105 g	113 g	143 g	150 g	180 ml
⅔	93 g	100 g	125 g	133 g	160 ml
½	70 g	75 g	95 g	100 g	120 ml
⅓	47 g	50 g	63 g	67 g	80 ml
¼	35 g	38 g	48 g	50 g	60 ml
⅛	18 g	19 g	24 g	25 g	30 ml

Useful Equivalents for Cooking/Oven Temperatures

Process	Fahrenheit	Celsius	Gas Mark
Freeze Water	32° F	0° C	
Room Temperature	68° F	20° C	
Boil Water	212° F	100° C	
Bake	325° F	160° C	3
	350° F	180° C	4
	375° F	190° C	5
	400° F	200° C	6
	425° F	220° C	7
	450° F	230° C	8
Broil			Grill

Useful Equivalents for Liquid Ingredients by Volume

¼ tsp			1 ml
½ tsp			2 ml
1 tsp			5 ml
3 tsp	1 tbsp		½ fl oz	15 ml
	2 tbsp	⅛ cup	1 fl oz	30 ml
	4 tbsp	¼ cup	2 fl oz	60 ml
	5⅓ tbsp	⅓ cup	3 fl oz	80 ml
	8 tbsp	½ cup	4 fl oz	120 ml
	10⅔ tbsp	⅔ cup	5 fl oz	160 ml
	12 tbsp	¾ cup	6 fl oz	180 ml
	16 tbsp	1 cup	8 fl oz	240 ml
	1 pt	2 cups	16 fl oz	480 ml
	1 qt	4 cups	32 fl oz	960 ml

Useful Equivalents for Dry Ingredients by Weight

(To convert ounces to grams, multiply the number of ounces by 30.)

1 oz	₁⁄₁₆ lb	30 g
4 oz	¼ lb	120 g
8 oz	½ lb	240 g
12 oz	¾ lb	360 g
16 oz	1 lb	480 g

Useful Equivalents for Length

(To convert inches to centimeters, multiply the number of inches by 2.5.)

1 in			2.5 cm	
6 in	½ ft		15 cm	
12 in	1 ft		30 cm	
36 in	3 ft	1 yd	90 cm	
40 in			100 cm	1 m

GLOSSARY

This glossary is a quick guide to some of the terms in this book that may be unfamiliar to you. While we've included the basics—what you need to know to get the most out of this book—many of these terms have more complex or nuanced meanings that come into play when you study plants and herbalism further.

A

aerial portions: aboveground plant parts (as opposed to roots)

alterative: supporting elimination pathways of the body (liver, urinary, skin, lymph, lungs, colon, etc.); for more information, see page 283

anodyne: serving to relieve pain

anther: the part of a flower's stamen that contains pollen

antimicrobial: broadly effective against a wide range of pathogens (bacteria, fungi, etc.)

antioxidant: inhibiting free radical damage and oxidative stress

antiseptic: serving to prevent the growth of pathogens

antispasmodic: working to relax muscular spasms

antiviral: able to negatively affect viruses; herbs do this in a variety of ways, including stimulating the host's immune system

aromatic: having a strong scent

astringent: able to tighten and tone mucosal tissues; for more information, see page 232

B

bitters: a bitter-tasting herbal preparation; often an extract made with alcohol

blood-building: strengthening or improving blood, often by increasing nutrients and/or red blood cell production

C

carminative: aromatic herbs that support digestion

catkin: a long inflorescence of small flowers that hangs from the branches of some plants

compress: an herbal preparation made by soaking a cloth in an herbal tea and then applying it to a specific area; often used for pain, rashes, and headaches

constitution: an individual's unique blend of energetic qualities as they relate to hot and cold and dry and moist

D

deciduous: shedding its leaves annually

decoction: an herbal preparation made by simmering (or sometimes boiling) herbs for an extended period demulcent: able to moisten and soothe mucous membranes; for more information, see pages 182–183

diaphoretic: supporting the fever process (see also: *relaxing diaphoretic*, *stimulating diaphoretic*)

digestive: promoting healthy digestion

diuretic: stimulating urination

dysmenorrhea: painful menstruation, usually involving uterine cramps

E

edema: a condition characterized by excess fluid trapped in tissues, which causes swelling

elixir: a plant extract often made with brandy and honey

emmenagogue: an herb that stimulates blood flow in the uterus; often used for amenorrhea

emollient: acting to soften and soothe skin and hair

ephemeral: short-lived plant that germinates when conditions are favorable

essential oil: a concentrated and naturally occurring volatile liquid that is obtained by distilling aromatic plants

evergreen: having leaves that remain throughout the whole year

expectorant: helping to expel excess mucus from the body (see also: *relaxing expectorant*, *stimulating expectorant*)

F

febrifuge: acting to support the fever process

fomentation: an herbal preparation made by soaking a cloth in an herbal tea and then applying it to a specific area; often used for pain, rashes, and headaches

G

glycerite: a plant extract that is glycerin based

gut flora: the variety of bacteria living the digestive tract

H

hepatic: affecting the liver

herbaceous: having a soft, not woody, stem

humus: dark, organic material in soil, made from decayed plant and animal matter

hydrosol: an aqueous solution that comes from steam-distilling aromatic plants, often a by-product of essential oils; also called floral water

I

immunomodulator: broadly supporting the immune system to make it more resilient

inflammatory modulator: acting to modulate inflammation (unlike pharmaceuticals that *inhibit* inflammation, including beneficial inflammation)

insulin resistance: a state of metabolic dysfunction in the body in which cells do not respond properly to the hormone insulin; can be a precursor to type 2 diabetes

in vitro studies: studies done in a controlled environment outside the living organism, such as in a petri dish

in vivo studies: studies done on a living organism, whether animal, human, or plant; we generally reference in vivo studies conducted on humans

L

laxative: acting to stimulate bowel movements

leukorrhea: excessive vaginal discharge

liqueur: a plant extract made with alcohol and sweetener

lymphagogue: acting to stimulate lymphatic flow and lymph production

M

menstruum: a solvent used to extract chemical constituents from herbs

mucilage: a viscous or gelatinous substance produced by plants; contains protein and polysaccharides

N

nervine: affecting the nervous system (see also: *relaxing nervine, stimulating nervine*)

nutritive: filled with nutrients

O

oxymel: an herbal preparation made with honey and vinegar

P

pastille: from the French word for "pill"; a small lozenge, often made by hand with powdered herbs and honey

poultice: a soft, moist mass of herbs applied to the body for a therapeutic effect

prebiotic: a substance high in carbohydrates that feeds the beneficial bacteria of the digestive tract (gut flora)

R

relaxing diaphoretic: an herb used when a person feels hot and tense but is not sweating; it opens up the periphery of the body and allows heat to escape (see also: *diaphoretic, stimulating diaphoretic*)

relaxing expectorant: an herb that increases healthy mucosal flow to address congestion that has become dried and stuck in the lungs (see also: *expectorant, stimulating expectorant*)

relaxing nervine: an herb that calms the nervous system; commonly used for people with high stress, anxiety, or difficulties with sleep (see also: *nervine, stimulating nervine*)

resin: a viscous, antimicrobial organic compound produced by plants in response to injury

rubefacient: a substance applied topically to increase blood circulation to an area; it causes the capillaries to dilate and increase blood circulation

S

saponins: a chemical compound found in plants that can produce a soaplike foam

sialagogue: stimulating saliva flow

spermatorrhea: excessive, involuntary ejaculation

stagnant digestion: condition in which the body has difficulty transforming food into the nutrients needed for good health; symptoms include a sensation of food sitting heavy in the stomach, bloating, nausea, decreased appetite, belching, flatulence, painful gas, and constipation

stimulating diaphoretic: an herb used when a person feels cold and is shivering; it spreads heat from the core of the body to the periphery, helping the body to warm up (see also: *diaphoretic*, *relaxing diaphoretic*)

stimulating expectorant: a substance that thins mucus to help expel it from the body; often spicy in nature (see also: *expectorant*, *relaxing expectorant*)

stimulating nervine: something that revs up the nervous system; some herbs do this through constituents like caffeine, and others have specific aromatic qualities that are stimulating in nature (see also: *nervine*, *relaxing nervine*)

stolon: a horizontal stem that can sprout new plants where nodes touch the soil; also called a runner

stratification: a process of treating seeds to mimic winter conditions needed to break dormancy and promote germination

styptic: acting to stop bleeding

succus: expressed juice of a plant

sucker: a plant sprout that arises at the base of the parent plant or from a bud on an underground root

T

tannin: a bitter, astringent polyphenol chemical found in plants; also called tannic acid

tea: a simple water extraction of an herb or spice, generally made with a small amount of herbs (1 teaspoon) and a short steeping time (5 to 10 minutes)

tincture: a plant extract that is often alcohol based

trophorestorative: supporting the health of a particular organ by restoring balance

V

vermifuge: an agent that helps to expel worms and other parasites from the body

vulnerary: useful in healing wounds

W

wildcrafting: identifying and harvesting plants in nature

RECOMMENDED RESOURCES

The best places to find herbs and other supplies are local grassroots herbalists, apothecaries, and plant nurseries or even small farms. If you aren't able to find something locally, we recommend the following resources. For a comprehensive list of resources, visit wildremediesbook.com/resources.

HERBS, SPICES, RAW INGREDIENTS, AND SUPPLIES

Mountain Rose Herbs: www.mountainroseherbs.com

Pacific Botanicals: www.pacificbotanicals.com

Zack Woods Herb Farm: www.zackwoodsherbs.com

Frontier Co-op: www.frontiercoop.com

Sustainable Herb Farms and Ethical Wildcrafters: www.herbalremediesadvice.org/Herb-Farms -Wildcrafters.html

SEEDS AND PLANTS

Strictly Medicinal Seeds: https://strictlymedicinalseeds.com

Crimson Sage Nursery: www.crimson-sage.com

Fedco Seeds: www.fedcoseeds.com

Richters: www.richters.com

BOOKS

De la Forêt, Rosalee. *Alchemy of Herbs: Transform Everyday Ingredients into Foods and Remedies That Heal* (Hay House, 2017).

Han, Emily. *Wild Drinks and Cocktails: Handcrafted Squashes, Shrubs, Switchels, Tonics, and Infusions to Mix at Home* (Fair Winds Press, 2015).

Brill, "Wildman" Steve. *Identifying and Harvesting Edible and Medicinal Plants in Wild (and Not So Wild) Places* (William Morrow, 1994).

Cech, Richo. *The Medicinal Herb Grower: A Guide for Cultivating Plants that Heal* (Horizon Herbs, 2009).

Elpel, Thomas J. *Botany in a Day: The Patterns Method of Plant Identification* (Hops Press, 2013).

Falconi, Dina. *Foraging and Feasting: A Field Guide and Wild Food Cookbook* (Botanical Arts Press, 2013).

Green, James. *The Herbal Medicine-Maker's Handbook: A Home Manual* (Crossing Press, 2000).

Herbalists Without Borders. *Start a Nourishing Community Garden* (Herbalists Without Borders, 2018); eguide available at www.hwbglobal.org.

Kimmerer, Robin Wall. *Braiding Sweetgrass: Indigenous Wisdom, Scientific Knowledge, and the Teachings of Plants* (Milkweed Editions, 2013).

Peterson Field Guides, including *A Field Guide to Medicinal Plants and Herbs of Eastern and Central North America* by Steven Foster and James A. Duke (Houghton Mifflin Harcourt, 2014) and *A Field Guide to Western Medicinal Plants and Herbs* by Steven Foster and Christopher Hobbs (Houghton Mifflin Harcourt, 2002).

Thayer, Samuel. *The Forager's Harvest: A Guide to Identifying, Harvesting, and Preparing Edible Wild Plants* (Forager's Harvest, 2006) and *Nature's Garden: A Guide to Identifying, Harvesting, and Preparing Wild Edible Plants* (Forager's Harvest, 2010).

Timber Press's regional foraging books, including *Midwest Medicinal Plants* by Lisa M. Rose (2017), *Mountain States Medicinal Plants* by Briana Wiles (2018), *Pacific Northwest Medicinal Plants* by Scott Kloos (2017), *California Foraging* by Judith Larner Lowry (2014), *Midwest Foraging* by Lisa M. Rose (2015), *Mountain States Foraging* by Briana Wiles (2016), *Northeast Foraging* by Leda Meredith (2014), *Pacific Northwest Foraging* by Douglas Deur (2014), *Southeast Foraging* by Chris Bennett (2015), and *Southwest Foraging* by John Slattery (2016).

WEBSITES

Rosalee de la Forêt's website: HerbsWithRosalee.com
Get more herbal tips and insights from Rosalee, including recipes, monographs, and more.

Emily Han's website: EmilyHan.com
Get recipes, learn about Emily's classes and events, and more.

LearningHerbs: LearningHerbs.com
Turn plants into herbal remedies that heal. The LearningHerbs blog is filled with easy recipes you can make at home.

American Herbalists Guild: americanherbalistsguild.com
This association of herbal practitioners offers free trainings and hosts an annual symposium.

Botany Everyday: botanyeveryday.com
A wonderful resource for herbalists interested in learning more about plant identification.

Cooperative Extension Services: nifa.usda.gov/cooperative-extension-system
Each U.S. state has a network of universities and offices that provide useful information about agriculture, food, the environment, and more. Local programs may include Master Gardeners, Master Naturalists, and Master Food Preservers, as well as soil-testing services.

Sustainable Herbs Program: sustainableherbsproject.com
Inspires and educates people about quality, sustainability, and fair trade in the botanical industry.

United Plant Savers: unitedplantsavers.org
United Plant Savers' mission is to protect native medicinal plants (and their habitat) of the United States and Canada, while ensuring an abundant renewable supply of plants for generations to come.

ENDNOTES

Introduction

1. Richard Louv, "No More 'Nature-Deficit Disorder,'" *Psychology Today*, January 28, 2009, https://www.psychologytoday.com/us/blog/people-in-nature/200901/no-more-nature-deficit-disorder.

2. G. N. Bratman et al., "Nature Experience Reduces Rumination and Subgenual Prefrontal Cortex Activation," *Proceedings of the National Academy of Sciences* 112, no. 28 (July 2015), doi:10.1073/pnas.1510459112.

3. P. Grahn and U. K. Stigsdotter, "Landscape Planning and Stress," *Urban Forestry & Urban Greening* 2, no. 1 (December 2003), doi:10.1078/1618-8667-00019.

Chapter 1: The Power of Plant Medicine

Epigraph: Thich Nhat Hanh, *Love Letter to the Earth* (Berkeley, CA: Parallax Press, 2012).

1. Yoel Melamed et al., "The Plant Component of an Acheulian Diet at Gesher Benot Ya'aqov, Israel," *Proceedings of the National Academy of Sciences of the United States of America* 113, no. 51 (2016), doi:10.1073/pnas.1607872113.

2. Kevin Spelman, "Ecological Pharmacology," YouTube video, April 11, 2013, https://youtu.be/-3j97uFYV68.

Chapter 2: Getting to Know Where You Live

Epigraph: Samuel Thayer, *Nature's Garden* (Bruce, WI: Foragers Harvest Press, 2010).

Chapter 3: Wildcrafting Principles

Epigraph: Rosemary Gladstar, *Planting the Future: Saving Our Medicinal Herbs*, ed. Rosemary Gladstar and Pamela Hirsch (Rochester, VT: Healing Arts Press, 2000).

1. M. Kat Anderson, *Tending the Wild: Native American Knowledge and the Management of California's Natural Resources* (Berkeley: University of California Press, 2005).

Chapter 4: Wildcrafting Practice

Epigraph: Craig Torres, quoted in Deborah Small, "A Southern California Native Cornucopia," Deborah Small's Ethnobotany Blog, July 15, 2011, https://deborahsmall.wordpress.com/2011/07/15/a-southern-california-native-cornucopia.

1. Robin Wall Kimmerer, *Braiding Sweetgrass: Indigenous Wisdom, Scientific Knowledge, and the Teachings of Plants* (Minneapolis: Milkweed Editions, 2013).

Chapter 5: Botany Basics

Epigraph: Robin Wall Kimmerer, *Braiding Sweetgrass* (Minneapolis: Milkweed Editions, 2013).

Chapter 6: Plants in the Kitchen

Epigraph: jim mcdonald, "Gathering your own Herbs," jim mcdonald, 2019, http://www.herbcraft.org/gathering.html.

Chapter 7: The Joy of Reconnection: Living Deeply with the Seasons

Epigraph: Bernd Heinrich, "A Naturalist's Journal," in Nathaniel T. Wheelwright and Bernd Heinrich, *The Naturalist's Notebook* (North Adams, MA: Storey Publishing, 2017).

Chapter 8: Chickweed

Epigraph: Rosemary Gladstar, *Medicinal Herbs: A Beginner's Guide* (North Adams, MA: Storey Publishing, 2012).

1. Guido Masé, "Plant Saponins," *A Radicle* (blog), September 23, 2105, http://aradicle.blogspot.com/2015/09/plant-saponins.html.

2. U.S. Department of Agriculture (hereinafter USDA), Agricultural Research Service, *Dr. Duke's Phytochemical and Ethnobotanical Databases*, 1992–2016, doi:10.15482/USDA.ADC/1239279.

3. Yu Shan et al., "Purification and Characterization of a Novel Anti-HSV-2 Protein with Antiproliferative and Peroxidase Activities from *Stellaria media*," *Acta Biochimica et Biophysica Sinica* 45, no. 8 (2013), doi:10.1093/abbs/gmt060; Lihua Ma et al., "Anti-hepatitis B Virus Activity of Chickweed [*Stellaria media* (L.) Vill.] Extracts in HepG2.2.15 Cells," *Molecules* 17, no. 7 (2012), doi:10.3390/molecules17078633.

Chapter 9: Dandelion Leaf and Flower

Epigraph: Juliet Blankespoor, "Dandelion," Chestnut School of Herbal Medicine Herbal Immersion Program, 2019, https://chestnutherbs.com/lesson/dandelion-taraxacum-officinale.

1. Anita Sanchez, *The Teeth of the Lion: The Story of the Beloved and Despised Dandelion* (Blacksburg, VA: McDonald & Woodward, 2006).

2. USDA Agricultural Research Service, *Dr. Duke's Phytochemical and Ethnobotanical Databases*.

3. Natalia Drabińska et al., "The Effect of Oligofructose-Enriched Inulin on Faecal Bacterial Counts and Microbiota-Associated Characteristics in Celiac Disease Children Following a Gluten-Free Diet: Results of a Randomized, Placebo-Controlled Trial," *Nutrients* 10, no. 2 (2018), doi:10.3390/nu10020201.

4. Helen Lightowler et al., "Replacement of Glycaemic Carbohydrates by Inulin-Type Fructans from Chicory (Oligofructose, Inulin) Reduces the Postprandial Blood Glucose and Insulin Response to Foods: Report of Two Double-Blind, Randomized, Controlled Trials," *European Journal of Nutrition* 57, no. 3 (2018), doi:10.1007/s00394-017-1409-z.

5. Bevin A. Clare, Richard S. Conroy, and Kevin Spelman, "The Diuretic Effect in Human Subjects of an Extract of *Taraxacum officinale* Folium over a Single Day," *Journal of Alternative and Complementary Medicine* 15, no. 8 (2009), doi:10.1089/acm.2008.0152.

6. Dariusz Jędrejek et al., "Evaluation of Antioxidant Activity of Phenolic Fractions from the Leaves and Petals of Dandelion in Human Plasma Treated with H_2O_2 and H_2O_2/Fe," *Chemico-biological Interactions* 262 (2017), doi:10.1016/j.cbi.2016.12.003.

7. Yafan Yang and Shuangshuang Li, "Dandelion Extracts Protect Human Skin Fibroblasts from UVB Damage and Cellular Senescence," *Oxidative Medicine and Cellular Longevity* 2015 (2015), doi:10.1155/2015/619560.

Chapter 10: Wild Mustard

Epigraph: Kami McBride, personal communication with authors, 2018.

1. Michele Anna Jordan, *The Good Cook's Book of Mustard: One of the World's Most Beloved Condiments, with More than 100 Recipes* (New York: Skyhorse Publishing, 2015).

2. Hayley Saul et al. "Phytoliths in Pottery Reveal the Use of Spice in European Prehistoric Cuisine," *PloS One* 8, no. 8 (2013), doi:10.1371/journal.pone.0070583.

3. Sahar Ghalandari et al., "Effect of Hydroalcoholic Extract of *Capsella bursa pastoris* on Early Postpartum Hemorrhage: A Clinical Trial Study," *Journal of Alternative and Complementary Medicine* 23, no. 10 (2017), doi:10.1089/acm.2017.0095.

4. Mahdis Naafe et al., "Effect of Hydroalcoholic Extracts of *Capsella bursa-pastoris* on Heavy Menstrual Bleeding: A Randomized Clinical Trial," *Journal of Alternative and Complementary Medicine* 24, no. 7 (2018), doi:10.1089/acm.2017.0267.

5. Anamika Singh and M. H. Fulekar, "Phytoremediation of Heavy Metals by *Brassica juncea* in Aquatic and Terrestrial Environment," in *The Plant Family Brassicaceae: Contribution Towards Phytoremediation*, ed. N. A. Anjum et al. (Dordrecht: Springer, 2012).

Chapter 11: Nettle

Epigraph: Sandra Lory, personal communication with authors, 2019.

1. Jo Robinson, *Eating on the Wild Side: The Missing Link to Optimum Health* (New York: Little Brown & Co., 2014).

2. USDA Agricultural Research Service, *Dr. Duke's Phytochemical and Ethnobotanical Databases*. Vesna Rafajlovska et al., "Determination of Protein and Mineral Contents in Stinging Nettle," *ResearchGate* 4 (2013), doi:10.7251/QOL1301026R.

3. Elif Özalkaya et al., "Effect of a Galactagogue Herbal Tea on Breast Milk Production and Prolactin Secretion by Mothers of Preterm Babies," *Nigerian Journal of Clinical Practice* 21, no. 1 (2018), doi:10.4103/1119-3077.224788.

4. P. Mittman, "Randomized, Double-Blind Study of Freeze-Dried *Urtica dioica* in the Treatment of Allergic Rhinitis," *Planta Medica* 56, no. 1 (1990), doi:10.1055/s-2006-960881.

5. N. Namazi et al. "The Effect of Hydro Alcoholic Nettle (*Urtica dioica*) Extracts on Insulin Sensitivity and Some Inflammatory Indicators in Patients with Type 2 Diabetes: A Randomized Double-Blind Control Trial," *Pakistan Journal of Biological Sciences* 14, no. 15 (2011), doi:10.3923/pjbs.2011.775.779; Saeed Kianbakht, Farahnaz Khalighi-Sigaroodi, and Fataneh Hashem Dabaghian, "Improved Glycemic Control in Patients with Advanced Type 2 Diabetes Mellitus Taking *Urtica dioica* Leaf Extract: A Randomized Double-Blind Placebo-Controlled Clinical Trial," *Clinical Laboratory* 59, no. 9-10 (2013), doi:10.7754/Clin.Lab.2012.121019; N. Namazi, A. Tarighat, and A. Bahrami, "The Effect of Hydro Alcoholic Nettle (*Urtica dioica*) Extract on Oxidative Stress in Patients with Type 2 Diabetes: A Randomized Double-Blind Clinical Trial," *Pakistan Journal of Biological Sciences* 15, no. 2 (2012), doi:10.3923/pjbs.2012.98.102; Nahid Khalili et al., "Silymarin, Olibanum, and Nettle, a Mixed Herbal Formulation in the Treatment of Type II Diabetes: A Randomized, Double-Blind, Placebo-Controlled, Clinical Trial," *Journal of Evidence-Based Complementary & Alternative Medicine* 22, no. 4 (2017), doi:10.1177/2156587217696929.

6. Alidad Amiri Behzadi, Hamid Kalalian-Moghaddam, and Amir Hossein Ahmadi, "Effects of *Urtica dioica* Supplementation on Blood Lipids, Hepatic Enzymes and Nitric Oxide Levels in Type 2 Diabetic Patients: A Double Blind, Randomized Clinical Trial," *Avicenna Journal of Phytomedicine* 6, no. 6 (2016), 686-695, PMID: 28078249; PMCID: PMC5206926.

7. Margret Moré et al., "A *Rosa canina—Urtica dioica—Harpagophytum procumbens/zeyheri* Combination Significantly Reduces Gonarthritis Symptoms in a Randomized, Placebo-Controlled Double-Blind Study," *Planta Medica* 83, no. 18 (2017), doi:10.1055/s-0043-112750.

8. Colin Randall et al., "Nettle Sting for Chronic Knee Pain: A Randomised Controlled Pilot Study," *Complementary Therapies in Medicine* 16, no. 2 (2008): doi:10.1016/j.ctim.2007.01.012; C. Randall et al., "Randomized Controlled Trial of Nettle Sting for Treatment of Base-of-Thumb Pain," *Journal of the Royal Society of Medicine* 93, no. 6 (2000), doi:10.1177/014107680009300607.

9. Jonathan Treasure, "Case History: Nettle Seed & Kidney Function," JonathanTreasure.com, accessed September 22, 2018, http://jonathantreasure.com/evidence-research-testimonials-case-history/case-histories/nettle-seed-kidney-function.

10. Mohammad Reza Safarinejad, "*Urtica dioica* for Treatment of Benign Prostatic Hyperplasia: A Prospective, Randomized, Double-Blind, Placebo-Controlled, Crossover Study," *Journal of Herbal Pharmacotherapy* 5, no. 4 (2005), doi:10.1080/J157v05n04_01.

11. Cathleen Rapp, "Special Saw Palmetto and Stinging Nettle Root Combination as Effective as Pharmaceutical Drug for Prostate Symptoms," *HerbalGram* 72 (2006).

12. Merrily A. Kuhn and David Winston, *Winston and Kuhn's Herbal Therapy & Supplements: A Scientific and Traditional Approach* (Philadelphia: Wolters Kluwer/Lippincott Williams & Wilkins, 2008).

Chapter 12: Plantain

Epigraph: Ian Opal Kesling, "Plantain (*Plantago* spp)," *HerbRally*, 2017, https://www.herbrally.com/monographs/plantain.

1. Ahmed Ali Romeh, Magdi Anwar Khamis, and Shawky Mohammed Metwally, "Potential of *Plantago major* L. for Phytoremediation of Lead-Contaminated Soil and Water," *Water, Air, & Soil Pollution* 227, no. 9 (2016), doi: 10.1007/s11270-015-2687-9; Ahmed Romeh, "Phytoremediation of Water and Soil Contaminated with Imidacloprid Pesticide by *Plantago major*, L.," *International Journal of Phytoremediation* 12, no. 2 (2010), doi:10.1080/15226510903213936.

Chapter 13: Violet

Epigraph: Tori Amos, "Cloud on My Tongue," track 10 on *Under the Pink*, Atlantic Records, 1994.

1. Graeme Tobyn, Alison Denham, and Margaret Whitelegg, *The Western Herbal Tradition: 2000 Years of Medicinal Plant Knowledge* (London: Churchill Livingstone, 2010).

2. Margaret Joan Roberts, *Edible & Medicinal Flowers* (Claremont: Spearhead Press, 2000).

3. Mohammad Ali Esmaeili et al., "Viola Plant Cyclotide Vigno 5 Induces Mitochondria-Mediated Apoptosis via Cytochrome C Release and Caspases Activation in Cervical Cancer Cells," *Fitoterapia* 109 (2016), doi:10.1016/j.fitote.2015.12.021; Yeon-Joo Kwak et al., "Fermented *Viola mandshurica* Inhibits Melanogenesis in B16 Melanoma Cells," *Bioscience, Biotechnology, and Biochemistry* 75, no. 5 (2011), doi:10.1271/bbb.100641.

4. Samantha L. Gerlach et al., "Anticancer and Chemosensitizing Abilities of Cycloviolacin 02 from *Viola odorata* and Psyle Cyclotides from *Psychotria leptothyrsa*," *Biopolymers* 94, no. 5 (2010), doi:10.1002/bip.21435.

5. Mohammad Javad Qasemzadeh et al., "The Effect of *Viola odorata* Flower Syrup on the Cough of Children with Asthma: A Double-Blind, Randomized Controlled Trial," *Journal of Evidence-Based Complementary & Alternative Medicine* 20, no. 4 (2015), doi:10.1177/2156587215584862.

6. jim mcdonald, "Violet Herb," Herbs with Rosalee, accessed October 11, 2018, https://www.herbalremediesadvice.org/violet-herb.html.

7. Hildegard von Bingen, *Hildegard von Bingen's Physica: The Complete English Translation of Her Classic Work on Health and Healing*, trans. Priscilla Throop (Rochester, VT: Healing Arts Press, 1998).

8. Zohre Feyzabadi et al., "Efficacy of *Viola odorata* in Treatment of Chronic Insomnia," *Iranian Red Crescent Medical Journal* 16, no. 12 (2014), doi:10.5812/ircmj.17511.

9. mcdonald, "Violet Herb."

Chapter 14: Elderflower

Epigraph: Darcy Williamson, *Healing Plants of the Rocky Mountains* (McCall, ID: From the Forest, 2002).

1. Cecilia Garza and James D. Adams, Jr., *Healing with Medicinal Plants of the West* (La Crescenta: Abedus Press, 2012).

2. Margaret Grieve, *A Modern Herbal* (New York: Dover, 1971).

3. Anna Jarzycka et al., "Assessment of Extracts of *Helichrysum arenarium*, *Crataegus monogyna*, *Sambucus nigra* in Photoprotective UVA and UVB; Photostability in Cosmetic Emulsions," *Journal of Photochemistry and Photobiology* 128 (2013), doi:10.1016/j.jphotobiol.2013.07.029.

4. Evlambia Harokopakis et al., "Inhibition of Proinflammatory Activities of Major Periodontal Pathogens by Aqueous Extracts from Elderflower (*Sambucus nigra*)," *Journal of Periodontology* 77, no. 2 (2006), doi:10.1902/jop.2006.050232.

Chapter 15: Mallow

Epigraph: Julie James, personal communication with authors, 2018.

1. Abdullatif Azab, "Malva: Food, Medicine and Chemistry," *European Chemical Bulletin* 6, no. 7 (2017), doi:10.17628/ecb.2017.6.295-320.

2. Elias Keyrouz et al., "*Malva neglecta*: A Natural Inhibitor of Bacterial Growth and Biofilm Formation," *Journal of Medicinal Plants Research* 11, no. 24 (2017), doi:10.5897/JMPR2017.6422.

3. S. Maryam Mirghiasi et al., "The Effect of *Malva neglecta* on the Reduction of Inflammatory Agents in Patients with Osteoarthritis," *Molecular Biology: Open Access* 4, no. 4 (2015), doi:10.4172/2168-9547.1000135.

4. Emanuela Cristiani et al., "Dental Calculus Reveals Mesolithic Foragers in the Balkans Consumed Domesticated Plant Foods," *Proceedings of the National Academy of Sciences of the United States of America* 113, no. 37 (2016), doi:10.1073/pnas.1603477113.

5. Alexis Soyer, *Pantropheon, or, History of Food, and Its Preparation, from the Earliest Ages of the World* (Boston: Ticknor, Reed, and Fields, 1853).

6. J. A. Duke, *CRC Handbook of Proximate Analysis Tables of Higher Plants* (Boca Raton: CRC Press, 1986).

Chapter 16: Mint

Epigraph: Brittany Wood Nickerson, *Recipes from the Herbalist's Kitchen* (North Adams, MA: Storey Publishing, 2017).

1. Z. Tayarani-Najaran et al., "Antiemetic Activity of Volatile Oil from *Mentha spicata* and *Mentha × piperita* in Chemotherapy-Induced Nausea and Vomiting," *Ecancermedicalscience* 7 (2013), doi:10.3332/ecancer.2013.290.

2. Brooks D. Cash, Michael S. Epstein, and Syed M. Shah, "A Novel Delivery System of Peppermint Oil Is an Effective Therapy for Irritable Bowel Syndrome Symptoms," *Digestive Diseases and Sciences* 61, no. 2 (2016), doi:10.1007/s10620-015-3858-7.

3. Naofumi Ohtsu et al., "Utilization of the Japanese Peppermint Herbal Water Byproduct of Steam Distillation as an Antimicrobial Agent," *Journal of Oleo Science* 67, no. 10 (2018), doi:10.5650/jos.ess18049; Rekha Raghavan et al., "Effectiveness of *Mentha piperita* Leaf Extracts against Oral Pathogens: An In Vitro Study," *Journal of Contemporary Dental Practice* 19, no. 9 (2018), doi:10.5005/jp-journals-10024-2378; Abderrahmane Houicher et al., "In Vitro Study of the Antifungal Activity of Essential Oils Obtained from *Mentha spicata*, *Thymus vulgaris*, and *Laurus nobilis*," *Recent Patents on Food, Nutrition & Agriculture* 8, no. 2 (2016), doi:10.2174/2212798408666160927124014.

4. Erin A. Connelly et al., "High-Rosmarinic Acid Spearmint Tea in the Management of Knee Osteoarthritis Symptoms," *Journal of Medicinal Food* 17, no. 12 (2014), doi:10.1089/jmf.2013.0189.

5. Seyedeh Zahra Masoumi et al., "Evaluation of Mint Efficacy Regarding Dysmenorrhea in Comparison with Mefenamic Acid: A Double Blinded Randomized Crossover Study," *Iranian Journal of Nursing and Midwifery Research* 21, no. 4 (2016), doi:10.4103/1735-9066.185574; Akram Heshmati et al., "The Effect of Peppermint (*Mentha piperita*) Capsules on the Severity of Primary Dysmenorrhea," *Journal of Herbal Medicine* 6, no. 3 (2016), doi:10.1016/j.hermed.2016.05.001.

Chapter 17: Prickly Pear

Epigraph: Damiana Calvario-Viana, personal communication with authors, August 26, 2019.

1. C. Roger Nance, *The Archaeology of La Calsada: A Rockshelter in the Sierra Madre Oriental, Mexico* (Austin: University of Texas Press, 2010).

2. Hannah Bauman and Ashley Schmidt, "Food as Medicine: Prickly Pear Cactus (*Opuntia ficus-indica*, Cactaceae)," *HerbalEGram* 12, no. 9 (September 2015).

3. Michele E. Lee, *Working the Roots: Over 400 Years of Traditional African American Healing* (Oakland: Wadastick Publishers, 2014).

4. Charles W. Kane, *Medicinal Plants of the American Southwest* (N.p.: Lincoln Town Press, 2011).

5. Michael Moore, *Medicinal Plants of the Desert and Canyon West* (Santa Fe: Museum of New Mexico Press, 1989).

6. Patricia López-Romero et al., "The Effect of Nopal (*Opuntia ficus indica*) on Postprandial Blood Glucose, Incretins, and Antioxidant Activity in Mexican Patients with Type 2 Diabetes after Consumption of Two Different Composition Breakfasts," *Journal of the Academy of Nutrition and Dietetics* 114, no. 11 (November 2014), doi:10.1016/j.jand.2014.06.352.

7. Michael P. Godard et al., "Acute Blood Glucose Lowering Effects and Long-Term Safety of Opundia™ Supplementation in Pre-Diabetic Males and Females," *Journal of Ethnopharmacology* 130, no. 3 (August 9, 2010), doi:10.1016/j.jep.2010.05.047.

8. Shagun Bindlish and Jay H. Shubrook, "Dietary and Botanical Supplement Therapy in Diabetes," *Osteopathic Family Physician* 6 (2014).

9 Abe Sanchez, "Nopales Tortillas," in *Cooking the Native Way* by the Chia Café Collective (Berkeley, CA: Heyday Books, 2018), 111.

10. Kane, *Medicinal Plants of the American Southwest*.

11. Ibid.

Chapter 18: St. John's Wort

Epigraph: Henriette Kress, *Practical Herbs 1* (Helsinki: Henriette Kress, 2013).

1. Daniel E. Moerman, *Native American Ethnobotany* (Portland: Timber Press, 1998).

2. Qin Xiang Ng, Nandini Venkatanarayanan, and Collin Yih Xian Ho, "Clinical Use of *Hypericum perforatum* (St. John's Wort) in Depression: A Meta-analysis," *Journal of Affective Disorders* 210 (2017), doi:10.1016/j.jad.2016.12.048.

3. David Winston, *Differential Treatment of Depression and Anxiety with Botanical and Nutritional Medicines* (2014), https://www.americanherbalistsguild.com/sites/default/files/Proceedings/winston_david_-_differ_treat-depression.pdf.

4. Amy Clewell et al., "Efficacy and Tolerability Assessment of a Topical Formulation Containing Copper Sulfate and *Hypericum perforatum* on Patients with Herpes Skin Lesions: A Comparative, Randomized Controlled Trial," *Journal of Drugs in Dermatology* 11, no. 2 (2012): 209–15.

5. Susan Arentz et al., "Combined Lifestyle and Herbal Medicine in Overweight Women with Polycystic Ovary Syndrome (PCOS): A Randomized Controlled Trial," *Phytotherapy Research* 31, no. 9 (2017), doi:10.1002/ptr.5858.

6. Sarah Canning et al., "The Efficacy of *Hypericum perforatum* (St John's Wort) for the Treatment of Premenstrual Syndrome: A Randomized, Double-Blind, Placebo-Controlled Trial," *CNS Drugs* 24, no. 3 (2010), doi:10.2165/11530120.

7. Harvey Wickes Felter and John Uri Lloyd, *King's American Dispensatory*, 18th ed., 3rd rev. ed. (Cincinnati: Ohio Valley Co., 1898).

8. Maryam Hajhashemi et al., "The Effect of *Achillea millefolium* and *Hypericum perforatum* Ointments on Episiotomy Wound Healing in Primiparous Women," *Journal of Maternal-Fetal & Neonatal Medicine* 31, no. 1 (2018), doi:10.1080/14767058.2016.1275549.

9. Sareh Samadi et al., "The Effect of *Hypericum perforatum* on the Wound Healing and Scar of Cesarean," *Journal of Alternative and Complementary Medicine* 16, no. 1 (2010), doi:10.1089/acm.2009.0317.

10. Martina C. Meinke et al., "In Vivo Photoprotective and Anti-inflammatory Effect of Hyperforin Is Associated with High Antioxidant Activity In Vitro and Ex Vivo," *European Journal of Pharmaceutics and Biopharmaceutics* 81, no. 2 (2012), doi:10.1016/j.ejpb.2012.03.002.

11. Anthony Booker et al., "St John's Wort (*Hypericum perforatum*) Products—An Assessment of Their Authenticity and Quality," *Phytomedicine* 40 (2018), doi:10.1016/j.phymed.2017.12.012.

12. Zoe Gardner and Michael McGuffin, *American Herbal Products Association's Botanical Safety Handbook*, 2nd ed. (Boca Raton: CRC Press, 2013).

13. Robin H. Fogle et al., "Does St. John's Wort Interfere with the Antiandrogenic Effect of Oral Contraceptive Pills?" *Contraception* 74, no. 3 (2006), doi:10.1016/j.contraception.2006.03.015.

14. Tuija H. Nieminen et al., "St John's Wort Greatly Reduces the Concentrations of Oral Oxycodone," *European Journal of Pain* 14, no. 8 (2010), doi:10.1016/j.ejpain.2009.12.007.

Chapter 19: Yarrow

Epigraph: Maria Noel Groves, *Body Into Balance* (North Adams, MA: Storey Publishing, 2016).

1. Guido Masé, "Herb Power: Find Your Wild Ally This Summer," *A Radicle* (blog), June 8, 2003, aradicle.blogspot.com/2013/06/herb-power-find-your-wild-ally-this.html.

2. Karen Hardy et al., "Neanderthal Medics? Evidence for Food, Cooking, and Medicinal Plants Entrapped in Dental Calculus," *Die Naturwissenschaften* 99, no. 8 (2012), doi:10.1007/s00114-012-0942-0.

3. 7Song, "Herb First Aid," https://courses.learningherbs.com.

4. Vanja Tadić et al., "The Estimation of the Traditionally Used Yarrow (*Achillea millefolium* L. Asteraceae) Oil Extracts with Anti-inflamatory Potential in Topical Application," *Journal of Ethnopharmacology* 199 (2017), doi:10.1016/j.jep.2017.02.002.

5. Maryam Hajhashemi et al., "The Effect of *Achillea millefolium* and *Hypericum perforatum* Ointments."

6. Michael Moore, *Medicinal Plants of the Mountain West* (Santa Fe: Museum of New Mexico Press, 2003).

7. Sedigheh Miranzadeh et al., "Effect of Adding the Herb *Achillea millefolium* on Mouthwash on Chemotherapy Induced Oral Mucositis in Cancer Patients: A Double-Blind Randomized Controlled Trial," *European Journal of Oncology Nursing* 19, no. 3 (2015), doi:10.1016/j.ejon.2014.10.019.

8. Aviva Jill Romm, *Botanical Medicine for Women's Health* (St. Louis: Churchill Livingstone, 2010).

9. Ensiyeh Jenabi and Bita Fereidoony, "Effect of *Achillea mille-folium* on Relief of Primary Dysmenorrhea: A Double-Blind Randomized Clinical Trial," *Journal of Pediatric and Adolescent Gynecology* 28, no. 5 (2015), doi:10.1016/j.jpag.2014.12.008.

10. John M. Scudder, *A Familiar Treatise on Medicine* (Moore, Wilstach & Moore, 1870); Finley Ellingwood, *American Materia Medica, Therapeutics and Pharmacognosy* (Portland: Electric Medical Publications, 1919); Felter and Lloyd, *King's American Dispensatory*.

Chapter 20: Apple

Epigraph: Michael Phillips, personal communication with authors, December 12, 2018.

1. Karen Carr, "Where Do Apples Come From? History of Apples," Quatr.us from Professor Carr Study Guides, September 17, 2018, https://quatr.us/food-2/where-do-apples-come-from.htm.

2. jim mcdonald, "Apple," jim mcdonald, accessed November 8, 2018, herbcraft.org, http://www.herbcraft.org/apple.html.

3. Athanasios Koutsos, Kieran M Tuohy, and Julie A Lovegrove, "Apples and Cardiovascular Health—Is the Gut Microbiota a Core Consideration?" *Nutrients* 7, no. 6 (2015), doi:10.3390/nu7063959.

4. Jo Robinson, *Eating on the Wild Side: The Missing Link to Optimum Health* (New York: Little Brown & Co, 2014).

5. Stephen B. Freedman et al., "Effect of Dilute Apple Juice and Preferred Fluids vs Electrolyte Maintenance Solution on Treatment Failure Among Children with Mild Gastroenteritis: A Randomized Clinical Trial," *JAMA* 315, no. 18 (2016), doi:10.1001/jama.2016.5352.

6. Robinson, *Eating on the Wild Side*.

7. Felter and Lloyd, *King's American Dispensatory*.

8. mcdonald, "Apple," jim mcdonald.

Chapter 21: Blackberry and Raspberry

Epigraph: Timothy Lee Scott, *Invasive Plant Medicine: The Ecological Benefits and Healing Abilities of Invasives* (Rochester, VT: Healing Arts Press, 2010).

1. Paweł Konieczyński and Marek Wesołowski, "Water-Extractable Magnesium, Manganese and Copper in Leaves and Herbs of Medicinal Plants," *Acta Poloniae Pharmaceutica* 69, no. 1 (2012).

2. Robinson, *Eating on the Wild Side*.

3. Ibid.

4. Han Saem Jeong et al., "Effects of *Rubus occidentalis* Extract on Blood Pressure in Patients with Prehypertension: Randomized, Double-Blinded, Placebo-Controlled Clinical Trial." *Nutrition* 32, no. 4 (2016), doi:10.1016/j.nut.2015.10.014; Han Saem Jeong et al., "Effects of Black Raspberry on Lipid Profiles and Vascular Endothelial Function in Patients with Metabolic Syn-

drome," *Phytotherapy Research* 28, no. 10 (2014), doi:10.1002/ptr.5154.

5. Jee Hyun An et al., "Effect of *Rubus occidentalis* Extract on Metabolic Parameters in Subjects with Prediabetes: A Proof-of-Concept, Randomized, Double-Blind, Placebo-Controlled Clinical Trial." *Phytotherapy Research* 30, no. 10 (2016), doi:10.1002/ptr.5664.

6. Han Saem Jeong et al., "Black Raspberry Extract Increased Circulating Endothelial Progenitor Cells and Improved Arterial Stiffness in Patients with Metabolic Syndrome: A Randomized Controlled Trial," *Journal of Medicinal Food* 19, no. 4 (2016), doi:10.1089/jmf.2015.3563.

7. Kai I. Cheang et al., "Raspberry Leaf and Hypoglycemia in Gestational Diabetes Mellitus," *Obstetrics and Gynecology* 128, no. 6 (2016), doi:10.1097/AOG.0000000000001757.

8. Felter and Lloyd, *King's American Dispensatory*.

9. Scott, *Invasive Plant Medicine*.

Chapter 22: Elderberry

Epigraph: Christophe Bernard, personal communication with authors, August 23, 2019.

1. Bernard Bertrand and Annie Bertrand, *Sous la protection du sureau*, 2nd ed. (Escalquens, France: Éditions de Terran, 2000).

2. Zichria Zakay-Rones et al., "Inhibition of Several Strains of Influenza Virus In Vitro and Reduction of Symptoms by an Elderberry Extract (*Sambucus nigra* L.) during an Outbreak of Influenza B Panama," *Journal of Alternative and Complementary Medicine* 1, no. 4 (1995), doi:10.1089/acm.1995.1.361.

3. Z. Zakay-Rones et al., "Randomized Study of the Efficacy and Safety of Oral Elderberry Extract in the Treatment of Influenza A and B Virus Infections," *Journal of International Medical Research* 32, no. 2 (2004), doi:10.1177/147323000403200205.

4. Evelin Tiralongo, Shirley S. Wee, and Rodney A. Lea, "Elderberry Supplementation Reduces Cold Duration and Symptoms in Air-Travellers: A Randomized, Double-Blind Placebo-Controlled Clinical Trial," *Nutrients* 8, no. 4 (2016), doi:10.3390/nu8040182.

5. Grieve, *A Modern Herbal*.

Chapter 23: Mullein

Epigraph: Maria Noel Groves, personal communication with authors, 2018.

1. Yan-Li Zhao et al., "Isolation of Chemical Constituents from the Aerial Parts of *Verbascum thapsus* and Their Antiangiogenic and Antiproliferative Activities," *Archives of Pharmacal Research* 34, no. 5 (2011), doi:10.1007/s12272-011-0501-9.

2. Christa Sinadinos, "Medicinal Uses of Mullein Root," *Medical Herbalism: A Journal for the Clinical Practitioner* 16, no. 2 (2011).

3. jim mcdonald, "Mullein," jim mcdonald, accessed September 26, 2017, http://www.herbcraft.org/mullein.html.

4. Moore, *Medicinal Plants of the Mountain West*.

5. A. Slagowska, I. Zgórniak-Nowosielska, and J. Grzybek, "Inhibition of Herpes Simplex Virus Replication by Flos Verbasci Infusion," *Polish Journal of Pharmacology and Pharmacy* 39, no. 1 (1987); M. Rajbhandari et al., "Antiviral Activity of Some Plants Used in Nepalese Traditional Medicine," *Journal of Evidence-Based Complementary & Alternative Medicine* 6, no. 4 (2009), doi:10.1093/ecam/nem156; S. M. Zanon et al., "Search for Antiviral Activity of Certain Medicinal Plants from Córdoba, Argentina," *Revista latinoamericana de microbiologia* 41, no. 2 (1999): 59–62.

6. Vladica Čudić, Dragoslava Stojiljković, and Aleksandar Jovović, "Phytoremediation Potential of Wild Plants Growing on Soil Contaminated with Heavy Metals," *Arhiv za higijenu rada i toksikologiju* 67, no. 3 (2016), doi:10.1515/aiht-2016-67-2829.

Chapter 24: Purslane

Epigraph: Sade Musa, personal communication with authors, November 27, 2018.

1. M. K. Uddin et al., "Purslane Weed (*Portulaca oleracea*): A Prospective Plant Source of Nutrition, Omega-3 Fatty Acid, and Antioxidant Attributes," *Scientific World Journal* 951019 (2014), doi:10.1155/2014/951019.

2. A. M. Sabzghabaee et al., "Clinical Effects of *Portulaca oleracea* Seeds on Dyslipidemia in Obese Adolescents: A Triple-Blinded Randomized Controlled Trial," *Medical Archives* 68, no. 3 (June 2014), doi:10.5455/medarh.2014.68.195-199; M. I. El-Saye, "Effects of *Portulaca oleracea* L. Seeds in Treatment of Type-2 Diabetes Mellitus Patients as Adjunctive and Alternative Therapy," *Journal of Ethnopharmacology* 137, no. 1 (September 2011), doi:10.1016/j.jep.2011.06.020.

3. O. Parry, F. Okwuasaba, and C. Ejike, "Preliminary Clinical Investigation into the Muscle Relaxant Actions of an Aqueous Extract of *Portulaca oleracea* Applied Topically," *Journal of Ethnopharmacology* 21, no. 1 (September 1987), doi:10.1016/0378-8741(87)90099-7.

4. S. Habtemariam, A. L. Harvey, and P. G. Waterman, "The Muscle Relaxant Properties of *Portulaca oleracea* Are Associated with High Concentrations of Potassium Ions," *Journal of Ethnopharmacology* 40, no. 3 (December 1993), doi:10.1016/0378-8741(93)90068-G.

5. Briana Wiles, *Mountain States Medicinal Plants* (Portland: Timber Press, 2018).

6. Gardner and McGuffin, *American Herbal Products Association's Botanical Safety Handbook*.

7. Ibid.

Chapter 25: Burdock

Epigraph: Cathy Skipper, personal communication with authors, 2018.

1. Leila Maghsoumi-Norouzabad et al., "Effects of *Arctium lappa* L. (Burdock) Root Tea on Inflammatory Status and Oxidative Stress in Patients with Knee Osteoarthritis," *International Journal of Rheumatic Diseases* 19, no. 3 (2016), doi:10.1111/1756-185X.12477.

2. Ke Huang et al., "Arctigenin Promotes Apoptosis in Ovarian Cancer Cells Via the INOS/NO/STAT3/survivin Signalling," *Basic & Clinical Pharmacology & Toxicology* 115, no. 6 (2014), doi:10.1111/bcpt.12270; Chia-Jung Hsieh et al., "Arctigenin, a Dietary Phy-

toestrogen, Induces Apoptosis of Estrogen Receptor-Negative Breast Cancer Cells through the ROS/p38 MAPK Pathway and Epigenetic Regulation," *Free Radical Biology & Medicine* 67 (2014), doi:10.1016/j.freeradbiomed.2013.10.004.

3. Shan Su, Xinlai Cheng, and Michael Wink, "Natural Lignans from *Arctium lappa* Modulate P-Glycoprotein Efflux Function in Multidrug Resistant Cancer Cells," *Phytomedicine: International Journal of Phytotherapy and Phytopharmacology* 22, no. 2 (2015), doi:10.1016/j.phymed.2014.12.009.

Chapter 26: Dandelion Root

Epigraph: Guido Masé, "Rise Up in Spring: Thinking Like a Plant," *Urban Moonshine*, last modified March 28, 2019, https://www.urbanmoonshine.com/blogs/blog/rise-up-in-spring-thinking-like-a-plant.

1. Peter Holmes, *The Energetics of Western Herbs: Treatment Strategies Integrating Western and Oriental Herbal Medicine*, rev. 4th ed., vol. 2 (Boulder: Snow Lotus Press, 2006).

2. Thomas Avery Garran, *Western Herbs According to Traditional Chinese Medicine: A Practitioner's Guide* (Rochester, VT: Healing Arts Press, 2008).

3. USDA Agricultural Research Service, *Dr. Duke's Phytochemical and Ethnobotanical Databases*.

4. Sophia C. Sigsteclt et al., "Evaluation of Aqueous Extracts of *Taraxacum officinale* on Growth and Invasion of Breast and Prostate Cancer Cells," *International Journal of Oncology* 32, no. 5 (2008), doi:10.3892/ijo.32.5.1085; Huanhuan Zhu et al., "Dandelion Root Extract Suppressed Gastric Cancer Cells Proliferation and Migration through Targeting LncRNA-CCAT1," *Biomedicine & Pharmacotherapy* 93 (2017), doi:10.1016/j.biopha.2017.07.007; Pamela Ovadje et al., "Dandelion Root Extract Affects Colorectal Cancer Proliferation and Survival through the Activation of Multiple Death Signalling Pathways," *Oncotarget* 7, no. 45 (2016), doi:10.18632/oncotarget.11485; John Tung Chien et al., "Antioxidant Property of *Taraxacum formosanum* Kitam and Its Antitumor Activity in Non-Small-Cell Lung Cancer Cells," *Phytomedicine* 49 (2018), doi:10.1016/j.phymed.2018.06.011; K. Menke et al., "*Taraxacum officinale* Extract Shows Antitumor Effects on Pediatric Cancer Cells and Enhance Mistletoe Therapy," *Complementary Therapies in Medicine* 40 (2018), doi:10.1016/j.ctim.2018.03.005.

5. Scott, *Invasive Plant Medicine*.

Chapter 27: Echinacea

Epigraph: Alice Cimino, personal communication with authors, December 12, 2018.

1. Noah Samuels et al., "Localized Reduction of Gingival Inflammation Using Site-Specific Therapy with a Topical Gingival Patch," *Journal of Clinical Dentistry* 23, no. 2 (2012).

2. Ellingwood, *American Materia Medica*.

3. S. M. Sharma et al., "Bactericidal and Anti-inflammatory Properties of a Standardized Echinacea Extract (Echinaforce): Dual Actions Against Respiratory Bacteria," *Phytomedicine* 17, no. 8-9 (2010), doi:10.1016/j.phymed.2009.10.022.

4. Andreas Schapowal, Peter Klein, and Sebastian L Johnston, "Echinacea Reduces the Risk of Recurrent Respiratory Tract Infections and Complications: A Meta-analysis of Random-

ized Controlled Trials," *Advances in Therapy* 32, no. 3 (2015), doi:10.1007/s12325-015-0194-4.

5. Manju Sharma et al., "Induction of Multiple Pro-inflammatory Cytokines by Respiratory Viruses and Reversal by Standardized Echinacea, a Potent Antiviral Herbal Extract," *Antiviral Research* 83, no. 2 (2009), doi:10.1016/j.antiviral.2009.04.009.

6. Karel Rauš et al., "Effect of An Echinacea-Based Hot Drink Versus Oseltamivir in Influenza Treatment: A Randomized, Double-Blind, Double-Dummy, Multicenter, Noninferiority Clinical Trial," *Current Therapeutic Research, Clinical and Experimental* 77 (2015), doi:10.1016/j.curtheres.2015.04.001.

7. James B. Hudson, "Applications of the Phytomedicine *Echinacea purpurea* (Purple Coneflower) in Infectious Diseases," *Journal of Biomedicine & Biotechnology* 2012 (2012), doi:10.1155/2012/769896.

8. Kevin Spelman, "The Pharmacodynamics, Pharmacokinetics and Clinical Use of *Echinacea purpurea*," accessed December 15, 2018, http://www.cecity.com/ncpa/2012_projects/echinacea_purpurea/article.htm.

9. Felter and Lloyd, *King's American Dispensatory*.

Chapter 28: Rose Hip

Epigraph: Leslie Lekos, personal communication with authors, 2018.

1. "Rose Hips for Oranges," *Canadian Medical Association Journal* 46, no. 4 (1942).

2. *Gloucester Citizen*, August 11, 1945.

3. S. N. Willich et al., "Rose Hip Herbal Remedy in Patients with Rheumatoid Arthritis—A Randomised Controlled Trial," *Phytomedicine* 17, no. 2 (2010), doi:10.1016/j.phymed.2009.09.003; K. Winther, K. Apel, and G. Thamsborg, "A Powder Made from Seeds and Shells of a Rose-Hip Subspecies (*Rosa canina*) Reduces Symptoms of Knee and Hip Osteoarthritis: A Randomized, Double-Blind, Placebo-Controlled Clinical Trial," *Scandinavian Journal of Rheumatology* 34, no. 4 (2005), doi:10.1080/03009740510018624.

4. Brian Chi Yan Cheng et al., "The Genus *Rosa* and Arthritis: Overview on Pharmacological Perspectives," *Pharmacological Research* 114 (2016), doi:10.1016/j.phrs.2016.10.029.

5. U. Andersson et al., "Effects of Rose Hip Intake on Risk Markers of Type 2 Diabetes and Cardiovascular Disease: A Randomized, Double-Blind, Cross-over Investigation in Obese Persons," *European Journal of Clinical Nutrition* 66, no. 5 (2012), doi:10.1038/ejcn.2011.203.

6. USDA Agricultural Research Service, *Dr. Duke's Phytochemical and Ethnobotanical Databases*; Inés Mármol et al., "Therapeutic Applications of Rose Hips from Different *Rosa* Species," *International Journal of Molecular Sciences* 18, no. 6 (2017), doi:10.3390/ijms18061137.

7. Vlasta Cunja et al., "Fresh from the Ornamental Garden: Hips of Selected Rose Cultivars Rich in Phytonutrients," *Journal of Food Science* 81, no. 2 (2016), doi:10.1111/1750-3841.13220; Jelena D. Nađpal et al., "Comparative Study of Biological Activities and Phytochemical Composition of Two Rose Hips and Their Preserves: *Rosa canina* L. and *Rosa arvensis* Huds," *Food Chemistry* 192 (2016), doi:10.1016/j.foodchem.2015.07.089;

Staffan C. Andersson et al., "Tocopherols in Rose Hips (*Rosa* Spp.) During Ripening," *Journal of the Science of Food and Agriculture* 92, no. 10 (2012), doi:10.1002/jsfa.5594; Lăcrămioara Oprica, Cristina Bucsa, and Maria Magdalena Zamfirache, "Ascorbic Acid Content of Rose Hip Fruit Depending on Altitude," *Iranian Journal of Public Health* 44, no. 1 (2015), PMID: 26060787.

8. Vlasta Cunja et al., "Frost Decreases Content of Sugars, Ascorbic Acid and Some Quercetin Glycosides but Stimulates Selected Carotenes in *Rosa canina* Hips," *Journal of Plant Physiology* 178 (2015), doi:10.1016/j.jplph.2015.01.014.

9. Cunja et al., "Frost Decreases Content of Sugars."

10. Sean Sherman with Beth Dooley. *The Sioux Chef's Indigenous Kitchen* (University of Minnesota Press, 2017). Copyright 2017 Ghost Dancer, LLC. All rights reserved. Reprinted by permission of Sean Sherman and the University of Minnesota Press.

Chapter 29: Citrus

Epigraph: Valerie Aikman-Smith, "Introduction," in Valerie Aikman-Smith and Victoria Pearson, *Citrus* (Berkeley, CA: Ten Speed Press, 2015).

1. Guohong Albert Wu et al., "Genomics of the Origin and Evolution of *Citrus*," *Nature* 554 (2018), https://www.nature.com/articles/nature25447.

2. Pinhas Spiegel-Roy and Eliezer E. Goldschmidt, *The Biology of Citrus* (Cambridge: Cambridge University Press, 1996).

3. R. Fatin Najwa and A. Azrina, "Comparison of Vitamin C Content in Citrus Fruits by Titration and High Performance Liquid Chromatography (HPLC) Methods," *International Food Research Journal* 24, no. 2 (2017): 726–33.

4. American Botanical Council, "Orange Peel, Bitter," *Herbal Medicine: Expanded Commission E Monographs* (2000).

5. Gardner and McGuffin, *American Herbal Products Association's Botanical Safety Handbook*.

Chapter 30: Cottonwood

Epigraph: Adrian White, "Cottonwood—Salves and Lore," *Iowa Herbalist*, January 25, 2014, https://iowaherbalist.com/2014/01/25/cottonwood-salves-and-lore.

1. Moore, *Medicinal Plants of the Mountain West*.

2. Ali Reza Rahimi, Maryam Emad, and Gholam Reza Rezaian, "Smoke from Leaves of *Populus euphratica* Olivier vs. Conventional Cryotherapy for the Treatment of Cutaneous Warts: A Pilot, Randomized, Single-Blind, Prospective Study," *International Journal of Dermatology* 47, no. 4 (2008), doi:10.1111/j.1365-4632.2008.03571.x.

3. Stéphanie Dudonné et al., "Phenolic Composition and Antioxidant Properties of Poplar Bud (*Populus nigra*) Extract: Individual Antioxidant Contribution of Phenolics and Transcriptional Effect on Skin Aging," *Journal of Agricultural and Food Chemistry* 59, no. 9 (2011), doi:10.1021/jf104791t.

4. Keum Young Lee, Stuart E. Strand, and Sharon L. Doty, "Phytoremediation of Chlorpyrifos by *Populus* and *Salix*," *International Journal of Phytoremediation* 14, no. 1 (2012), doi:10.1080/15226514.2011.560213.

5. Moore, *Medicinal Plants of the Mountain West*.

6. E. Kadocsa, I. Bittera, and M. Juhász, "[Aeropollinologic and Allergologic Studies for the Clarification of 'Poplar Tree Hay Fever']," *Orvosi hetilap* 134, no. 38 (1993), PMID: 8414453; Ali Ince et al., "Allergenic Pollen in the Atmosphere of Kayseri, Turkey," *Asian Pacific Journal of Allergy and Immunology* 22, no. 2-3 (2004), PMID: 15565949.

7. Kristiina Aalto-Korte et al., "Allergic Contact Dermatitis from Salicyl Alcohol and Salicylaldehyde in Aspen Bark (*Populus tremula*)," *Contact Dermatitis* 52, no. 2 (2005). doi:10.1111/j.0105-1873.2005.00506.x.

Chapter 31: Evergreen Conifers

Epigraph: Danielle Prohom Olson, "Comfort & Joy: The Healing Power of Conifers," *Gather Victoria*, November 8, 2015, https://gathervictoria.com/2015/11/08/recipes-for-comfort-joy-the-healing-powers-of-conifers.

1. Tanya M. Barnes and Kerryn A. Greive, "Topical Pine Tar: History, Properties and Use as a Treatment for Common Skin Conditions," *Australasian Journal of Dermatology* 58, no. 2 (2017), doi:10.1111/ajd.12427.

2. Ain Raal, Katrin Nisuma, and Andres Meos, "*Pinus sylvestris* L. and Other Conifers as Natural Sources of Ascorbic Acid," *Journal of Pharmacy & Pharmacognosy Research* 6, no. 2 (April 2018): 89–95.

3. K. Y. Kim and H. J. Chung, "Flavor Compounds of Pine Sprout Tea and Pine Needle Tea," *Journal of Agricultural and Food Chemistry* 48, no. 4 (2000), doi:10.1021/jf9900229.

4. Moore, *Medicinal Plants of the Mountain West*.

5. Barnes and Greive, "Topical Pine Tar."

6. Katja Swift, "Foraging for Pine Resin," *AromaCulture* (December 2017).

7. Florence Williams, *The Nature Fix: Why Nature Makes Us Happier, Healthier, and More Creative* (New York: W.W. Norton & Company, 2018).

8. Qing Li et al., "Acute Effects of Walking in Forest Environments on Cardiovascular and Metabolic Parameters," *European Journal of Applied Physiology* 111, no. 11 (2011), doi:10.1007/s00421-011-1918-z; Qing Li et al., "A Day Trip to a Forest Park Increases Human Natural Killer Activity and the Expression of Anti-cancer Proteins in Male Subjects," *Journal of Biological Regulators and Homeostatic Agents* 24, no. 2 (2010), PMID: 20487629.

9. Robert L. Barnes and Charles R. Berry, "Seasonal Changes in Carbohydrates and Ascorbic Acid and White Pine and Possible Relation to Tipburn Sensitivity" *Research Note* SE-124 (1969), U.S. Department of Agriculture, Forest Service, Southeastern Forest Experiment Station, https://www.srs.fs.usda.gov/pubs/3462.

Chapter 32: Willow

Epigraph: Stephany Hoffelt, personal communication with authors, 2018.

1. Arto Miettinen et al., "The Palaeoenvironment of the 'Antrea Net Find,'" *Iskos* 16 (2008): 71–87.

2. J. Vlachojannis, F. Magora, and S. Chrubasik, "Willow Species and Aspirin: Different Mechanism of Actions," *Phytotherapy Research* 25, no. 7 (2011), doi:10.1002/ptr.3386.

3. Kerry Bone and Simon Mills, *Principles and Practice of Phytotherapy* (Edinburgh: Churchill Livingstone, 2013).

4. Mohd Shara and Sidney J. Stohs, "Efficacy and Safety of White Willow Bark (*Salix alba*) Extracts," *Phytotherapy Research* 29, no. 8 (2015), doi:10.1002/ptr.5377; B. Uehleke et al., "Willow Bark Extract STW 33-I in the Long-Term Treatment of Outpatients with Rheumatic Pain Mainly Osteoarthritis or Back Pain," *Phytomedicine* 20, no. 11 (2013), doi:10.1016/j.phymed.2013.03.023; B. Schmid et al., "Efficacy and Tolerability of a Standardized Willow Bark Extract in Patients with Osteoarthritis: Randomized Placebo-Controlled, Double Blind Clinical Trial," *Phytotherapy Research* 15, no. 4 (2001), PMID: 11406860.

5. Henriette Kress, *Practical Herb Cards* (Helsinki: Henriette Kress, 2017).

6. Felter and Lloyd, *King's American Dispensatory*.

INDEX

Note: Page numbers in *italics* indicate recipes.

ACKNOWLEDGMENTS

Just as the microbes and mycelium nourish the soils, an enormous network of beings brought this book into fruition.

We wrote this book in deep gratitude for all that we've received from this life on earth, including the plant world and all the interconnected webs that run through it.

A big thank you to the entire team at LearningHerbs. To John Gallagher for supporting the vision of this book from day one. To Kimberly Gallagher for her valuable feedback. To Jan Bosman for his design refinements on the cover. And to Deb Winters, Karin Rose, Jenny Barandich, Kathy Szabo, Li Wong, Nahanni Hartwood, and Savhanna Winters for all of their behind-the-scenes work.

Thank you to Hay House for taking on this project! To our editors, Nicolette Salamanca Young and Mary Norris, for helping to refine our vision. To Julie Davison for the beautiful interior, and Karla Baker for the gorgeous cover.

The outline for this book was created during a beautiful stay on the shores of the Pacific Ocean in La Push, Washington. Thank you to the Quileute Tribe for their hospitality.

We outlined the book using the powerful tools we learned from Victoria Labalme and the Rock the Room® system. We are continually inspired by Victoria's work. We are also deeply grateful for the teachings of Dr. Robin Wall Kimmerer, especially her book *Braiding Sweetgrass*.

Thank you to early readers Kat Sanchez, Mobi Warren, Traci Picard, Susan Marynowski, and Xavier de la Forêt for their valuable feedback, and to 7Song for his help with the botanical illustrations. Thank you to Marc Williams and "Wildman" Steve Brill for editing suggestions.

The recipes were thoroughly tested, reviewed, and improved by our volunteer recipe testers. Thank you to Val Paul for orchestrating the whole endeavor! And thank you to our testers: Abbie White, Abigail Salyards, Amanda Mayther, Amy E. Davey, Amy Norton, Angel Luther, Angela Wilcox, Annette Naber, Beckie Rhodes, Beth Southwick, Britta Vance, Catherine Seavey Hurd, Christine Borosh, Cindy Christ, Cote Garceau Saez, Danika Hinton, dorothy swanson, Ellen Demotses, Emily Leigh, Fiona Wolff, Giovanna Becker, Gretchen Beaubier, Haley Otway, Heather Nocton Davis, Jana House, Janice Driver, Jennifer Schneller, Jennifer Warnick, Jerilynn Bedingfield, Jessica Lockwood, Jessica A. Thomas, Jet Eccleston, Katrina L. McNulty, Keisha O. Forbes, Leanne Morris, Lora Krall, Lori Hutchison, Lydia Lynne Koltai, Melanie Isles, Patricia káyə stəbtábul', Furgason, Renée Otte, Rhiannon Servini, Sherri DuPriest Hooks, Stephanie Kapadia, Sue O'Bryan, Teresa Roark, Torey Lee, Tracey S. Curtis, Trudy Born, Vanessa Nixon Klein, and Wendy Joubert. Thanks to Colleen Codekas for sharing the violet vinegar.

Thank you to jim mcdonald, Rebecca Altman, and the team at The Sioux Chef for allowing us to use their tasty recipes.

It was important for us to include inspiring stories about some of the many ways people are working with their communities. Thank you to Joyce Bergen, Lexi Koch, Lorna Mauney-Brodek, Lottie Spady, Nance Klehm, Sandra Warriors Pistol Bullet, and Steph Zabel for their time, energy, and contributions.

The vibrance within these pages comes from the plants, insects, and animals that inspired the images! Thank you to EA and Rachelle from Weymuller Photography who got us both out from behind the camera. And to Ganna Tiulkina who exquisitely brought our visions of botanical art to life. Thanks to Tom Forker for the beautiful nature photo. Matt Burke lent his expertise, both with the camera and in teaching Rosalee some more tips and tricks in photography. (Thank you to Emily, Mara, and Felix for coming all the way from Australia to help with the photoshoot.) Thank you to the Richardson-Kennedy Family (Russell, Karimah, and Rayah) and the Cendre-da-Suh family (Martin, Jenny, Margot, and Iggy) for being such wonderful models. Gregory Han masterfully edited our photos to give us the beautiful final images in this book.

We also want to give our appreciation to the family of Ellen Hutchins for the use of the seaweed print in the Introduction. If you ever find yourself in County Cork, Ireland, in late August, don't miss the Ellen Hutchins Festival!

ACKNOWLEDGMENTS FROM ROSALEE

As soon as I published my first book, people started asking when I would publish my second. I was fairly adamant that one book was enough for me. Later that year, I traveled to Ireland for a retreat with my friend Kat Koch. After a soul-enlivening week, Kat helped me to meet with a musician who's been inspiring me for over 25 years: Tori Amos. My conversation with Tori planted a seed, which quickly germinated into the idea for this book. Moments later, I knew I only wanted to write that book with Emily by my side.

Working with Emily has been one of the most fun and rewarding collaborative experiences of my life. She brought beauty, refinement, and, very importantly, insects, to this book. Countless times we finished each other's sentences or thought of the same idea at the same time, but her unique perspectives also have helped me to grow

as both an herbalist and as a person. I often think of Emily when I hear these (paraphrased) lyrics from another favorite musician, Ani DiFranco, "There is strength in the differences between us, and comfort where we overlap."

Back to Tori Amos (a familiar phrase for me): it was her presence and willingness to give back to her fans that stoked the initial sparks for this book. And while it's surprisingly difficult to use lyric quotes in a book, Tori's team made it possible for us to quote one of my very favorite songs in the Violet chapter. Thank you! Also, thank you to EWFs for pointing me in the right direction to get permission.

So many herbalists have helped inspire me and inform me through their books, articles, conference presentations, or during personal conversations. It would be impossible to list everyone here, so I send out a blanket of gratitude to all who walk this path and who take the time to share what they've learned from the plants. I also want to thank my students and readers for their inquisitive questions, stories, and feedback which informs and influences my own path forward.

I also want to thank Jon Young of the 8 Shields Institute and the Kamana Naturalist Training program for first teaching me about the sit spot and many other naturalist practices that continue to influence me decades later.

My friends are the roots that sustain me. I am blessed to have too many to acknowledge here, but I especially want to mention the following: Thank you to Rebecca Altman for her unwavering support and invigorating conversations. To jim mcdonald for surviving the great calamity and for continuing to inform and inspire both my approach to herbs and life. Thank you to the whole Channing crew for all the nourishing food as well as for constantly reminding me about what's important in this life: love, friendship, and celebration. Big hugs to Susie for her continued friendship and for sharing the magic of the bees.

To Jess for her loving friendship. And to my dad, Pako, who always supported me, whether I was protesting in the streets or mixing up strange herbal concoctions (code 3 dad).

The land I now call home is filled with botanical diversity, fascinating creatures (humans included), and wonder-filled vistas. Thank you to all the caretakers and co-creators of this place, especially the Methow People and those that continue to protect this precious valley.

Monsieur Quincampoix grudgingly put up with the writing of this book. He nonchalantly stood by during photo shoots, waited somewhat patiently to be petted while I was writing or testing recipes, and while he seems generally unimpressed at the idea of books, he nevertheless offered lots of purring support in my lap after long days.

Of all the blessings of my life, l'autre chat, my husband, Xavier, remains my greatest treasure. Neither this book, nor many aspects of my life, would be possible without his support. He's the one who's cooking our meals and maintaining our homestead when I am wrapped up in the herbal world. Without complaint he cleans up my recipe creation kitchen explosions and even helps me dig deep roots in dry, hard soils. He's also the one I return to every day for love, wisdom, and inspiration.

ACKNOWLEDGMENTS FROM EMILY

I offer acknowledgement and gratitude to the ancestors, including those in my own lineage, those who have cared for the Tongva land where I live, and those plants, animals, microorganisms, and other beings who came before us.

Thank you to my teachers, who are too numerous to list, but especially Hoang Ho, Michelle Denyer, Mobi Warren, Philip Phillips, Vuong Coi, Eleanor Han, Bruce Warren, Alma Jane Warren, Thich Nhat Hanh, Cesar Chavez, and Felipe Barajas. Nonhumans have been some of my greatest teachers, from ancient granite rock in the Texas Hill Country to piles of coyote scat in the Southern California sage scrub. Each day I am grateful for the teachings and kinship of the spider stretching their legs across a yarrow flower, or the lichen growing ever so slowly around an oak twig.

Thank you to Rosalee for being my collaborator, teacher, and friend. I could never have imagined what a marvelous journey we've been on together and am grateful to you (and Tori) for sparking it.

And finally, thank you to Gregory, Eames, Eero, and the flora and fauna of Mt. Washington for supporting, inspiring, amusing, and uplifting me while I worked on the book. Gregory, I am endlessly appreciative of your partnership and love.

ABOUT THE AUTHORS

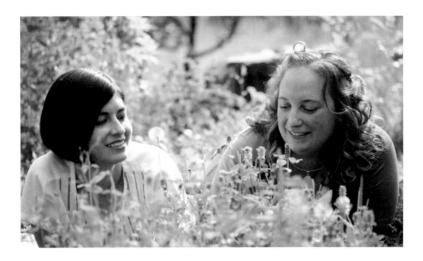

Rosalee de la Forêt, RH, is passionate about inspiring you to enjoy plants every single day, whether it's marveling their beauty or using their gifts as food and medicine. She is the best-selling author of the book *Alchemy of Herbs*, the education director for LearningHerbs, and a registered herbalist with the American Herbalists Guild. In addition to writing books, Rosalee teaches online courses about herbs, including Taste of Herbs, Herbal Cold Care, and Apothecary. Rosalee lives in a log cabin in the northeastern cascades of Washington State with her husband. She's an avid gardener and excels at cuddling up with her cat and a good book. See more of Rosalee's articles and recipes at www.HerbsWithRosalee.com.

From teaching nature workshops to creating botanical cocktail recipes, **Emily Han** helps people slow down, nurture their senses, and cultivate their connection to the earth. Her work as a naturalist, herbalist, writer, and educator focuses on intersections of nature, culture, and food. She is the author of *Wild Drinks & Cocktails*, the communications director for LearningHerbs, and co-founder of the International Food Swap Network. Emily is a Certified California Naturalist and Master Food Preserver. She lives Los Angeles with her husband, Gregory. As citizen scientists, their claim to fame is discovering two previously unknown populations of snails in their backyard. To learn more, visit EmilyHan.com.

The authors will donate a portion of their annual proceeds from this book to organizations committed to a world that encompasses the Wild Remedies Ideals.

Hay House Titles of Related Interest

YOU CAN HEAL YOUR LIFE, the movie, starring Louise Hay & Friends
(available as a 1-DVD program, an expanded 2-DVD set, and an online streaming video)
Learn more at www.hayhouse.com/louise-movie

THE SHIFT, the movie,
starring Dr. Wayne W. Dyer
(available as a 1-DVD program, an expanded 2-DVD set, and an online streaming video)
Learn more at www.hayhouse.com/the-shift-movie

Cultured Food in a Jar: 100+ Probiotic Recipes to Inspire and Change Your Life, by Donna Schwenk

Feeding You Lies: How to Unravel the Food Industry's Playbook and Reclaim Your Health, by Vani Hari

Grow a New Body: How Spirit and Power Plant Nutrients Can Transform Your Health, by Alberto Villoldo

Hungry for More: Satisfy Your Deepest Cravings, Feed Your Dreams and Live a Full-Up Life, by Mel Wells

Joy's Simple Food Remedies: Tasty Cures for Whatever's Ailing You, by Joy Bauer

All of the above are available at your local bookstore,
or may be ordered by contacting Hay House (see next page).

We hope you enjoyed this Hay House book. If you'd like to receive our online catalog featuring additional information on Hay House books and products, or if you'd like to find out more about the Hay Foundation, please contact:

Hay House, Inc., P.O. Box 5100, Carlsbad, CA 92018-5100
(760) 431-7695 or (800) 654-5126
(760) 431-6948 (fax) or (800) 650-5115 (fax)
www.hayhouse.com® • www.hayfoundation.org

Published in Australia by: Hay House Australia Pty. Ltd.,
18/36 Ralph St., Alexandria NSW 2015
Phone: 612-9669-4299 • *Fax:* 612-9669-4144
www.hayhouse.com.au

Published in the United Kingdom by: Hay House UK, Ltd.,
The Sixth Floor, Watson House, 54 Baker Street, London W1U 7BU
Phone: +44 (0)20 3927 7290 • *Fax:* +44 (0)20 3927 7291
www.hayhouse.co.uk

Published in India by: Hay House Publishers India,
Muskaan Complex, Plot No. 3, B-2, Vasant Kunj, New Delhi 110 070
Phone: 91-11-4176-1620 • *Fax:* 91-11-4176-1630
www.hayhouse.co.in

Access New Knowledge.
Anytime. Anywhere.

Learn and evolve at your own pace
with the world's leading experts.

www.hayhouseU.com

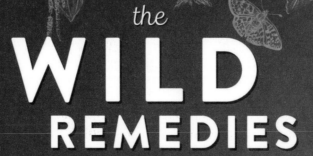
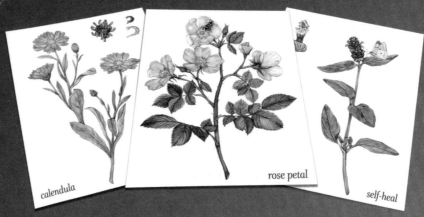

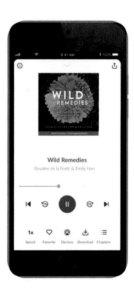